In   a   nder

'*The Wonder Down Under* is set to do for the vagina what Guilia   ders'
Gut did for our digestive system.'

– *Stylist*

'This new guide should be on every woman's shelf.'

– *Emerald Street*

'Tells you everything you need to know.'

– *Fabulous*

'A vital publication – it deserves to be a hit.'

– *The Press Association*

'You appear to have a world map between your legs, with many unknown tracks. This book is your *Lonely Planet* guide for *down under*. Travel all over the world!'

– *Women's Health*, Dutch edition

'It is one thing to share research and facts; it is another thing entirely to engage a young audience. The authors succeed at both . . . Behind the research, facts and footnotes, there is a genuine desire to intrigue us, engage us, advise us – and make us less embarrassed about – our own genitals . . . One can only hope this book is purchased for school libraries across the world – and maybe even becomes part of the science curriculum.'

– Ellen Sofie Lauritzen, Morgenbladet

'A pleasure . . . Dahl and Brochmann shatter myth after myth, all in language that is factual, easily understandable, engaging, uplifting and witty at the same time – this book is quite simply absolutely brilliant.'

– Faedrelandsvennen

'Demystifies female genitals in detail . . . *The Wonder Down Under* is a complete   ly matters: to be more   de São Paulo

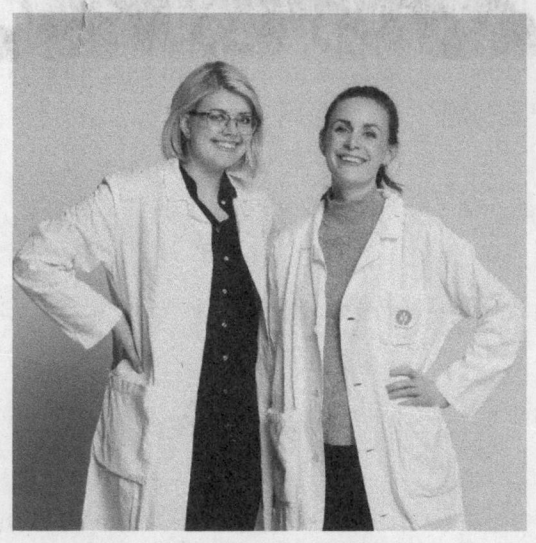

Photograph © Anne Valeur

Based in Oslo, Norway, Dr Nina Brochmann and Dr Ellen Støkken Dahl have, for several years, worked as educators in sexual health advising young people and minority groups. In 2015, they started their blog *Underlivet* ('The Genital Area'), with the aim of dispelling myths around female sexual health.

DR NINA BROCHMANN
DR ELLEN STØKKEN DAHL

THE WONDER
DOWN UNDER

The ultimate guide to female health and empowerment

Translated by
Lucy Moffatt

First published in Great Britain in 2018 by Yellow Kite
An imprint of Hodder & Stoughton
An Hachette UK company

First published in paperback by Yellow Kite in 2019

Originally published in Norway as *Gleden Med Skjeden* in 2017 by H. Ascheoug & Co. (W. Nygaard) AS, Oslo, Norway
Published in agreement with Oslo Literary Agency

1

Copyright © 2017 H. Ascheoug & Co. (W. Nygaard) AS

Illustrations by Hanne Sigbjørnsen

English translation by Lucy Moffatt

The publisher would like to thank Dr Elizabeth Owen for consulting on medical practices in the UK.

The rights of Dr Nina Brochmann and Dr Ellen Støkken Dahl to be identified as the Authors of the Work have been asserted by them in accordance with the Copyright, Designs and Patents Act 1988.

A CIP catalogue record for this title is available from the British Library

Paperback ISBN 978 1 473 66689 4
Ebook ISBN 978 1 473 66691 7

Typeset in Minion Pro by Palimpsest Book Production Ltd, Falkirk, Stirlingshire

Printed and bound by Clays Ltd, Elcograf S.p.A.

Hodder & Stoughton policy is to use papers that are natural, renewable and recyclable products and made from ~~wood grown in sustainable forests. The logging and manufacturing~~ processes are exp...origin.

T...LA.

CONTENTS

PREFACE

Threading condoms onto white polystyrene penises was how we first met, early in the autumn of 2011. We were both first-year medical students at the University of Oslo, Norway, and had just signed up to become volunteer sex-education teachers with an organisation run by medical students. Little did we know that this encounter, and the ensuing friendship, would culminate in a project that would ultimately travel far outside of little Oslo, reaching readers across the world. Back then, we were just two curious and enthusiastic nerds, eager to spread proper condom technique.

Over the next couple of years, we travelled around in Norway as sex-ed teachers, working with groups of teenagers, sex workers and refugees. We were teaching them the essentials about their bodies and a healthy sex life. We drew ovaries and testicles on chalkboards, discussed sexual consent through role plays and had the teenagers create their personal wish list for their sexual debuts. It was wonderful and meaningful work, but what overwhelmed us was the number of questions and concerns people had. There was so much anxiety, shame and insecurity around our most intimate body parts. Sometimes it felt like we could have spent a whole day just answering questions: do I look normal down there? Does discharge mean I have a sexually transmitted disease? How can I be sure that I bleed on my wedding night? After a while, it just didn't feel like we were doing enough. To answer each of these questions in person would take a lifetime.

The solution was to start a blog called *Underlivet* ('The Genitals'), to reach out to a larger audience. We wanted to give girls and women a sense of wonder and pride in their incredible bodies. Our goal was to provide research-based, sound medical information, written in an accessible and funny way. No moralising, no embarrassment – just an honest and trustworthy resource.

Before long, *Underlivet* had become one of the most read health blogs in Norway, giving us the courage to write the book you are holding in your

1

hands right now. It came out in Norwegian in January 2017 and now, less than a year later, it is being translated into 30 languages, from Korean to Polish, from Russian to Dutch. As it was written primarily with a Scandinavian audience in mind, some of the medical practices and statistics we cover may differ slightly to those in different parts of the world. Where possible, we've explored the conventions of other countries but there remains some Norwegian statistics, particularly in the chapters on sex. We decided to keep these, as the numbers are fairly similar in most European countries. Furthermore, the main message of our book is really not about numbers, but about sparking pride in the female body, and the acceptance of individual sexuality.

It is fantastic – and slightly terrifying – to know that our debut book is reaching so many people, and we are happy in the knowledge that women and girls in all corners of the world will get to read what we have to say, because we strongly believe that good sexual health is important. On the other hand, it also saddens us. The interest in our book shows us that information on this subject is scarce. It means that women all over the world have serious questions and few sources to turn to. We are saddened because we wish the reality were different. But we guess it shouldn't have come as a surprise. Scandinavia is, after all, known for its openness regarding sexuality, so if *we* have these questions, everybody else must have them too.

Men and boys will certainly find invaluable (and most likely surprising) information contained here, but it's chiefly you women we're writing this book for – especially the many of you who are unsure as to whether your bodies work the way they should, things look the way they should and you feel the way you should. We hope this book will give you the confidence you need. We're also writing for those of you who are happy and proud with how things are, but simply want to learn more about the amazing wonder down under – because we believe that much of the key to good health (sexual and otherwise) lies in an understanding of how it all works.

When women make choices about their own bodies and sexuality, they do so within a larger context. Cultural, religious, and political forces regulate these choices, whether it's a matter of contraception, abortion, sexual identity or sexual practices. In autumn 2016, for instance, we read newspaper articles about the hypersexualised behaviour of teenagers in some Norwegian high schools.[1] Merciless social pressure to fit in meant that 16-year-old girls were feeling compelled to overstep their own sexual boundaries – so drastically in some cases that we could scarcely believe what we were reading. It's hair-raising to think that 18-year-old boys can think it's okay to use their superior age to get younger girls to give blow jobs to ten boys in a row, but that is exactly what was happening. As Norwegian newspaper *VG* wrote at the time, this is a culture in which 'the distinction between consensual sex and assault has grown dangerously thin'.[2] In recent decades, we have seen the increased sexualisation of youth culture, particularly of girls, not just in Norway, but all over the world. And for many young women, growing up in this environment means enduring any number of unpleasant sexual experiences that they then struggle with later in life.

It shouldn't be this way.

We want women to be able to make independent choices from a point of self-confidence and self-assurance, armed with all the facts. And we want these choices to be based on sound medical knowledge – not gossip, misunderstandings or fear. Sexuality and sexual health must be demystified, and we must take ownership of our bodies. This book will give you the opportunity to make sensible and well-informed choices that suit *you*.

Perhaps you're wondering: why should I bother reading a medical book written by two Norwegian students, one of whom hasn't even finished medical school yet? And as we were writing the manuscript for the Norwegian edition of this book, we asked ourselves the very same question plenty of times. And this is why we approached its creation, and particularly that of the foreign editions, with a healthy dose of humility, taking inspiration from the example of German medical student Giulia Enders who achieved resounding success with her book, *Darm mit Charme* (published in English as *Gut: The Inside Story of Our Body's Most Underrated Organ*). The rhyming title of our book even pays homage to the German title of hers. Enders' book transformed intestines and faeces into topics people could discuss on prime-time talk shows. She paved the way for us, showing how medicine can be made understandable and funny, and – most importantly – how we can talk about our most intimate body parts without even a whiff of shame.

As medical students, we have certain advantages that nobody can take

3

away from us: we are curious, we are young and we have the nerve to ask the 'stupid' questions. We don't have professional reputations to jeopardise and we haven't (yet) spent so much time among the ranks of doctors that we've forgotten how to speak plainly to people.

Many times, when we were working on the book, we found that we too had fallen victim to the myths surrounding the female sex organs. And there are a lot of these myths. The ones about the hymen are perhaps the most persistent, and continue to place girls the world over at risk. Yet few doctors trouble themselves about this little body part. Some even help to perpetuate the myths by checking girls' genitals on behalf of their parents. In our quest for answers, we often found that senior gynaecologists would dismiss our questions about the hymen as uninteresting or unimportant. This is unacceptable, given its implications in many women's lives. Our TEDxOslo talk 'The Virginity Fraud', which debunks the most common misperceptions on the hymen, has now had over 2 million views, and our inboxes continue to be filled with personal stories from women who have fallen victim to the fallacies.

Another myth is that hormonal contraception is unnatural and dangerous. This misunderstanding leads to unplanned pregnancies for thousands of girls and women who choose to use unreliable contraceptive methods instead. We understand that people are confused and afraid of the side-effects, and we are sick and tired of seeing people in the medical community dismiss such concerns without providing proper explanations. That is why we have devoted plenty of space here to a thorough discussion of contraception. We review the most important research on possible side-effects, such as mood swings and low libido. Where there is uncertainty, we are open about it, but our primary aim is to reassure you. Serious side-effects are, in fact, extremely rare, and there is little evidence that depression or a decreased sex drive are problems that affect a large proportion of women using hormonal contraceptives. There are always exceptions, but we hope that after reading this book you'll be able to distinguish between what is and is not usual.

Other myths, while not directly harmful, reflect the fact that even in this intrinsically female arena, when it comes to medical research it is still very much a man's world. Hearing women complain that they never have 'vaginal

4

orgasms' reminds us of just how much our understanding of female sexuality has been coloured by men's needs over the centuries. There *is no* 'vaginal orgasm' as such – just orgasms as a result of different types of stimulation, all of which are equally delightful. We hope that by reading this book and becoming better informed, women can stop feeling inferior for needing other forms of stimulation besides penetration in order to achieve orgasm.

These are just a few of the things you will read about in *The Wonder Down Under*. We look forward to you joining us on a journey through the female sex organs, from the vulva to the ovaries, and learning lots, just as we did while working on the book. The most important thing for us is that after reading it you'll be able to relax. After all, a body is just a body; we all have one, and it offers us joys and challenges alike throughout our lives. Be proud of what your body achieves and be patient with it when it struggles.

Happy reading!

Nina and Ellen
Oslo, Norway
2017

THE GENITALS

Our genital area is, perhaps, our most intimate body part. It is our close companion from the moment we burst into the world from our mother's vagina and first see the light of day. In nursery we delighted in comparing innie and outie pee-pees. Then, with the onset of puberty, came the first, dark hairs on our crotch. We all remember our first period, whether the moment was filled with pride or terror. Perhaps you began to masturbate and found you could make your body curl up in pleasure. Then came your sexual debut, with all that it entails in the way of vulnerability, curiosity and desire. Perhaps you already have children, and so experienced the enormous changes that your sex organs undergo, and the miracles they are capable of performing. Your genitals are part of you. It's about time you got to know them better.

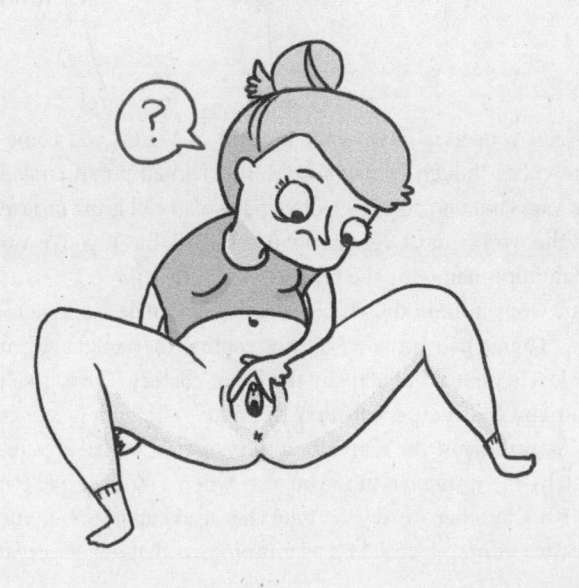

VULVA – THE WONDER DOWN UNDER

Stand naked in front of the mirror and take a good look at yourself. Your genital area begins low down on your belly, with a fatty area that covers the front of your pubic bone. This soft area is called the mound of Venus, and it becomes covered in hair during puberty. The fatty cushion is larger for some women than others, so in some women the pubic area protrudes slightly from their belly, whereas others have flatter variants – both are quite normal.

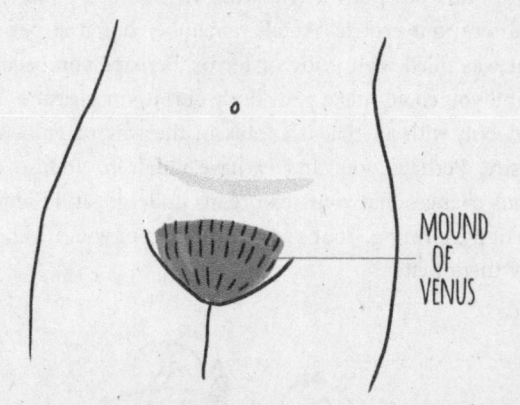

MOUND OF VENUS

If you run your gaze down your mound of Venus, you come to what we call the vulva, though it may also be nicknamed pussy, cookie jar, snatch, flower, vag, cunt and so on – Norwegians also call it the mouse. *Vulva* may not be the world's most commonly used word, but if you're a woman that's the anatomical name for the bit between your legs.

Some women think the visible part of the female sex organs is called the vagina. 'There's hair growing on my vagina', they might say, or 'You have such a lovely vagina', but actually that's not correct. The vagina doesn't have any hair and it isn't especially easy to see it – although it is of course totally lovely. Vagina is just the name for a part of your sexual apparatus, or more accurately, the muscular tube you use when you have penetrative sex or give birth – in other words, the tube that leads up to the uterus (see p. 11). The reason we're so focused on terminology is that our sex organs are about so much more than just the vagina, no matter how much pleasure we get out of it! Most people who refer to the female genitalia as the vagina mean vulva, and it's the vulva we'll begin with in our description of the fantastic female sex organs.

So what does the vulva look like?

The vulva is formed like a flower, with two layers of petals, known as labia (the Latin for lips). And believe it or not, it wasn't us who came up with the flower metaphor. When looking at the different parts, it makes sense to start from the outside and work our way in.

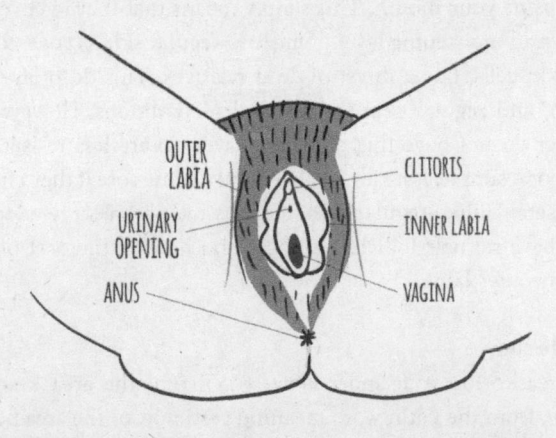

The labia are there to protect the sensitive parts that lie further in. The outer labia (labia majora), which are thicker than the inner ones, are full of fat and work a little like air bags or shock absorbers. Although they may be long enough to cover the inner labia, they can also be very narrow. Some women just have two small dents in their skin that frame the rest of the vulva on either side.

The outer sides of the labia majora are covered in regular skin. Like the rest of the skin on your body, it's full of sebaceous glands, sweat glands and hair follicles. In addition to hair, which is a great thing, it is also possible to get spots and eczema on your outer labia, which isn't so great. Sadly, skin will be skin. The inner side of this layer is lined with mucous membranes like the inner labia.

The inner labia are often longer than the outer labia, although not always. They may be full of crinkles and folds, like a princess skirt made of tulle. Stand looking at yourself in the mirror. In some women, the inner labia protrude markedly from the outer labia; others need to spread aside their outer labia in order to see them. In contrast to the fatty outer labia, the inner labia are thinner and highly sensitive. They aren't as sensitive as the clitoris, which is the most sensitive place on your body, but they are full of nerve endings, so it can feel very good to touch them.

The inner labia don't have regular skin. Instead, they are covered with a mucous membrane – you'll have seen mucous membranes before, for example inside your mouth. This simply means that they're covered with a protective and moistening layer of mucus. Regular skin is covered in a layer of dead skin cells, like a duvet of dead relatives. This dead layer provides protection, and regular skin thrives in dry conditions. However, mucous membranes do not have this protective layer, so are less resistant to wear and tear. For example, long inner labia may become sore if they chafe against tight trousers. Unlike regular skin, mucous membranes prefer to be moist and they have no hair follicles, so there's no hair on the part of the vulva inside your outer labia.

The vestibulum

If you spread aside your inner labia, you'll find the area known as the *vestibulum*, from the Latin word meaning vestibule, or the area between the entrance to a building and its interior. If you are the kind of person who goes to the theatre or the opera, the vestibule is the place where you eat cake and drink champagne in the interval. It's the splendid entrance hall with columns and soft red velvet curtains. A woman's vestibulum doesn't have any columns to speak of, but it's an entranceway nonetheless and we would argue that it has the same velvety grandeur. You'll find two holes here: the urinary and the vaginal openings. The urinary opening, or urethra, lies between the clitoris, which is located right at the front, where the labia meet, and the vagina, which is closer to the anus (the 'other' hole).

Few people have a conscious relationship with their urinary opening, even though we all use it several times a day. In fact, some people think there isn't a separate hole for urine, but that we are like men, who have just one hole for two things: sperm and urine. That isn't so – the urethra has its own opening. We don't pee with our vaginas, although it's easy to misunderstand this, even if you've seen loads of female genitalia. The urinary opening can be very difficult to find even if you look for it with a mirror. It is tiny and there are often a lot of small folds of skin around the hole, but she who seeks shall find.

VAGINA – THE AMAZING EXPANDING TUBE

Unlike the little urinary opening, the much larger vaginal opening should be easy to find. The vagina is a narrow muscular tube 7–10 centimetres in length, which leads from the vulva to the uterus. Most of the time this tube is compressed so that the back and front walls are squeezed up against one another. This helps keep you waterproof. Imagine that! Your vagina is highly elastic in all directions – a bit like a pleated skirt. If you examine it with your fingers, you'll notice how ridged it is. When you feel horny, it expands both length- and widthwise.

The muscles around the vagina are strong, as you'll notice if you stick a finger into your vagina and then clench it tight. Like other muscles, these ones – the pelvic-floor muscles – become stronger when you exercise them.

The inside of the vaginal wall is covered with a moist mucous membrane. Most of the moisture is not produced in glands, but seeps straight through the vaginal walls from the interior of the body. There are no glands in the vaginal wall itself, but a bit of secretion comes from glands in the cervix (the entrance to the uterus – see p. 28). There is always moisture present in the vagina, but when you are horny, you become even wetter than usual. More fluid seeps in through the vaginal wall when extra blood flows to the whole of the genital area. You'll notice the increased blood supply to your genitals because your clitoris and inner labia will become engorged. The fluid produced when you are horny reduces the friction in your vagina when you masturbate or have sex. Less friction means less damage to the vaginal wall, which can often take quite a pummelling during sex. It's not unusual to have a bit of bleeding from small tears in the vaginal wall after sex, and then you may feel a bit sore. Luckily, it's quite harmless. The vaginal wall is good at repairing itself.

In addition to the moisture that comes through the vaginal wall, some mucus comes from two glands located just behind the vaginal opening, one on either side towards your bottom. Known as Bartholin's glands, after the Danish anatomist Casper Bartholin, they produce a slick fluid that helps lubricate the vaginal opening. Bartholin's glands are oval, the size of peas and can be troublemakers. If the little tube through which they dispatch their mucus becomes blocked, a vulval cyst can form. This is detectable as a small, hard lump to one side of the vulva, like a little balloon. If the cyst becomes infected, it can turn into a painful business, but the problem can be fixed with minor surgery. There's some disagreement over how important Bartholin's glands are for lubrication of the vagina.[1] Women who've had the glands removed following problems with cysts still experience an increase in vaginal moisture when they're turned on.

The famous 'G-spot'

Apparently some way into the vagina on the anterior wall, in other words, towards the bladder and stomach, lies a spot that is popular in the sex columns of women's magazines. We're talking now about the G-spot, named after the German gynaecologist, Ernst Gräfenberg, who discovered it in the 1940s. Researchers have been discussing and searching for the G-spot ever since, and it is still pretty controversial. They are uncertain what it is, and its existence as a separate anatomical entity hasn't even been proved yet.

The G-spot is described as an extra-sensitive point in the vagina, and some women say they can achieve orgasm just by stimulating it. The G-spot can be stimulated by making a 'come-hither' gesture with a finger. Imagine a Disney witch trying to lure you towards her – that's the movement you're after. According to some women, stimulation of the G-spot feels better than or different to stimulation elsewhere in the vagina. As you may have noticed, the vagina itself is not especially sensitive compared with the vulva and especially the clitoris. Sensitivity is highest in the vaginal opening and lessens further up.

The media often treat the G-spot as if it were a separate anatomical structure. It is especially easy to gain this impression if you read sex columns or sexual self-help books. A British review article from 2012 examined research claiming that the G-spot is a separate area of the vagina and concluded that the proof was sparse. Most research on the G-spot is based on questionnaires in which women themselves describe it. The review article mentioned above also stated that many of the women who believe in the G-spot had difficulty pointing it out on themselves. The researchers also report that studies based on imaging techniques have failed to find any separate structure capable of producing orgasm or sexual pleasure in women, other than the clitoris.[2]

One hypothesis about the G-spot is, in fact, that it is not a separate physical structure, but simply a deep-lying inner part of the clitoris that is stimulated during sex, *directly through the vaginal wall*. In 2010, a group of researchers published a study in which they had observed the anterior vaginal wall of a woman while she had vaginal sex with her partner. They used ultrasound to see what was happening and searched for the G-spot. They didn't find it, but concluded that the inner parts of the clitoris lie so close to the anterior vaginal wall that the clitoris may be the answer to the G-spot mystery.[3]

Some studies claim that the G-spot is important for achieving a squirting orgasm, and this leads us to another theory that the G-spot may be linked to a group of glands located between the urethra and the anterior vaginal wall.[4] Known as Skene's glands, they are the female equivalent of the male prostate, a walnut-sized gland that surrounds the urethra between the bladder and the penis. Skene's glands are associated with female ejaculation, or squirting orgasms, as they produce liquid that may be released during orgasm – just like the prostate.

It's odd that an area as accessible as the vaginal wall should be so shrouded in mystery. Especially when there's so much scribbling about the G-spot. We wait with bated breath for more high-quality research on the female body.

CLITORIS – AN ICEBERG

Now, perhaps you were surprised just now when we mentioned the *inner parts* of the clitoris. Which inner parts we hear you say? After all, most texts say that the clitoris is the size of a raisin and is located on the uppermost part of the vulva, neatly positioned at the point where the outer labia meet. But this little button is just the tip of an iceberg. In the deep darkness of the pelvic area, an organ lies hidden that exceeds all your wildest imaginings.

Although anatomists have known since the 1800s that the clitoris is a largely subterranean organ,* this is far from general knowledge. While the male penis is described in detail in anatomies and textbooks, the clitoris has remained a curiosity. As late as 1948, *Gray's Anatomy* chose not to label the clitoris. Nor has the male-dominated medical world been particularly interested in conducting further research on the clitoris. There is still disagreement over what forms part of the clitoris and how it works. In a medical context, this is startling.

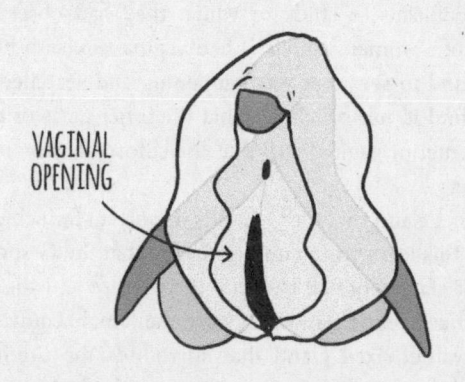

VAGINAL
OPENING

It's a tiny part of the story

What we do know is that what most people describe as the clitoris is only a fraction of a large organ that extends into the pelvis, and down along either side of the vulva.[5] If we had X-ray specs, we would see that the clitoris complex is shaped like an upside-down Y. The little raisin, called the *glans* or *head* of the clitoris, is right at the top and the only visible part. It may be anything from 0.5 to 3.5 centimetres long, but appears smaller because it is partly covered by a little hood.[6] Below the head is a shaft that descends through the body at an angle, like a boomerang, before splitting

---

* The anatomist Georg Ludwig Kobelt described the inner construction of the clitoris in the 1840s and concluded that the male and female sexual organs shared the same building blocks.

into two 'legs', which lie on either side of the genital area, buried beneath the labia.

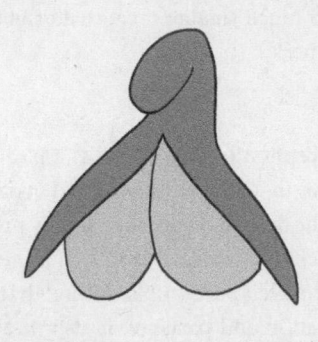

Each of the legs contains erectile tissue, the *corpus cavernosum*, which fills with blood and becomes engorged during arousal. Between these two legs there are two extra bodies of erectile tissue, the *bulbi vestibuli*, which surround the vaginal and urinary openings.

For those of you who were especially attentive in science classes, this description may be ringing some bells – but wasn't it the man's penis that had a head, shaft and erectile tissue? The principal source of female pleasure, the clitoris, is a well-kept secret, in stark contrast to the erect penis, which is conspicuous to say the least. It may, therefore, seem surprising that the clitoris and the penis are two versions of the same organ.

In fact, the genital tracts of male and female embryos are identical until the 12th week of pregnancy. They are dominated by a kind of mini-penis (or giga-clitoris!) known as *the genital tubercle*, which has the potential to develop into either a female or male sexual organ. Since the penis and the clitoris both develop from the same basic structure, the two organs share many similarities of form and function.

The head of the penis is, in fact, the same as the clitoral button, which is why both are given the same name – *glans*. The glans is the most sensitive spot on both the female and male body. It is estimated that the female and male glans both contain more than 8,000 sensory nerve endings. A sensory nerve ending receives information about pressure and touch, and sends signals to the brain, where it is interpreted as either pain or pleasure. The more nerve endings there are, the more nuanced and powerful are the signals the brain receives. Nonetheless, the head of the clitoris is a great deal more sensitive than the head of the penis because the nerve endings are concentrated into a much smaller area: that's right, in fact, the concentration is 50 times higher![7]

Pleasure or pain

Unfortunately, the perception of the clitoris as a pleasure button may have led some men to believe that all pressure is good pressure. If a bit of simple pressure doesn't elicit the desired result, they simply press harder and harder. But that's not how the clitoris works. It is so rich in nerve endings that even the tiniest variation in touch is perceptible. Although this offers undreamt-of possibilities for stimulation and pleasure, it also means that the transition from pleasure to pain or outright numbness is tiny. Over the long term, hard pressure can cause the nerve endings to simply refuse to send signals on to the brain: the clitoral button is switched to 'mute'. If that happens, the clitoris has to be left in peace until it's ready to start talking again. In other words, it's a bit like hooking up: if you try too hard, things often go wrong.

The man's erectile tissues make the penis hard when they become engorged with blood. So, it goes without saying that the woman's erectile tissues should do exactly the same. When we are aroused, the clitoral complex can swell to double its normal size.[8] It is, quite simply, an impressive erection. Since the clitoral legs and the *bulbi vestibuli* lie beneath the labia and around the urinary and vaginal openings, this can make the vulva look larger during arousal. In addition, the vestibulum and the inner labia take on a darker, purplish-red colouring owing to the blood that gathers there.

And the similarities don't stop there. Men like to boast about 'morning glory' and nightly erections, but women get them too. In a study conducted at the University of Florida in the 1970s, two women with large clitorises were studied and compared with men. The study found that the women had just as many nightly 'erections' during deep sleep as the men.[9] Another study found that women had 'erections' up to eight times a night, for a combined period of 1 hour, 20 minutes![10]

As you'll have gathered, there's a lot we didn't learn about the clitoris in our science classes. This proud organ has been overlooked, undervalued and hidden away for far too long. Only when we realise how the clitoris extends to encompass all areas of our pelvic region will we be able to understand what a marvellous instrument of pleasure we're equipped with.

BLOODY VIRGINITY

For thousands of years, different cultures have been extremely concerned with virginity – not men's, but women's. A man cannot be a Madonna or a whore, pure or impure, but a woman can, and 'luckily', vaginal bleeding on the wedding night can reveal what kind of a woman she is.

A lot of people use the term 'pop her cherry' to suggest that a woman who hasn't had sex before can be popped like a bottle of champagne. It's as if her vagina is as different before and after her sexual debut as a bottle of Moët and Chandon is with and without its cork. As you may have gathered from our tone, that is not the case.

The idea of virginity is widespread in popular culture. For Jessica the vampire in *True Blood*, every sex act is her first and she has to bleed time after time. Doubt surrounds Queen Margaery Tyrell in *Game of Thrones* – is she really still *pure* after marrying king number three? Classic literature also describes virginity and bleeding. 'Damn!' Norwegian novelist Sigrid Undset's character Kristin Lavransdatter might have said, as the blood ran down her thigh in the film we saw about her in our literature classes. Instead, she said something along the lines of: 'Who will want a flower whose bloom has been ripped off?' as she wept bitterly in the arms of her lover, Erlend. As a man, Erlend had no need to weep as he had no virtue to lose.

The idea that the woman is an innocent flower, and that '*taking her virginity*' is the same as ripping the head off a flower is even encoded in medical language. The bleeding that is supposed to occur when a woman has sex for the first time is called 'deflowering' – the whole business is indescribably old-fashioned.[11] It's almost as if men from different cultures and different historical eras ganged up to find ways of controlling and limiting woman's sexuality and her ability to make decisions about her own body.

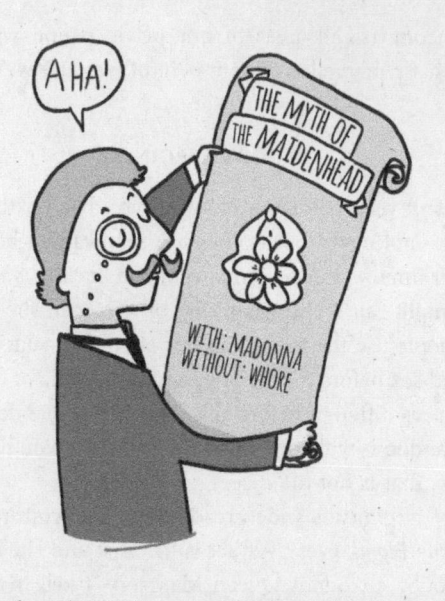

As you'll have gathered, it's time to talk about the *hymen*, that mythical structure in the vaginal opening that can still cost women the world over their honour or even their lives based solely on antiquated traditions and misinformation. It's unbelievable that men and women are still differentiated in this way and that something as wonderful and positive as sex could mean ruination for women without having any consequences for men. When you consider, on top of this, that the concept of the hymen and the associated bleeding is based on myths, the whole thing is too stupid for words.

The hymen has traditionally been presented as a kind of seal of chastity which, as myth has it, will be broken and bleed when the woman first has sexual intercourse, and only then. This bleeding has been used as proof of virginity – a proof so important for people that it used to be customary to hang the blood-stained sheet out to dry after the wedding night, so that the whole neighbourhood could see that everything had been as it should. The myth of the hymen says: if you bleed after sexual intercourse, people will know that you haven't had sex before; and equally, that if you don't bleed, you've already had sex. But this myth, like most others, is totally wrong.

Belief in this myth is perpetuated by the widespread perception of the

18

hymen as a membrane. When you hear the word 'membrane' perhaps you picture a taut sheet of plastic kitchen film that will split if you poke a hole in it. Pop! But if you've ever looked at your genitalia in a mirror, you'll know there isn't a sheet of plastic kitchen film over your vagina, even if you haven't had sex before. But don't let's allow one myth to be replaced by another. Lately we've heard a lot of talk to the effect that 'the hymen doesn't exist'. While it's true that there isn't a seal keeping the vagina shut, that doesn't mean there isn't an anatomical structure that is the cause of the misunderstanding.

There is a fold of mucous membrane

Just inside the vaginal opening there is an encircling fold of mucous membrane that lies up against the vaginal wall like a ring. It's this little ring that's traditionally been called the virginal membrane, the maidenhead and such like – we call it the hymen. Although these words all mean the same thing, virginal membrane is such a misleading term that it is better to avoid it.

All women are born with a hymen, but that doesn't mean it's any use to them. It is the female equivalent of male nipples. It has no function and is just a leftover from our embryonic existence.

The hymen has both depth and breadth. In other words, it isn't thin like plastic wrap, it's thick and robust. In pre-pubescent girls, it is usually smooth and shaped like a doughnut with a hole in the middle. Then the body's hormonal orchestra takes the stage and, like so many other parts of the body, the hymen changes in puberty. By the time puberty ends, it has often become crescent shaped. It's broadest at the rear, towards the anus, and still encircles the vaginal wall, but now has a bigger hole in the centre.[12] That's how it is in theory at least. In reality, there's no single way a hymen should look. Most women have a circular hymen with a hole in the middle. Some are even and smooth, others are wrinkled and indented, but this is not a sign of sexual activity. Some women have hymens with strands stretched across the vaginal opening, so that they look more like an 'ø' than an 'o'. Hymens can also look like sieves, with lots of small holes instead of one big hole in the middle. Yet others look like small fringes on the vaginal wall. A small minority of girls have a hymen that does cover the whole of the entrance to the vagina. These girls often have a fairly rigid, tough membrane, and this is a variant that spells trouble, because of course the menstrual blood has to have a way out! Women with this type will often only discover the problem when they have their first period. If the menstrual blood gets trapped inside the vagina, it can cause severe pain and will require surgery. This rare variant is the closest it gets to the myth of the hymen as a seal.[13]

Whatever form the hymen takes, it is flexible and elastic (except in those rare cases where it covers the entire opening), and it is the narrowest point of the vagina. The vagina has a dramatic ability to expand and then contract again – you can, after all, get a baby out through it. So, the hymen should also be able to expand. But although it is elastic, it won't necessarily be elastic enough for sexual intercourse. It's a bit like a rubber band that can be stretched so far, but snaps if you pull too hard on it.

When you have vaginal sex for the first time, the hymen is stretched along with the rest of the vagina. For many women the hymen is elastic enough to ensure that all goes well, but for others, it can tear and bleed a little. In other words, some women bleed the first time they have sex and others don't. It all depends on how elastic their hymen is. Women who have an unusual-shaped hymen with a part that stretches across the vaginal opening like an 'ø' will find that this part must often tear to make way for a penis or fingers.

It's difficult to be certain just how many women have hymens that bleed when they have sex for the first time. There's some statistical material, but the numbers vary. Two different studies we've looked at reported that 56 per cent and 40 per cent of all women, respectively, bleed when they have consensual vaginal sex for the first time. This is far from all women, but it's still a high proportion.[14]

Both studies interviewed women about the first time they had sexual intercourse. So, we can't possibly know for sure whether it was the hymen that bled, even though it is the vagina's narrowest point, or whether the blood came from elsewhere. As we noted in the section about the vagina (see p. 11), it's both possible and normal for bleeding to occur as a result of small tears in the vaginal wall if people have slightly rough sex, aren't wet enough or tense up the muscles around their vagina because they're nervous. This can happen the first time a woman has sex or on several occasions.

Have you heard about virginity tests?

Another important part of the myth about the hymen involves virginity tests, which rely on the belief that it is possible to tell from looking at a woman's genitalia whether or not she has had sexual intercourse. Apparently the Virgin Mary underwent a virginity test, and the same is said of Joan of Arc and many other women from different conservative environments in modern times.

Now and again, we hear about doctors who are still carrying out virginity tests on young women at the request of their parents, who want proof that their daughters are intact[15] – despite the fact that experts in forensic medicine deem such tests to be irrelevant.[16] We also hear of doctors issuing virginity certificates to terrified young women who are afraid of the consequences if there's no bleeding on the wedding night.

However, it is usually impossible to see any difference between the hymens of girls who have had sex and those who haven't.[17] This renders the whole business of virginity testing absurd. And although the hymen may be damaged during sexual intercourse if it's severely stretched, the damage won't necessarily be permanent. It turns out that, in many cases, the hymen can heal without any visible scarring.[18]

Much of the research on the hymen and the way it changes after a woman's sexual debut comes from surveys of women and girls who have been exposed to sexual abuse. A Norwegian review article reports that what were previously thought to be suspect changes in children's hymens – for example a wide opening[19] or narrow brim – are now interpreted as entirely non-specific findings and not as proof of sexual abuse.[20] These variations in the hymen can also be found among children who haven't been exposed to sex abuse. The authors of the article are, incidentally, careful to note that the lack of a relevant finding doesn't prove that a child has *not* been exposed to sexual abuse.

On the whole, it's not possible to find out whether or not a woman has had sex by looking between her legs. The hymen is not a guarantee for those who haven't had sex, nor is there one variant for those who've had sex and another for those who are still 'virgins'. Like other body parts, the hymen's appearance varies according to the individual. Sorry, but virginity tests don't work.

Unfortunately, this information about the hymen is not generally known.

Women still resort to surgery to guarantee that they'll bleed on their wedding night – hymenoplasty, as it's called. In Norway, the private Volvat clinic in Oslo offered this surgery until as recently as 2006.[21] It stopped doing them after seeking the Council for Medical Ethics' view on the practice. The council objected to the procedure because it becomes a kind of quick fix or replacement for a proper solution to the problem: cultural change.[22] But it still exists in some countries – in the UK it is available privately. On the internet, it's possible to buy fake membranes containing theatrical blood for around US$30, which guarantee that you can 'kiss your deep dark secret goodbye' and get married with confidence.[23] Incidentally, Egyptian politicians suggested prohibiting imports of this product in 2009.[24]

Why do women feel they need to resort to these kinds of solutions instead of informing people that the absence of bleeding does not equate to the absence of virginity? And why is it so important for some societies to have proof that women remain 'intact' until they get married? The bleeding must become less significant, virginity tests must be abandoned once and for all, but most importantly we must jettison the idea that virginity itself is important.

The problem is that it is difficult to find reliable information about the hymen – and, not least, to distinguish what is right from what is less right or wrong. In our quest for knowledge about the hymen, we found little information that was accessible, available to most people and correct, too. We found a great deal of research literature – despite the fact that the hymen is barely mentioned in the gynaecology textbooks most commonly used in medical school – and we encountered some of the same myths again. We still have masses of questions. It's hair-raising to think that doctors have shown so little interest in a structure that can, in the worst of cases, cause modern women to lose their honour or their lives. Worse still, the little information that is available doesn't reach the people who need it. We all have an important job to do here. It's just a matter of getting started.

THE OTHER HOLE

Known as the place where the sun don't shine, this crinkly, brown orifice is often overlooked in discussions about women's genitals, but the only thing separating the vagina and the 'other hole' is a thin wall. Being in such close quarters, it is unavoidably connected to the vagina, the vulva and many women's sexual self-image.

This hole, correctly called the *anus*, is a formidable ring of muscle designed to keep gas and faeces in their place until we're ready to get rid of them. This has clearly been a vital task since time immemorial, as our body comes equipped with not just one, but two sphincters in a row. If one of them lets us down, we have an extra backup.

The inner sphincter is controlled by what is known as the autonomic nervous system – the part of the nervous system we don't have conscious control over. When the body notices that the rectum is beginning to fill up with faeces, signals go out telling the inner sphincter to relax. This is the defecation reflex, which we experience as a sudden urge to find the nearest toilet. If we had only this primitive reflex, we would be pooing all the time, the way babies do, but we humans are social creatures. The outer sphincter – the one you can feel if you put a finger in your butt and clench – is the top dog. It's a voluntary muscle, which ensures that you can hold off until circumstances allow you a little privacy. If you keep clenching for long enough, your body takes the hint and the primal instincts realise they've lost. The faeces discreetly withdraws back up into the gut and patiently awaits a better occasion. The poo window, as we like to call it, has closed for the time being.

The anus is the dark corner of the genital area, but fortunately there's more to it than just crap. The area around and just inside the anus is full of nerve endings just waiting to be stimulated. Some people find it expands the dimensions of their sex life if they invite it to join the party. Others may content themselves with acknowledging that it's a beautiful system, and send it a few affectionate thoughts from time to time.

HAIRY TIPS

Being a woman means having hair on your crotch – as far as nature's concerned, that is. In puberty, thin dark hairs begin to appear on the mound of Venus and alongside the labia. Gradually, they spread and multiply until in the end a dense, triangular meadow of hair spreads all the way back to the anus, and generally spills over a bit to the inner thighs, crossing the famous bikini line.

Aesthetic ideals of hairless or well-coiffed vulvas have become fashionable again in recent years – a source of anxiety and problems for many women. A lot of people worry that hair removal results in more hair, darker hair or even causes the hairs to grow faster. For many years, we were also terrified that our bikini lines would grow uncontrollably in all directions if we weren't careful with the razor. For the same reason, many a teenage boy has regularly borrowed his dad's razor and shaved his bum fluff in the hope that a manly moustache will sprout and conceal his acne. Happily for us, but unhappily for the teenage boy, this is total nonsense.

Genes and hormones determine how much body hair you'll have and when it grows.[25] Everyone is born equipped with all the hair follicles they'll ever have – around 5 million. Some of them, for example those around your sex organs and in your armpits, are especially hormone-sensitive. In puberty, the body explodes with sex hormones, causing these hormone-sensitive follicles to enlarge and produce thicker, darker hair. The pattern for hormone-sensitive follicles varies from one person to the next, which explains why some men have dense fur on their back, while others barely have a hair on their chest. Although it feels otherwise, you don't grow any more hair in puberty; it's just that the soft, downy fluff gradually transforms into 'grown-up' hair. Shaving doesn't stimulate hair growth or change, it's simply that people often start to shave when their hair growth is still in the process of change so they think it was caused by shaving.

Some people also think the hairs become thicker and stiffer or grow more quickly when they shave. That isn't possible either, although it really can feel that way when you're sitting there the day after shaving with pubes like a porcupine. Hair mostly consists of dead material. All the hair that's visible above the skin is dead protein; the only life to be found is down inside the follicle. Even if you do cut your hair, the follicle has no way of knowing it; the dead only speak in *Ghosthunters*! In the real world, the follicle keeps on producing hair at the same rate as before, blissfully ignorant of the fact that you are ruthlessly mowing down everything it manages to produce. Also, the size of the follicle is what determines how thick the hair grows – however much you shave, the size of the follicle won't change. That said, the hair can feel stiffer just because it is shorter when it grows out. Normal hair that's left to its own devices wears thinner and thinner towards the tip and that's why it feels soft. When we shave, we cut the hair at its thickest point – close to the surface of the skin. So, when it grows out again, the tip is thicker for a while.[26]

To remove or not to remove?

We may curse (or treasure) our body hair, and, as we've said its distribution is genetically preordained. If you opt to do something about the hair growth, though, that is your choice. The hair on your body definitely has a function, but it certainly isn't so important that you'd be better off not removing it if that's what you want to do. But it is worth knowing that the hairs help heighten sexual sensitivity. If your partner strokes you lightly over your pubic hair, the bending of the hairs will send a signal to the follicles, which will pass the message on to your nervous system.[27] Hair follicles are connected to many nerve endings, so without the hair you lose a part of the sensory experience.

Throughout history, different forms of hair removal have been normal practice for both sexes. Nowadays, you can shave, wax, epilate or use hair-removal cream, to name the temporary solutions. For the most part, the choice is a matter of taste, although there are certain differences.[28]

Epilation and waxing can lead to thinner hair growth because the follicles become damaged over time when you rip the hairs out by the root. The disadvantage is that thinner hairs find it harder to penetrate the skin, which can lead to ingrown hairs and inflammation of the follicles. But hair-removal cream 'dissolves' the part of the hair that lies above the surface of the skin by destroying the protein structure of the hair. Since the follicle isn't affected, people often have fewer problems with ingrown hairs after using the creams.

There are a lot of names for the main problem with hair removal: razor bumps, ingrown hairs and *pseudofolliculitis barbae*.[29] When you remove hair, especially if it's curly, it can turn back on itself and begin to grow down into the skin. The body registers this ingrown hair as a foreign body and this triggers an inflammation in the follicle, like a little spot. If you're unlucky or if you pick the spot-like bump, you may develop a bacterial infection as well. Then it may become painful and swollen, and often results in scarring.

Advice about bump-free hair removal abounds in the media. And we swallow the beauty experts' advice hook, line and sinker: after all, a clean-shaven crotch with ingrown hairs and spots is hardly a pretty sight. But do you really need that £65 cream the waxing salon is trying to sell you or the special razors for women that come in at around £5 per blade?

Unfortunately, you're throwing your money away. If you're really bothered by ingrown hair and follicle infections, it's worth trying hair-removal cream instead of the other methods. If you prefer epilating, waxing or shaving, it's important to pay attention to hygiene. Wash the area well before you start. People who are prone to follicular infections would do well to rinse the area with disinfectant or apply disinfectant lotion after hair removal. You can buy these products over the counter at chemists, or even the supermarket, and they're far cheaper than the specialist products sold in fancy bottles at the salons.

Finally, it's important to point out that if you do get an ingrown hair or an infection you should avoid squeezing because that can lead to scarring. What's more, in a worst-case scenario the infection may spread. It's even possible to get such a serious infection in the follicle that it can grow to the size of a grape. In that case, you should consult a doctor who may need to drain the abscess and can prescribe antibiotics if necessary.

THE FIVE COMMANDMENTS OF SHAVING

1. Don't shave against the hair or stretch your skin. If you pull your skin taut and shave against the hair, you'll get the smoothest and softest result, since you'll be cutting the hairs beneath the surface of the skin. Unfortunately, that makes it easier for the hairs to become embedded in the skin as they grow, resulting in inflammation of the follicle.

2. Always use a clean, sharp razor blade, preferably a new one. It's tempting to use razor blades several times because they're so expensive, but that's a false economy. A sharp blade leaves the hair more cleanly cut, allowing it to grow out more easily without becoming embedded in the skin. You also have to use less force, which helps prevent irritation and razor bumps. In addition, a used blade may be dirty and the bacteria can get into the follicles, which may become infected.

3. Use (cheap) razor blades with a single blade. Razor blades come in new, ever-fancier versions, with ever-increasing numbers of blades and, as a result, ever-higher prices. The message is generally 'a closer shave'. Perhaps surprisingly, this results in more ingrown hairs, because the additional blades cause the hairs to be cut beneath the surface of the skin. What's more, the cost means women don't change blades as often as they should, so that the they become blunt and covered in bacteria. So, you're no better off. Men's razor blades are often cheaper, so it may be worth buying them instead.

4. Use plenty of warm water. Dry shaving should be avoided at all costs. Dry hair is stiff and therefore harder to cut; you need to use more force to get a good result, and that will irritate your skin more, increasing the likelihood of red bumps and inflammation. A warm shower is an effective way of getting softer hair. Shaving foam has the same effect if you leave it to work for five minutes before you shave, although it has little effect the way most people use it (quick on, quick off).

5. Mild exfoliation. Washing the area with gentle, circular movements, either with an exfoliating glove or a grainy exfoliating wash, can eventually help work the ingrown hairs free from the skin. Don't rub too hard because that can lead to more irritation and skin inflammation.

INTERNAL SEX ORGANS – THE HIDDEN TREASURES

It can be easy to forget that the female sex organs are much more than just the vulva and vagina. Beneath the layers of skin, fat and muscle lies a set of soft, hidden body parts that include the internal sex organs.

Let's start the journey in. If you stick a finger 7 to 10 centimetres into your vagina, you'll feel a soft little projection, with the same consistency and shape as the tip of a nose – just a little bigger. That's the neck of the uterus or the *cervix*: the entrance to the uterus. From the vagina, the cervix looks like a flattened hemisphere. At first glance, it doesn't look like an exit or entrance at all, but right in the middle of it there's a tiny little hole called the mouth of the uterus. This is the start of a narrow passage 2 to 3 centimetres in length, which leads to the interior of the uterus. It is through this thin passage that the menstrual fluids seep out. Discharge also comes out of here. In fact, this small passageway is where most of the discharge is produced.

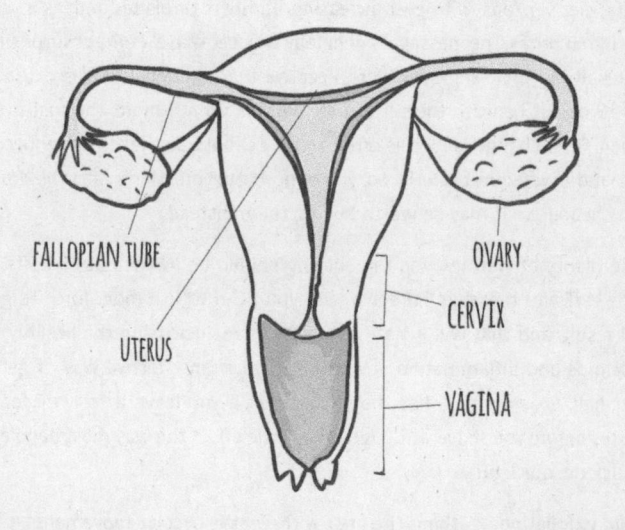

FALLOPIAN TUBE

OVARY

CERVIX

UTERUS

VAGINA

A lot of people wonder about sex and the uterus. Many people think the passage from the vagina to the uterus is wide open. We've often been asked: 'If you have sex when you're pregnant is it possible for the penis to hit the baby?'

If you've read Haruki Murakami's novel, *Kafka on the Shore*, you may have enjoyed the paragraph where a woman felt the man's sperm spraying against the walls of her uterus, implying that the penis was inside the woman's uterus when the man ejaculated.[30] The simple fact is that you can't get a penis into a uterus. The cervix isn't open, it's closed. In any case, the vagina is more than deep enough to accommodate most penises, since it is elastic both breadth- and depthwise. It simply isn't necessary to go further in.

Our impression is that most women aren't aware of their own cervix, and that isn't so surprising really. They can't see it and there's no guarantee that a woman has felt it or even knows that it's there. But the cervix deserves all the attention you can give it – for the sake of your health. The cervix is a part of the body where young women can be struck by cancer (see p. 235). In addition, it's often the place where many of the symptoms of sexually transmitted infection manifest themselves (see pp. 207–22).

What about the uterus?
The cervix is important, but it's actually just a small part of a larger organ, the womb or *uterus*. The uterus is usually a small organ the size of a fist. It's about 7.5 centimetres long and weighs no more than 70 grams, but if you're pregnant it expands dramatically. After all, it needs to become big enough to carry one (or more) growing embryos right up to term. It looks like an upside-down pear, with the cervix as the thin part the stalk grows out of.

In most women, the uterus is tipped forward, towards the navel, at roughly 90 degrees to the vagina. That's one more reason why a penis can never get into the uterus: it can't bend when it's erect, because if it did, it would break. The penis is no contortionist! Around 20 per cent of women have a backward-leaning uterus, which works just as well. It's a bit like the way some people have blue eyes and others have brown – they can still see just as well.

The uterus is hollow, but not in the same way that a barrel is hollow, because it doesn't contain air. Its anterior (front) and posterior (back) walls are pressed tightly up against each other – just like the vaginal walls – with a thin layer of fluid between them. The uterus has a very thick muscular wall, which contracts like a dishcloth being wrung out, for example, to push menstrual fluid out through the narrow passage in the cervix. When you get menstrual pains, it feels as if you're having cramps in your abdomen or your back, but the pains come from the uterus itself, as it works to push out the blood and mucus.

The wall of the uterus has several layers, and the innermost layer, the endometrium, is a mucous membrane, which changes enormously over the course of the menstrual cycle and plays a central role in menstruation. This layer grows thick every month and if you don't become pregnant, it's expelled from the uterus. It's worth remembering the name endometrium because it's related to a condition that bothers a lot of women: *endometriosis.* This is a disease in which the uterine lining grows in other areas of the body as well as the inside of the uterus. Among other symptoms, this condition is responsible for extra painful periods. You'll learn more about endometriosis later in the book (see p. 190).

Think of the uterus as a triangle with one corner pointing downwards and thin tubes projecting from each of the upper corners. Known as the Fallopian tubes, they extend 10 centimetres to either side and their purpose is to carry the egg from the ovaries down into the uterus. At the end of each tube are small finger-like projections called *fimbriae* that stretch out towards the ovaries to catch the eggs they release. Fertilisation of an egg by the sperm takes place in one of the Fallopian tubes, and the fertilised egg then floats into the uterus, where it fastens itself to the endometrium so that it can grow.

About the ovaries
The ovaries are like small bags or sacs. We have two of them, one on either side of the uterus, and they have two tasks. The first is to store and mature the eggs, which are the woman's sex cells, the second is to produce the hormones that control our cycle.

Unlike men, women don't produce new sex cells over the course of their life. At birth,* when we first see the light of day, we have about 300,000 eggs.[31] But these eggs are not yet mature. The ones we are born with are, in fact, precursors of fertile eggs. These pre-eggs are already formed by the fifth month of the embryo's life. Up until puberty, when the menstrual cycle starts up, these pre-eggs will rehearse for their future task. They begin to mature in batches, but since they don't receive the ovulation signal from

---

* New research suggests that there might be some production of new eggs after birth, but this is still quite contentious in the medical community.

the brain, they simply end up dying. In massive numbers. By the time we reach puberty, we've lost over a third of our eggs to these practice runs and are left with an exclusive group of around 180,000 eggs. By the time we are 25, we have approximately 65,000 left. These eggs must patiently await their turn, and will mature and be released one menstrual cycle after another.

Now perhaps you're thinking it's peculiar that we have 180,000 eggs at the start of puberty. We're obviously not going to have periods that many times over the course of our lives, so what are we doing with tens of thousands of eggs? The truth – and this came as a surprise to us as well – is that we can actually use up to 1,000 eggs every single month, not just one. The number used each month varies and slows down significantly the older we are. That's how the numbers add up if you've tried to do the maths. In other words, the difference between our eggs and the man's sperm isn't as vast as it's often made out to be. For women, as for men, multiple sex cells fight a hard battle among themselves for the right to try and make a baby. So, every month a battalion of eggs begin to mature, but only one exclusive egg matures enough to make it through security and is selected to be released from the ovary. The rest are brutally rejected and destroyed.[32]

Several times, we've come up against an interesting question about hormonal contraception: will contraception that prevents ovulation make your eggs and fertility last longer? After all, it sounds logical that it would be worth the body's while to save the eggs until you were ready to use them to make a baby instead of chucking them out every month through menstruation. Unfortunately, it doesn't work that way. Hormonal contraception only prevents that one, selected egg from being released from the ovary each month; it doesn't prevent the maturation of the 1,000 monthly pre-eggs. You'll lose just as many eggs each month, no matter which type of contraception you use.[33]

At 45 to 55, we reach the age of menopause, a phase of life in which the female body undergoes just as many, and equally dramatic, changes as it did in puberty. The most important one is that we cease to be fertile – we have quite simply used up our egg reserves. The age at which the menopause begins varies from one woman to the next and its timing is largely determined by genetics. What's more, some women naturally have more eggs than others. Men, on the other hand, continue to produce several million sperm cells a day until the moment their hearts stop beating. Their fertility has no best-before date, although the sperm often diminishes in quality over the years.* Mick Jagger, at the age of 73, became a father for the eighth time in 2016, with his much younger model girlfriend – the world is unfair.

As we mentioned, the ovaries also produce hormones. The most important and best known of these are oestrogen and progesterone. These hormones alter our bodies in the different phases of life, and they control the menstrual cycle in collaboration with several different hormones from other areas including the brain. But we'll come back to that again later.

GENDER, GENDER AND GENDER

For many people, the word *gender* contains an opposition: woman-man, girl-boy. When you hear the question, 'what is a man?' or 'what is a woman?' you may think it's easy to answer; because of course a man is a person with a man's body, and a woman is a person with a woman's body. *The Wonder Down Under*, for example, is a book about people who have a vagina and other female sex organs, so that must mean it's a book about women, mustn't it?

It's hardly surprising you might think this way, but it's not actually that simple. Whether we are women or men is not only determined by our sex organs or our body shape. What's more, the physical difference between the sexes is much smaller than you think.

In this section, we'll focus on three factors that are involved in determining just what gender we are: our chromosomes, which we refer to here as *genetic gender*; our bodies, or *biological gender*; and psychological factors, or *psychological gender*. We are not saying that these are the only factors that constitute 'gender'. We can also talk about social and cultural factors of course. But since this is a medical book, we've opted to focus on the genetic, physical and psychological.

Genetic gender – a cookery book
Have you ever seen a picture of a DNA (or deoxyribonucleic acid to give it its full name) strand? If you zoom in with a gigantic microscope, it looks

---

* The quality of sperm cells also deteriorates with age. In other words, the man's age influences the couple's fertility and the child's risk of congenital disease.

like a ladder that's been twisted into a spiral. But the rungs on the DNA ladder aren't like the ones on the stepladder you use when you're changing a light bulb in your flat. In relation to its width, which is less than microscopic, the DNA ladder is insanely tall and it has very special rungs.

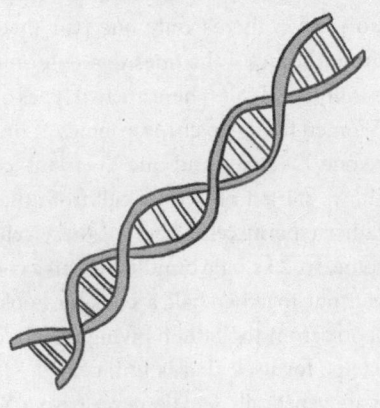

The rungs on the DNA ladder are made of substances that we can compare to letters. On each rung there are two letters. Together, they can be read as codes or mini recipes. Each recipe encodes a protein that carries out a specific task in the body. In combination, we call the codes for several proteins a gene. Our genes determine whether we have blue or brown eyes, two or three legs, wings and tails or big brains. In conjunction, all these codes are a bit like a cookery book filled with recipes for absolutely every component we need specifically to make *us*. The posh name for this kind of cookery book is a genome. Our genome is our own unique genetic recipe.

At the centre of every single cell in the body there's a complete cookery book for the person the cell comes from, meaning that there are around 3 metres of DNA strands in every cell. This is what the police rely on when they use blood, sperm, nails or skin cells to look for criminals. If you take a totally random cell from another person, for example Norwegian Prime Minister, Erna Solberg, this cell will, in theory, contain all the information you need to build a new version of her – in other words, a clone. But how can a whole, 3-metre long cookery book fit into something as small as a cell? Well, the long DNA strands are coiled into densely packed bundles, just like yarn, so that everything fits in. In each cell we have 46 such bundles, known as chromosomes, which combine to constitute the whole genetic code, or the entire cookery book. The chromosomes are organised into pairs, so the 46 chromosomes are made up of 23 pairs. Within each pair, one bundle comes from our mother and one from our father.

When it comes to gender, there's only one pair that counts: the 23rd, which are the sex chromosomes – the ones that determine whether we are male or female genetically speaking. There are two types of sex chromosome, known as X and Y. Women have two chromosomes of the same type, coded XX, while men have one X variant and one Y variant, coded XY.

As you may recall, we started off with a cell from the mother (egg cell) and one from the father (sperm cell). Each of these cells contained half a set of each chromosome, so, 23 single bundles or half a cookery book. When you make a baby, you put together half a cookery book from the mother and half a cookery book from the father, giving the child a whole cookery book containing a recipe for itself that is unique.

Since people who are genetically female never have a Y chromosome, just two Xs, an egg cell will always contain an X version of the sex chromosome. This is the mother's contribution to the embryo's 23rd chromosome pair. The mother will never be able to offer a Y. However, the father's sex cell, the sperm cell, may contain either an X or a Y. Around half of the sperm cells contain an X chromosome and the rest will have a Y. If a sperm cell containing a Y combines with the egg, the embryo will be a boy, because the code is XY. If a sperm cell containing an X combines with the egg, the embryo will be a girl, coded XX.

So, it is always the man who 'decides' whether the child will be a boy or a girl. Historically there has been a great deal of pressure on women to 'give men sons'. You may have read about this in relation to frustrated kings waiting for their queen to produce a suitable heir, who historically must *of course* be a man. Although in the UK this is no longer the case. These days we know better. It's pure chance whether the child is a girl or a boy; there's a 50/50 chance every time,* depending on which sperm cell from the man combines with the egg. The woman's egg cell has no influence over the child's gender.

---

*   Actually it isn't exactly 50/50. For one reason or another, slightly more boys than girls are born when Mother Nature gets her way.

What we can conclude from all this is that if the 23rd chromosome pair contains two X chromosomes, the embryo's cookery book says: 'to be developed into a female'. If the 23rd chromosome pair contains both types of chromosome, X and Y, the cookery book says: 'to be developed into a male'.

This all seems nice and easy and, with these recipes in mind, you may have the impression that gender is just a matter of 'either/or'. But, as you'll soon see, that's far from the case. In fact, men's and women's sex organs are incredibly similar, and many in-between things can come about in the process of reaching a finished sex organ. We often tend to focus a bit too hard on the differences, but after all, we have more between our legs than just a 'hole or a tail'.

Now, it's also true that one thing or another can go awry, both with the chromosomes and the individual genes in the DNA, and as a result the recipe can come out wrong. And a mistake in a recipe means that the result will also be different – it's a bit like adding a teaspoon of pepper instead of a teaspoon of sugar. It may still taste good, but it's definitely different from what you'd expected.

People can also be born with too many or too few sex chromosomes, and what gender does that make them? What gender is X, XXX or XXY? That's a good question. As you've probably realised by now, there's no such thing as YY, because it's impossible for two sperm cells to make a baby together. To get to the bottom of all this, we need to talk a bit about how our sex organs develop, and that makes this a good moment to introduce the second aspect of gender: *physical gender*.

Physical gender – body and sex organs

So far, we've seen that the egg cell and the sperm cell combine and, if nothing goes wrong, we're left with an XX or an XY recipe – a female or a male. In spite of that, the boy and girl embryos are no different from one another at the start. At the outset, the embryos are, in fact, *absolutely identical,* regardless of their chromosome combination. An embryo always starts off with gender-neutral genitalia, which have the potential to become both female and male sex organs, and the embryo's internal sex organs can just as easily become testicles as ovaries.

For simplicity's sake, we'll focus mostly on the external sex organs here. This is how they look right at the beginning.

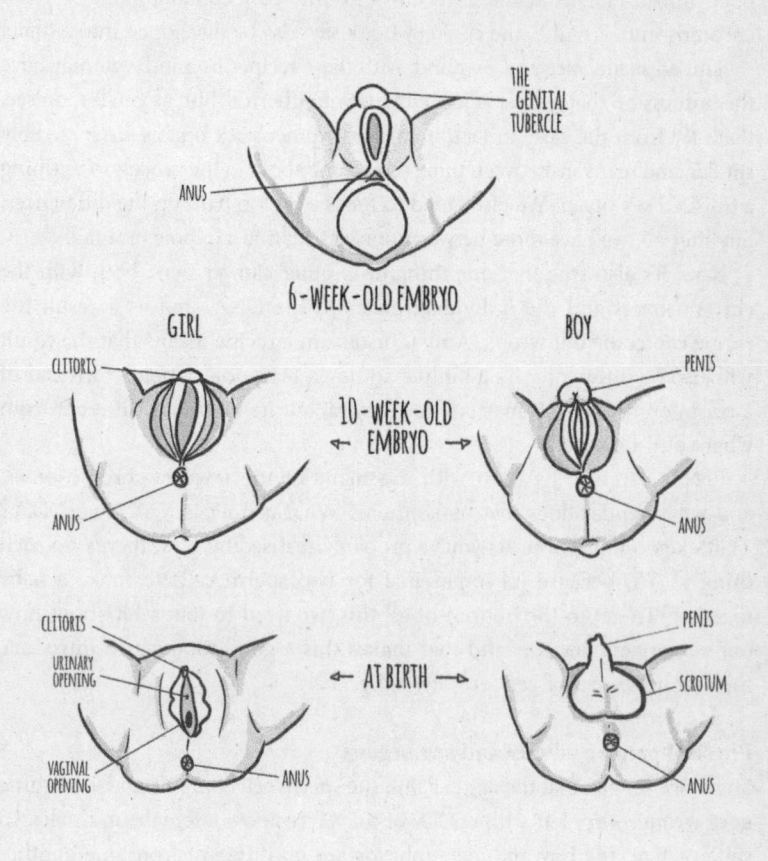

THE
GENITAL
TUBERCLE

ANUS

6-WEEK-OLD EMBRYO

GIRL

BOY

CLITORIS

PENIS

10-WEEK-OLD
← EMBRYO →

ANUS

ANUS

CLITORIS

PENIS

URINARY
OPENING

← AT BIRTH →

SCROTUM

VAGINAL
OPENING

ANUS

ANUS

Uppermost in the genital area lies the genital tubercle. It looks a bit like a mini-penis, doesn't it, or perhaps a clitoris? In fact, it can become either.

For the gender-neutral embryonic genitalia to develop into male sex organs, the embryo needs everything to go according to plan over the course of just a few critical days pretty early in the pregnancy. The embryo must be influenced by male sex hormones at precisely the right time. The most important hormone in this game is testosterone, which is only produced if the embryo has a Y chromosome. If this embryo isn't influenced by testosterone – most often because of an error in one or more of the boy embryo's genes – the genital area automatically forms into a vulva. And that leaves you with a *genetic* boy who has the sex organs of a girl.

In other words, the vulva is what all embryos come equipped with unless a special counter-command is issued. Some men have taken this to mean that they 'have something extra', whereas women are more basic – a white T-shirt compared with a fancy party top, say, although you can interpret it as you wish. However, you could just as easily say that women are the primary and fundamental sex, and it's men who are the variant, *the second sex*. But, hang on a minute… wasn't that women, too?

Look again at the illustration of gender development on the previous page. As we said earlier, the little knob at the top of the embryo's genital area, the genital tubercle, can become either a penis or a clitoris. If you know a bit about the penis and if you read the section on the clitoris earlier in the book (see p. 13), you'll certainly have realised that the two have a lot in common.

This is particularly important for women who are stressed out by the size of their clitoral glans. We're fed the idea that the clitoris is a sweet little button, but the outer parts may well stick out a long way. That doesn't mean you're more like a man! Clitorises come in different sizes, just like penises, which can be anything from 7 to 20 centimetres long. A shorter penis doesn't make a man a woman.

But back to our embryo. In the male, the urethra fuses with the penis, while the female urethra becomes a separate unit. Folds form on either side of the growing clitoris-penis. These can become either the male scrotum or the outer labia (labia majora). For the folds to become a scrotum, they must fuse together in the middle. To become labia, they do not need to fuse, but just to grow a little.

If you don't believe us when we say that a man's external genitalia are very much like our own, you should take a good look between the legs of the next man you see naked. As you'll see, his scrotum is divided in two by a neat, thin line, just like a seam. And guess what – it is a seam! This is where the 'labia' have fused together to become a scrotum. The penis is nothing but an overgrown clitoris with an inbuilt urethra. Imagine shrinking it massively, shifting the urethra a bit further down and dividing the scrotum in two, and you'll get a kind of vulva. Wow! That's pretty cool, but don't go cutting up your cutie or any other men you happen to meet. Men need their scrotums to keep their testicles in. Having said that, this is pretty much what surgeons do when they perform gender-confirmation surgery from a male to a female body; we'll come back to *that* later.

Now we can return to the question of chromosomal error. We have already said that all embryos without a Y chromosome become physically women, while all those with a Y chromosome are influenced by testosterone so that the foetus becomes physically male. Or wiped out, according to the popular cartoon series, *Y: The Last Man*. Well, it may not be so.

These are theoretical cases, but if a given foetus is coded X or XXX, its cookery book will say it's a woman. If it has Y or XXY coding, the recipe will point towards male development. But as in other cookery books, the result isn't always as described in the recipe. It is possible to develop into a woman, physically speaking, even if you are genetically a man – and vice versa!

Some foetuses that are *genetically male* may have difficulty responding to the testosterone produced in the body. In the absence of testosterone, they'll become female on the outside, with a vulva between their legs instead of a penis and scrotum. Varying gradations of this condition exist. Some people may be born without a uterus and with testicles between their legs rather than ovaries in their belly, even though they have a vulva. It's also possible to end up with external genitalia that have developed to a point somewhere in between the penis–balls complex (male sex organs) and the vulva.

There are children born every year who cause the midwife to scratch his or her head when the parents ask if it's a boy or a girl. The fact is, the midwife may not be able to give them an answer. These types of diagnosis may be called intersex,* which simply means 'in-between sex'.

The example we described earlier, where there is no correspondence between the genetic gender and the outer sex organs, is another type of intersex. Intersex can therefore take many forms. It may be that external genitalia do not match a gender, or that the external and internal genitalia correspond to different genders or even both genders.

Many children who are born intersex undergo surgery at birth, which brings us to a sad history lesson. Previously, all children who were born with 'ambiguous' external genitalia were surgically assigned female. In the first place, people thought this would be fine because gender was seen as being dependent on nurture. As long as you brought the child up in a given gender, it would feel itself to be that gender. If a child was given dolls and pink clothes, that would do the trick. Nature or nurture, as the saying goes.

Secondly, surgeons thought it was easier to achieve a good outcome if they made a vulva than if they made a penis and balls. The surgeons, who were of course men themselves, felt that the person couldn't have a good life with a small, only semi-functional penis, whereas a semi-functional vulva wouldn't be a problem for women. After all, sex was most important for men. The result was that they made *physical* girls out of children who, *genetically* and *psychologically*, were boys. Many lives have been ruined in this way.

This has caused many surgeons to change their practice dramatically. Doctors now carry out more in-depth examinations to determine gender, so that the child will probably end up with a body that is the 'right gender' after surgery. They no longer operate on a baby at birth, but often take several years to examine the child first.

There has been some debate around this kind of treatment. Many people think these children shouldn't have any surgery, but should be allowed to decide for themselves what they want to do once they reach adulthood. The people who take this view think the entire idea that everybody must fit into

---

* There are many views about the term 'intersex'. It may be used to describe a group of medical conditions or an identity. We think it's a good term for describing physical variants between male and female development, but we know that people prefer different terms when they are talking about themselves.

the boy or girl mould is wrong in principle. Why isn't it acceptable to be something in between? Why can't we just bring up children as 'they' and let them discover their own sexual identity over time? This brings us to the third aspect of gender: *psychological gender*.

Psychological gender – a question of identity

This question is more difficult to explain through biology, because our psychological gender is a question of identity: what we think about ourselves and who we are. It is personal, and only you can know what is right for you.

Many important things are overlooked because we think far too much about what is 'normal'. For most people, the three factors all point towards *one gender*. We feel as if we're women, we look like women between our legs and our genes confirm that we are women. But the fact that most of us experience things one way doesn't mean it's the same for *everybody* – a lesson humanity is constantly having to learn over and over again.

When your son says he's a girl, only wants to wear dresses and prefers his big sister's Barbie collection to a train set and football, it's easy to insist that it's just a phase, but that isn't necessarily true. Nor is it a given that a person must be 'feminine' or prefer dolls to football in order to be a girl. Psychological gender is not the same as personality and need not be based on traditional gender roles. Nonetheless, it is quite possible for a person's psychological gender to differ from their genital and genetic gender. We often use the terms *trans* or 'born in the wrong body' about people with a different gender to the one indicated by their bodies and their genes.

So, what is trans? The word 'trans' comes from the Latin, meaning 'through', 'to cross' or 'to change', as in *to transcend*. The term is used to describe a person who identifies as a gender different from the one he or she belongs to genetically or physically. People may also call themselves trans if they don't identify with a specific gender, but not everybody feels the need for this kind of label. Trans is often marked with an asterisk, as *trans** to show that it is a broad term encompassing many things. It may, for example, be worth asking a transperson what they prefer to be identified as: he, she or *they* – or something else entirely? You won't necessarily know in advance, so ask if you're wondering. People who aren't trans are called *cis,* a Latin prefix meaning on the same side as something – the opposite of 'to cross'.

A transwoman is a person who was born in a male body, but who is nonetheless a woman, and who may wish to change her body so that her physical and psychological genders match. A transman is a person who was born in a female body, but identifies as a man. Many transpeople know from childhood that they belong to a gender that doesn't match their body. This may seem terrifying to parents, in the same way that other unknown things seem terrifying. So, it's important for us to talk about trans and raise awareness about it. If parents suspect their child has been 'born in the wrong body', the child can be referred to a paediatrician. If appropriate, the child can eventually be given gender-confirmation treatment, with the help of hormones and surgery.

Fortunately, most people are becoming more used to trans, generally through popular culture. The actor Laverne Cox in *Orange is the New Black* (2013) and Caitlyn Jenner, of Kardashian family fame, are among those who have put trans on the map in recent years. In Norway, the series *Born in the Wrong Body* has attracted a lot of attention, and several transpeople have actively engaged in the social debate. The Norwegian physican and sexologist Esben Esther Pirelli Benestad, who identifies as genderfluid and prefers the term *they*, and, a bit more recently, Luca Dalen Espseth, a transman, are among those showing children and young people that they're not alone in being trans.

In conclusion
There are (at least) three factors that determine which gender we belong to. The ones we have dealt with here are genetic, physical and psychological gender. Gender need not be binary. We may have chromosomal differences that mean we don't have the typical chromosome combination of XX or XY. We may have genetic errors that have formed us into something in between woman and man in the physical development of our sex organs. It is also possible for your psychological gender to differ from the genital and genetic gender you were born with. In other words, gender isn't as simple as it might seem. We hope this overview has sparked your curiosity and made you a little more open to the mosaic of possibilities that gender presents.

Discharge, periods and other gore

Like the other orifices in our bodies, the vagina is an exit and not just a place for putting things into. Out of it come screaming babies, blood, mucus and gore. This makes it a source of immense joy and embarrassment, and gives us ways of finding out if there's anything wrong down there. Then there are the hormones – the signal substances that run the whole show. The time has come to talk about the slightly less tangible parts of our sexual apparatus.

DOUCHEBAGS AND DISCO MICE

Discharge. Let the word roll around on your tongue. It's an odd word that calls to mind plumbing systems and sewage pipes. Discharge is most familiar to us as the slick, milky or yellowish-white stain that makes a regular appearance in our knickers after puberty. It's what makes our knickers 'dirty'. Perhaps it's hardly surprising discharge isn't a hot topic or something we discuss at top volume. It seems kind of icky. And yet, at the same time, the very thought of a moist vagina is enough to put a twinkle in most straight men's eyes. But, what is discharge? Is there any difference between the different types of moisture down there? And why should we bother thinking about discharge in the first place?

Let's get one thing straight right away: all healthy girls who've reached puberty will find discharge in their knickers every single day. It's a fluid that seeps out of our vaginas continuously from the very first day our sexual organs come under the influence of a hormone called oestrogen at the onset of puberty. Some of the discharge comes from glands in the cervix. The walls of the vagina don't have any glands, but a lot of fluid seeps through them, mingling with fluid from the cervix and from glands at the opening of the vagina, including the Bartholin's glands (see p. 12).

Normally, between a half and a whole teaspoonful of discharge will seep out over the course of the day, although this varies depending on the individual woman as well as the point she is at in her menstrual cycle.[1] Some women using hormonal contraception find that their discharge levels increase, as do pregnant women. The consistency of the discharge will also vary, ranging from a runny liquid to a slimy, thread-like substance that looks like egg white just before ovulation.

Discharge isn't just normal, it's a must. It makes the vagina into a self-cleaning tube. Its purpose is to keep the vagina clean and to flush out unwelcome guests such as fungi and bacteria, as well as dead cells from the surface of the mucous membrane. In addition, it usually contains masses of good lactic-acid bacteria, known as *lactobacilli*, which produce – yes, you've guessed it – lactic acid. That's what gives the discharge its slightly acidic taste and smell.

Even more importantly, the lactic acids create the low pH that is absolutely essential to a healthy vagina – in other words, an acidic environment. Most of the bacteria that cause disease can't thrive in an acidic environment. In addition, lactic-acid bacteria prevent potentially harmful bacteria from finding the conditions they need to grow, because they're all competing for the same space and nutrients. The result is that infections are prevented. In short, discharge keeps our vaginas healthy.

At the same time, discharge lubricates the mucous membranes and keeps them moist. Dry mucous membranes are easily torn and once that happens, problems quickly follow. Just think what your mouth would be like without spit. Without discharge, the mucous membranes in the vagina tear and you can get little sores. Sex becomes a nightmare and the likelihood of sexually transmitted infections also increases because the body's outer barrier has been damaged. In other words, discharge isn't some dirty thing that should be flushed out of our vaginas, but an important ally.

Discharge is not a sign of poor hygiene

The problem is, people think discharge is icky – as if it were a sign of being dirty or having poor hygiene. Very few girls will leave their used knickers lying around or hanging out in the bathroom. In some environments, things have gone so far that women think the vagina should be flushed clean of discharge. Perhaps you've never thought about where the insult 'douchebag' comes from. Nor had Nina until she moved to the US, bought herself a bottle of intimate wash at the shop and left it in the communal shower-room in the dorms. After a while, a sniggering fellow student told her she should remove it because the rumours were already flying around about the Norwegian girl with the douchebag. 'Douchebag?' said Nina, a bit confused. She was told that *everybody* believed she was squirting perfumed soapy water into her vagina using a kind of bulb syringe – apparently a common practice among sex workers and many other women. Nina tried to explain that it was just regular vaginal wash, pH 3.5 and all that, but she quickly gave up trying to convince her fellow students. Nice girls must never, for God's sake, draw attention to the fact that their genitals need the occasional wash. Even admitting that you washed your genitals can be taboo, as if it might give away the great secret of discharge. Nina left the bottle in the showers.

Our genitals are happiest with warm water or a mild, intimate soap. You should never use ordinary soap to clean inside them because it can easily cause your vulnerable mucous membranes to dry out or become irritated. Itching and burning down below are often caused by using products that are too strong, or simply by washing too much. You should never flush out your vagina as this can increase the likelihood of infections.

What reason could women have for feeling they need to flush out their vaginas? For many, it's probably to do with smell. A lot of women we've spoken to are anxious about whether they smell 'normal' down there. They say they worry whether colleagues can detect the smell of their vaginas when they're sitting side by side at a meeting, or refuse to let their sex partners go down on them in case they find their scent a turn-off.

Healthy genitals do smell
That's just the way it is. Fresh discharge has a mildly acidic smell and taste because it contains lactic acid. What's more, our vulva and groin are amply equipped with sweat glands. Tight trousers, knickers made of synthetic fabric and crossed legs create a nice, warm environment between our legs. Over the course of a long day, you will therefore, naturally enough, sweat a great deal there, too. The combination of an entire day's worth of discharge and sweat, together with a dash of residual urine creates a characteristic

odour. In our circle of female friends, we use the Norwegian term '*discomus*', meaning 'disco mouse'. This describes the distinctive smell your genitals – your *mouse* – gives off after a long night on the dance floor, or a trip to the gym for that matter. It doesn't exactly smell bad, but it certainly can smell pretty intense.

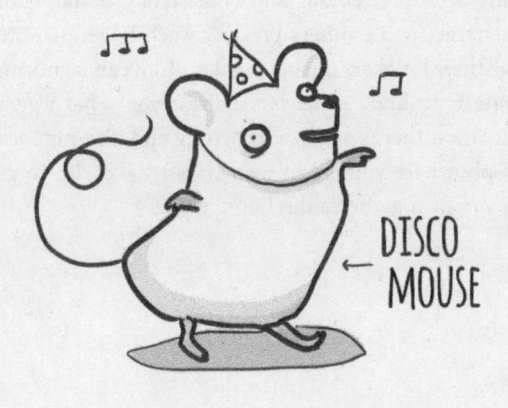

DISCO MOUSE

The smell and quantity of discharge can vary according to what phase you're at in your menstrual cycle. Our sex hormones seem to influence our body's ability to rid itself of an evil-smelling substance called *trimethylamine*, which is what can cause that classic smell of rotten fish. It has been observed that, among healthy women, the body has 60–70 per cent less capacity to rid itself of this substance just before and during menstruation.[2] That could explain why even healthy women may find their genitals give off a fishy smell around the time of their period.

The scent of our genitals is one of our most intimate odours. As you'll have gathered, it's quite normal for them to smell a bit, especially at the end of a long day; but as a rule, they shouldn't smell 'bad', if you get what we mean. A bad smell may be a sign of infection and is a good reason to pay a visit to your doctor. If you've been for a check-up and your odour problems aren't caused by an infection, it may be a good idea to wear loose trousers or skirts, change your underwear over the course of the day and take proper (but not excessive!) care of your hygiene.

As you'll have realised, discharge is closely associated with the wellbeing of your sex organs, so it's hardly surprising that, with a little observation, it can tell us a lot about the situation down under. Discharge can change as a result of both infections and imbalances in the vaginal flora, but substantial changes also occur during a normal menstrual cycle.

In other words, it's important to get to know what normal discharge is like – in terms of odour, colour and consistency. Some women produce very little discharge, while others produce such large quantities that they have to change their knickers during the day. Both can be normal. The most important thing is to know what is usual for you. That way, you can not only work out when there's something wrong and it's time for a trip to the doctor, or simply where you are in your menstrual cycle. To give you a bit of a hand, we've put together a discharge guide.

DISCHARGE GUIDE

DISCHARGE YOU SHOULD CHECK WITH A DOCTOR

• A copious, runny discharge that is greyish-white with a fishy smell can be a sign of bacterial vaginosis, which is an imbalance in the vaginal normal flora.

• A thick, lumpy white discharge with a normal odour may be a sign of yeast infection.

• An increased flow of discharge, generally yellowish-white in colour, may indicate infections such as chlamydia, mycoplasma or gonorrhoea. The latter produces a more yellowish-green discharge than the first two.

• Copious amounts of runny, foaming discharge that is yellowish-green in colour and evil smelling may be a sign of a trichomoniasis.*

• Copious amounts of whitish, possibly grainy discharge with a normal smell may be a sign of overproduction of lactobacilli, especially if you also have itching and groin pain too.

• Discharge mixed with blood when not on your period – everything from small brown spots to pink, dark or fresh blood in the discharge – may be caused by a sexually transmitted infection or abnormal cells in the cervix. You should always get any unexplained bleeding checked by a doctor.

NORMAL CHANGES THAT ARE NO CAUSE FOR CONCERN

• Slimy egg white that you can stretch between your fingers can mean ovulation is imminent.

• Increased amounts of discharge that is the same odour, colour and consistency as usual can result from hormonal contraception or pregnancy.

---

* Trichomonas vaginalis is a little parasite that causes trichomoniasis. This disease is rare in Norway, but is one of the most common sexually transmitted infections worldwide. Some people may suffer intense itching of the vulva and vagina, as well as evil-smelling discharge and a burning sensation when passing water, while others don't notice a thing. The infection is not dangerous and is treated with Metronidazole, a special type of antibiotic.

PERIODS – HOW TO BLEED WITHOUT DYING

Periods come roughly every month. Sometimes they're painful, sometimes they're embarrassing and take you by surprise, but most times everything goes smoothly. Although we could quite happily manage without vaginal bleeding each month, menstruation can be a huge relief in certain situations – *Phew! You weren't pregnant this time either.*

Menstruation takes up a large share of our lives. If you bleed once a month and your period lasts five days each time, you'll have up to 60 days of bleeding each year. If you have periods for 40 years, that means you'll have 2,400 days (or six-and-a-half years) of menstruation over the course of your life! As you'll have gathered, we ought to talk a lot more about this bleeding, especially since it can involve a bunch of crappy challenges like PMS (pre-menstrual syndrome, which we'll come back to later), embarrassing situations and severe pain.

These challenges may be bad enough, although modern-day women have minimal problems compared with the troubles faced by our sisters in days gone by before sanitary towels, tampons, the menstrual cup and painkillers were invented. In those days, women crocheted or knitted cotton sanitary towels, which had to be boiled and hung out to dry after every use. Around the world, menstruation is still a major challenge. PMS pales into insignificance when you hear about girls having to give up school because of their monthly bleeding, or girls who use dirty cloths and develop infections because they don't have access to the clean disposable products that are taken for granted in the West. Menstruation is an often-overlooked barrier to genuine equality for the women of the world. Think about that next time you're in the shop buying your tampons.

Let's focus on the bleeding itself

Most of us know that the blood is connected to fertility. Menstruation demonstrates that you have an internal cycle and that your body has the capacity to bear a child. But what is it that's actually bleeding and where is the wound? Why does the colour change from brown to red, and why is it lumpy?

The blood comes because the womb, or uterus, was ready to receive a fertilised egg, but failed to do so this time around. The uterus readies itself for pregnancy by increasing the amount of endometrium or mucous membrane – in other words, the inner wall, or lining, of the uterus. If an egg is fertilised it will attach itself to this lining, which nourishes the tiny growing creature by supplying it with the mother's blood. When no fertilised egg arrives, the body no longer has any need for the thick layer of mucous membrane, so the whole lot is expelled and 'bleeds' away. This is what causes the slimy consistency of the period blood. Some of the lumps are quite simply scraps of the expelled mucous membrane; the flow is not pure blood from an open wound.

Many women become worried if their menstrual blood is a different colour or consistency to what they have previously experienced, but there's nothing abnormal about having blood that is either red and fresh or brown and clotted. The colour and consistency of your period can vary from one cycle to the next, or from day to day within the same period, because blood coagulates. Blood changes colour and consistency when it's outside the blood vessels. It is red and runny when it is very fresh. When the menstrual blood is bright red and runny, this means it has flowed out of the uterus rapidly and has not had time to coagulate, or clot. By the same token, brown, clotted blood is a bit older. If you have heavier bleeding, it's often fresher, because then it's easier for the uterus to squeeze it out. If you have very light bleeding, the blood may remain inside the uterus and congeal a bit, but the body still gets rid of this too, all on its own – blood does not build up inside you.

A period is neither unhygienic nor dangerous. It consists of blood and mucus and it's up to you how you feel about that. If you want to, there's nothing to stop you having sex while you're bleeding, but do remember contraception. The fact that you're menstruating doesn't mean you're protected against pregnancy or infection by sexually transmitted infections.

Now that you know what a period is, perhaps you'll understand why we don't usually bleed when we're pregnant. Because the menstrual blood consists of the mucous membrane that lines the inside of the uterus when we're pregnant, of course we want to keep it, so that the foetus won't 'bleed' away. A hormone called progesterone, which you'll soon read more about, helps us keep it in place.

Are periods necessary, you may ask?

Hold on a minute, though. You've learnt what a period is, but do we need it? As you may have noticed, most other female animals don't bleed every single month. A lot of people think female dogs on heat are having periods, but that bleeding is something quite different. Bitches bleed from their vaginas when they're ovulating and can become pregnant; they don't bleed from the uterus like we do. In fact, periods are a rarity we share only with a couple of human-like apes and some other odd creatures, including a type of bat. In other words, menstruation itself is not necessary to produce offspring.

This is pretty stupid. Why should humans in particular have to waste extra energy making a new uterine lining month after month, again and again, only to see it bleed away to nothing? What's up, Darwin?

You've probably heard the terms evolution and natural selection. Over the history of any species, individuals with random genetic traits that prove advantageous to them have been particularly successful in transmitting their genes. As a result, these traits dominate in the generations that follow. This is how humans and animals have developed over the millennia. Unlike most other mammals, we humans ended up with periods. But does that mean that periods themselves constitute an advantage? Not according to American biologist Deena Emera. Her theory is that periods are not an *adaptive advantage*, but a non-*adaptive consequence*.[3]

Emera thinks periods are a consequence linked to an adaptive advantage that we don't notice in our day-to-day lives: something that we might call spontaneous mucous-membrane growth.* The uterine lining grows, as you now know, to provide board and lodging for the fertilised egg. In animals that do not have periods, the mucous membrane only grows when a fertilised egg is present. In other words, the maternal body responds to the cry for help from the fertilised egg by building a uterine lining in which it can live. However, things are a bit different for humans as the mucous membrane grows every month without a fertilised egg being present.

When the lining of the uterus in humans and other menstruating species

---

* This is a simplification of the term 'spontaneous decidualisation', which Emera uses in her article. The decidualisation process actually involves more than mucous-membrane growth.

doesn't receive a fertilised egg, it is expelled, because there is a cost attached to maintaining extra tissue we don't need. We get periods, which can therefore be described as a consequence of growth of the mucous membrane. Animals that do not have this have no superfluous tissue to get rid of each month, so do not have periods – they only produce the lining of the uterus when they need it.

So what is the advantage of mucous-membrane growth?

The theories presented by Emera are based on the idea that the mother and foetus just do not have shared interests. In fact, it is conceivable that the mother and the foetus have been engaged in an arms race over the course of our evolution, in which the foetus develops traits that give it access to more of the mother's resources. The mother, for her part, develops traits that allow her to hold back resources she needs for her own survival.

Against this backdrop, Emera presents two theories about why mucous-membrane growth is an advantage for humans.

The first is that the growth of the uterine lining protects the mother against an aggressive, invasive foetus. And – yes, you guessed it – the foetuses of menstruating species are extra aggressive compared with those of species that don't have periods. These foetuses have no scruples. They run amok, breaking into their mother's bodies like parasites demanding energy and nourishment. Since the human has already produced a layer of mucous membrane, this seems to have an extra-protective effect against the invading foetus. You can think of it as the mother having prepared a shield to gain better control over what resources the foetus will have access to and what she'll keep for herself.

Another theory is that the mother's body can register the quality of the foetus when the fertilised egg attaches itself to the finished mucous membrane. As you will read in greater detail later on in the book, far from all fertilised eggs end up as babies. Many foetuses are spontaneously aborted at a very early stage because there's something genetically wrong with them. It would be stupid for the mother to waste energy carrying to term a foetus that isn't viable. If her body can detect this through the lining of the uterus, it can conserve valuable strength by expelling faulty ones early on.

The advantageous aspect of periods is therefore not the period itself, but the mucous-membrane growth of which the period is a consequence. Mucous-membrane growth is not, in fact, something we require each month, but is only needed for the establishment of a pregnancy. Many people assume that it's important to have bleeding, that it's healthy to have periods, but that's not true. If we cut out the monthly mucous-membrane growth, there's no longer any point in having periods. Periods are a consequence and the bleeding is not healthy in itself. It simply implies a monthly blood loss.

As Danish journalist Lone Frank pointed out in an article about Emera's research, we modern human beings are very different from our forebears, who developed monthly menstruation hundreds of thousands of years ago.[4] While modern women have around 500 cycles over the course of their lives, primitive women would only have had around 100. Why? Well, because they spent much of their lives pregnant or breastfeeding, in the absence of reliable contraception.

Opting out of periods with the aid of contraception is no more unnatural for us than opting out of having a couple of extra children. Today we have the possibility of choosing whether we want to have children at all, and we can control how many we have. Periods have no intrinsic biological value for modern women.

There are many myths attached to periods

There's a lot of talk about how periods determine what you can and can't do. But what do periods actually mean to you and your everyday life? Are there some things you should avoid? Is your yoga instructor right, for example, to advise you against doing headstands while your bleeding is at its worst?

We asked a yoga instructor why you shouldn't do headstands during your period. 'It's not good for the blood to run back into your belly,' he said. In a way he's right. It's apparently not unusual for small amounts of menstrual blood to run up through the Fallopian tubes and out into your abdomen when you have your period. Many stressed surgeons have experienced this, finding blood in the bellies of menstruating women they're operating on without detecting any bleeding wound. It isn't dangerous for menstrual blood to find its way into the belly, though. Your body quickly tidies it all up.

Many people also believe that certain activities such as standing on your head can cause you to bleed more, but that isn't true either. As we have said, periods are simply the expulsion of the endometrium. You lose no more or less endometrial growth by standing on your head, having sex or running around the place. Over the course of one period, the only thing that bleeds out is the existing endometrial wall. However, the thickness of the wall, and therefore also the amount that must come out, may vary a bit from time to time.

Unless certain activities bother you because they cause you pain, you can do exactly what you want when you have your period. You can stand on your head, run a marathon, go swimming or have sex – it's up to you. Some women even find that physical activity relieves menstrual pains.

But is it really true that we don't bleed more as a result of having sex? When we were writing this chapter at a café in Oslo it occurred to us that we'd both heard stories from female friends about dramatic and traumatic bleeding that literally caught them with their pants down. There in the arms of a new male acquaintance they experienced their heaviest ever menstrual bleeding. In one case, the girl was woken up, lying in a pool of blood, by a terrified lover who didn't know whether she was dead or alive. *Hello! Helloooo!? Should I call 999?.* The incident happened at his house – and the sheets, they had been white. In another case, the unexpected bleeding started in the very midst of the act, resulting in a scene reminiscent of a slaughterhouse or a 1972 slasher movie. What in heaven's name had happened? We had to look into this.

It turns out there is no conclusive explanation for what causes these monster bleeds, but there are several theories that may make sense if you know a bit more about how the body works.

The first is what we call the cramps theory. As we know, muscle contractions in the uterus are what push out the period blood, but cramps can also be caused by other things too. Sometimes uterine cramps aren't bad at all. What we're talking about here is the orgasm, the sexual climax in which the entire sexual apparatus, including the uterus, contracts in fabulous waves. It's possible that an orgasm may kick-start a period that's imminent.

The second is the hormone theory. When we have sex, the body releases a hormone called oxytocin, often referred to as the pleasure hormone. Oxytocin plays an important role in various processes in the body. Among others, it's involved in triggering childbirth. Oxytocin stimulates contractions, so it's pretty serious stuff. As if the orgasm alone wasn't enough, oxytocin can also cause the uterus to contract, thereby pushing out blood.

A third possible explanation is that a bit of menstrual blood may accumulate inside the vagina and only come out when the 'floodgates' open during sex. As you may recall, the vagina contains many folds in which blood can gather. What's more, when you're relaxed, the vagina isn't an open tube, but a tightly compressed one, whose anterior and posterior walls are squeezed together.

One charming myth that has been doing the rounds since the early 1970s is that women's periods synchronise when they live for a long time under the same roof. Our bodies supposedly have a telepathic power that causes us to bond through cramps and chocolate cravings. It was a Harvard psychologist who believed she had proved this after studying the menstrual cycles of women living in the same dorm at college in the USA.[5] Evolutionary researchers pounced on it, taking the view that there was a benefit to women menstruating and ovulating at the same time: men wouldn't be tempted to hop from one woman to another but would form stable couple relationships instead.[6] As many as 80 per cent of all women apparently believe in the myth of synchronised periods.[7]

But no matter how cute it sounds, more recent research shows that we've been had. Studies of lesbian couples,[8] Chinese women living in dorms[9] and West African women placed in 'menstrual huts' showed no synchronicity.[10] Although we may seem to be menstruating in sync, this is because there's considerable variation in cycle length from one woman to the next. If you and your best friend menstruate at the same time, it's most likely just a matter of chance and not, sadly, a sign that you have a special bond.

DON'T BLEED ON THE SOFA! ALL ABOUT SANITARY TOWELS, TAMPONS AND MENSTRUAL CUPS

As long as you have access to sanitary products, your monthly bleeding needn't prevent you from doing the stuff you like or want to do. And the risk of bleeding on your friend's sofa is also significantly lowered if you stem the flow with something.

The most common hygiene products are disposable: sanitary towels and tampons. Over the past few years, the menstrual cup has been making headway as a favourite for many women. There are a lot of reasons for this, including economics, the environment and comfort. It's entirely up to you what you choose. It's a matter of taste and your situation.

Sanitary towels
Women have used different types of sanitary towels ever since we crept out of the cradle of civilisation. One very early (and funny) description of a sanitary towel is to be found in a story about the first known female mathematician. Hypatia, a Greek who lived in around 400CE, is said to have become so sick of a pushy admirer that she threw her bloody rag at him to put him off.[11] History does not relate whether or not it was successful.

Modern sanitary towels have a self-adhesive strip on the underside so that you can attach them to your underwear, and they absorb the menstrual fluids as they seep out of your vagina. Many different-sized towels are available, from tiny thong panty liners to big, soft night-time towels. The benefit of sanitary towels over tampons is that you don't risk bacteria growth in your vagina. It's therefore advisable to use towels where the risk of infection is especially high – for example, in situations where it is easier for bacteria to make their way into the uterus because it is more open, such as just after you've had an intra-uterine device inserted, and after an abortion or childbirth.

Tampons
A tampon is a small, bullet-shaped object made of absorbent material that you insert into your vagina when you have your period. The advantage of having menstrual protection inside the vagina is that it makes it easier to do exercise, and especially to go swimming. Although the word comes from the French 'tampon' meaning plug, it doesn't work by keeping the blood inside your vagina. Instead, the tampon collects the blood by absorbing it. Tampons aren't a new invention by any means, but they haven't always come individually wrapped in plastic. Women in Ancient Egypt used to insert soft papyrus into their vaginas as menstrual protection.

Today, tampons come in different sizes and with or without applicators. You choose the size according to how much you're bleeding. But there's no point using bigger tampons to avoid having to change them as often, as tampons are supposed to be changed frequently; the normal recommendation is to change it at least every three to eight hours, or more often. To avoid bacteria growth, it's important to wash your hands thoroughly before and after changing one.

We've heard masses of tampon stories over the years. One classic involves inserting two tampons at once or 'losing' a tampon in your vagina. *Help*, a lot of people think, *now it's going to disappear into my body*. But the idea of a tampon finding its way into your abdomen is as much a myth as the idea of a contact lens making its way into your brain through your eye. As you now know, the vagina is an almost closed tube (see p. 11). The tiny little passage that runs through the cervix and into the uterus is so narrow that even the smallest tampon could never manage to make its way through. The cervix is not an open passage leading into the uterus and nothing can vanish into your abdomen by way of your vagina. Oddly enough, though, things can hide away in the innermost crannies of the vagina and that's why the tampons come equipped with a string so that you can pull them out again.

If you're worried that a tampon has got too far into your vagina, you can try to push it out. Squat and then bear down as if you're going to have a poo. Use your fingers to feel around for it. Since the vagina is no more than 7 centimetres long, it's usually possible to fish out the tampon yourself. If you can't do it, you need to get yourself to your GP – ASAP. Everything that goes into your vagina must come out again. If you think you're the first person to go to her doctor with this problem, you can set your mind at rest.

Menstrual cup

The menstrual cup is a hygiene product that doesn't absorb blood, but collects it instead. It's a soft silicon beaker that you fold together and insert into your vagina. Once inside, the cup unfolds with its open end towards the cervix, so that the blood is collected, and the rim presses against the vaginal wall to hold it in place. Since the menstrual cup is not a disposable product, hygiene is especially important. It must be emptied, rinsed and possibly washed with a mild vaginal rinse at least once every 12 hours. In between each period, it's a good idea to clean the menstrual cup by placing it in boiling water to kill any bacteria.

The advantage of the menstrual cup is, primarily, that you can use it for longer periods at a stretch than tampons. At the same time, it's perfectly fine to do exercise and go swimming wearing one, because it sits inside your vagina. You can use the same cup for years on end, up to a decade, which also makes it a cheap and environmentally friendly alternative. One menstrual cup can replace the thousands of tampons and sanitary towels that end up in landfills.

You've probably heard about toxic shock

You'll certainly have seen the warnings about using tampons. In every single box of tampons, there's a little pamphlet warning against a frightening thing called toxic shock syndrome (TSS), also popularly known as tampon disease. Can you really get seriously ill from using tampons?

Toxic shock syndrome is a rare bacterial infection that attacks the entire body. Tampon use is a risk factor for developing it because the warm, blood-soaked tampon in the vagina makes a cosy breeding ground for bacteria. If you're careless with your hygiene when inserting a tampon and then leave it in for too long, you may be extremely unlucky – which is also why it's best not to leave a tampon in for more than eight hours. It takes time for the bacteria to propagate and make their way into the body, so the likelihood of it happening mainly arises if you forget you've got a tampon in your vagina. Correct tampon use is not a risk factor.

If you get TSS, you'll notice something is wrong. The symptoms can be fever, a rash, a sore throat, vomiting, diarrhoea and confusion; you'll feel really unwell. Incidentally, you should always pay attention to any severe and unexpected symptoms of illness. If you think you've got TSS, it's vital to go and see a doctor quickly, because the infection becomes steadily worse over time and can progress rapidly. In the worst situation, it can be life-threatening.

But just because TSS is linked to tampon use, that doesn't mean it's dangerous to use tampons. TSS is a serious disease, but it's also very rare. The number of cases of TSS that are caused by tampon use has diminished dramatically since highly absorbent tampons were taken off the market. Today, only around half of the cases of TSS are linked to menstruation. It's also possible to contract TSS from seriously infected wounds and after surgery. In other words, it's quite possible to contract TSS without using tampons, and men can also get it, so perhaps 'tampon disease' isn't the best name for it.[12]

When it comes to TSS and the menstrual cup, we don't know very much yet because little research has been done on the subject. The menstrual cup is a relatively new phenomenon. So far, at least one case of TSS linked to the menstrual cup has been reported worldwide.[13] So we don't yet know whether the menstrual cup is better or worse than tampons when it comes to this infection. Regardless, it's a good idea to pay attention to hygiene.

PMS – THE PAIN-AND-MURDER SYNDROME

'What's the matter – got your period?' It's a classic control technique. Sometimes people find it's a lot easier to write women off as incompetent, hormonal or grouchy than to take us seriously. This 'period technique' isn't just a sexist way of running women down, it's also wrong, from a strictly physiological point of view. Errors of this kind must be cleared up in the name of popular education. If people will insist on using crappy control techniques on us, they could at least get their physiology right. As you may have noticed with your own body, it's not during the days of bleeding that you're most affected psychologically by your menstrual cycle. The problems actually begin *before the bleeding starts*. We're referring, of course, to the well-known if somewhat vaguely defined syndrome, PMS.

PMS or premenstrual syndrome (sometimes known as premenstrual tension) may be crappy, but on the whole it's something we can live with. And although it can cause minor problems, PMS isn't a valid reason to write women off in any way whatsoever. Women aren't grouchy, incompetent or 'hormonal' because we have a menstrual cycle. Of course, it's possible to be appalling and unprofessional regardless of what gender you identify as, we're not disputing that, but that's an entirely different matter.

What exactly is PMS?

PMS is an umbrella term used to describe all the ailments that may arise in the days leading up to your period. They can involve almost anything at all in the way of physical and psychological symptoms: pain, irritability, depression, bloating, mood swings, weeping, anxiety and acne; the list is a long one. Women may also experience a worsening in pre-existing illnesses, such as migraine, epilepsy or asthma. The problems arise in the phase of the menstrual cycle that falls between ovulation and menstruation, what's known as the premenstrual, or luteal, phase. When the period finally arrives, the pressure may be relieved and the symptoms may evaporate during the first days of bleeding.

There are no specific examinations that can be used to diagnose PMS. A doctor will not be able to tell that you have PMS through carrying out a gynaecological examination, for example. This makes diagnosis a bit difficult. Your experience of the symptoms is what determines whether or not you have it. Minor symptoms in the run-up to your period do not merit the diagnosis, and pretty much all women suffer from these. It's not as if you need a diagnosis just because you have a female body. As many as 85–95 per cent of all women have mild PMS-like symptoms in the days leading up to their period.[14]

In order to be diagnosed with PMS, your symptoms must be so severe that they are a physical or psychological hindrance to your everyday life. Of course, it depends on the individual how bad the symptoms need to be to become a hindrance. You can expect some symptoms, but there has to be a limit. Some women are totally incapacitated by their symptoms and that's certainly not the way it should be. As well as being of a certain severity, the symptoms must occur during most cycles; in other words, you must have them pretty much every single month. Moreover, of course, the symptoms must stop and start at the times typical for PMS: they must start in the premenstrual phase and stop when your period arrives. Around 20–30 per cent of all women have symptoms that qualify as mild or moderate PMS.[15]

Women who have the most severe symptoms are generally assigned a diagnosis where the criteria are stricter than for PMS – although the same symptoms are still involved – called premenstrual dysphoric disorder, or PMDD. In such cases the symptoms have definitely crossed the line from manageable to unbearable and PMDD applies to 3–8 per cent of all women.[16] There is also a condition known as premenstrual depression in which some women suffer serious signs of depression, such as suicidal thoughts, every single cycle – and this can obviously be dangerous. The three conditions overlap somewhat.

Although periods last from puberty to menopause, PMS may not last as long. PMS symptoms can start at any time after your first period, but many women have several PMS-free years in the beginning. Most women who suffer from PMS get it by their early 20s and the symptoms typically continue throughout their reproductive lives. Some women's symptoms become more severe later in life, and as a result they do not seek medical help until they are in their 30s or 40s. However, when you finally reach menopause, your PMS story is history.[17]

We don't know what causes PMS. Different theories propose everything from higher sensitivity to shifts in the body's hormone levels to neurological or even cultural causes.[18] All women experience hormone swings during their cycle, but why some suffer PMS or PMDD while others are symptom-free is unknown. Perhaps we'll find a cause over time.

Most women don't need medical treatment for PMS and the most important part of it is to avoid medicalising minor ailments that probably stem from natural hormonal swings. As we said earlier, most people have minor ailments. As a rule, PMS is something you can live with and there are alternatives available for people with unbearable problems.

Where people suffer severely, treatment is directed at the individual symptoms, which may vary considerably. If you become depressed or suffer from anxiety, you'll be offered a different treatment to someone with severe pains. For some people, oestrogen-based hormonal contraception can help, allowing them to skip their periods entirely. Other women who suffer primarily from psychological problems may benefit from anti-depressants. Those who have pain can use painkillers.

Back to those sexist comments

Let's go back to the people who resort to sexist control techniques when they speak to women. No matter what you believe, it simply isn't true that women with PMS lose their minds or capacity to respond rationally in the days before their periods. And if you absolutely must be oafish enough to comment on where a woman is in her menstrual cycle and use it against her, don't say: 'What's the matter – got your period?' but 'What's the matter, are you about to have your period in a few days' time?' It doesn't have quite the same ring, but it's important to get your physiology straight if you will insist on insulting somebody.

THE WHEEL OF ETERNITY – HORMONES AND THE MENSTRUAL CYCLE

Every month, most fertile women experience an inner, hormone-driven cycle. We're talking about the menstrual cycle here. Most of us know a little about it: at some point or another an egg arrives, there's a possibility we may become pregnant if we have sex at the right (or wrong) time and our period tells us that we aren't pregnant.

Do we actually need to know any more? We've seen plenty of medical students snap their book shut when they reach the chapter about the menstrual cycle, so why should you bother to read about it? First and foremost, it'll be useful for you; secondly, it's pretty exciting; and thirdly, we promise to make this much easier to grasp than your average textbook author would.

If all of us knew a bit more about how the minuscule signal substances known as hormones direct us through the menstrual cycle, it would be easier to understand a whole lot of things that all women relate to in their everyday life. We get questions about this all the time – 'How does hormonal contraception work?' 'What on earth is a fertile window and when does it happen?' 'What controls our menstruation and what's the mechanism behind various female diseases?'

Hormones – the substances that steer our vessel

We ended the section about the internal sex organs with the ovaries and the hormones that are produced there: oestrogen and progesterone, the female sex hormones. Now it's time to go into greater detail.

Oestrogen has acquired an undeservedly bad reputation lately. All we hear about is the risk of thrombosis, mood swings, breast cancer and other scary stuff, but oestrogen is a fantastic hormone. It's responsible for the things we have traditionally associated with womanliness. Tits, bum, hips – they're all down to oestrogen. Oestrogen is what keeps the vaginal walls moist and thick so that sex feels pleasurable and it's what makes our uteruses capable of bearing children. It also keeps facial hair and spots at bay. In fact, transwomen use oestrogen treatment to alter the fat distribution on their bodies from the typical male to the typical female distribution. Out with the male pot belly, in with tits and hips. It's pretty incredible what this little hormone can do.

If you've got a feel for language, you can probably work out what progesterone's all about, too. 'Pro' means for and 'gestation' means pregnancy. Progesterone therefore means 'for pregnancy'. We need masses of progesterone when our bodies are preparing to receive a fertilised egg, which happens every single month. Progesterone stops the uterus from contracting and pushing out a potentially fertilised egg. In addition, it makes the lining of the uterus an awesome place to live, with masses of blood and mucus from glands to nourish our future offspring.

Two other hormones are needed to control our menstrual cycle. They come from a pea-sized structure under the brain that's shaped like a scrotum and is called the pituitary gland. As sex-writers, we see sex organs everywhere.

The pituitary gland produces two reproductive-system hormones called the follicle-stimulating hormone (FSH) and the luteinising hormone (LH). Put briefly, the FSH deals with maturation of the egg. The egg lies inside a cluster of cells known as a follicle, which accounts for the name, follicle-stimulating hormone. The luteinising hormone is best known for triggering ovulation. The male pituitary gland actually produces precisely the same hormones, but for once the hormones have been named for the function they perform in the female body. Since this is highly unusual in the world of medicine, we think it's extra cool.

So far so good. Now that you've got to know the hormones, which are, after all, the stars of this show, it's time to take a look at the cycle itself.

Menstrual cycle – 28 days again and again and again!
To understand the menstrual cycle it's useful to draw a circular timeline. Although the length of a cycle can vary from one woman to the next – and even from one period to the next for individual women – we use a model cycle of 28 days for simplicity's sake, since 28 can be neatly divided into four weeks. However, it's quite normal for a cycle to be anything from 23 to 35 days long.

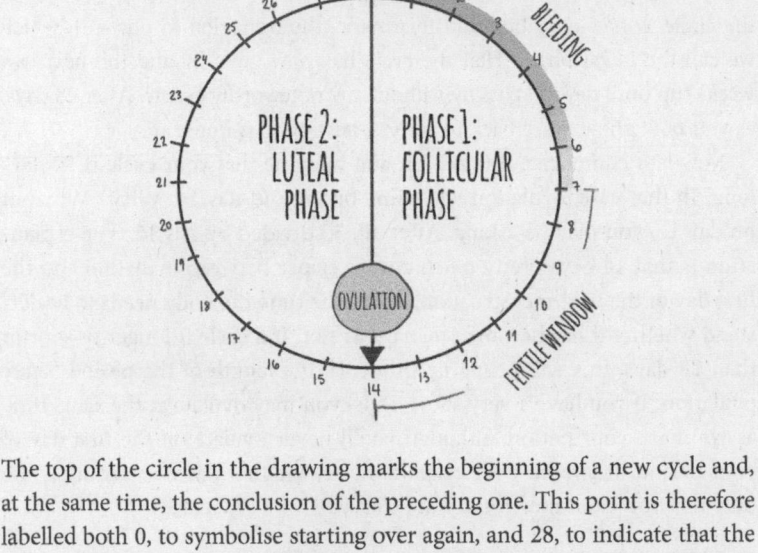

The top of the circle in the drawing marks the beginning of a new cycle and, at the same time, the conclusion of the preceding one. This point is therefore labelled both 0, to symbolise starting over again, and 28, to indicate that the same point marks the end of the last day, and the conclusion of the previous cycle. The start of one cycle is therefore always simultaneous with the end of the previous cycle. Your menstrual cycle is a wheel of eternity!

Many people find this difficult to understand. How can the beginning and the end happen at the same time? It's easier to grasp if we compare the menstrual cycle with something that's very familiar to us. Because this is exactly the same thing that happens with a clock when we pass from one day to the next. The moment a clock strikes midnight, the time on a digital clock is both 24:00, to mark the last hour of the day that is ending, and 00:00 to mark a new beginning. The clock moves from one day to the next and on the stroke of midnight, you are in both days at once. There isn't a gap between two, and the same goes for the menstrual cycle.

It's easy to notice the beginning of a new cycle, because that's when you begin to bleed. The bleeding can normally last up to a week, so the first seven days in the cycle.

To keep things straightforward, the menstrual cycle is often divided into two phases. When you start a new menstrual cycle, you're in what's known as the follicular phase. This is the time when a follicle containing an egg ripens and prepares itself for ovulation. On around day 14, marked by the bottom of the circle, comes ovulation and this marks the transition to phase II, which we call the luteal phase. Half the cycle has now gone by and the next two weeks (up until day 28) pass by without any noteworthy events. After 28 days, as you now know, we're back to zero. A new cycle is under way.

Now let's complicate things a bit and imagine that your cycle is 30 days long. In that case, ovulation will come on around day 16. What? Why not on day 15, you may be asking. After all, 30 divided by 2 is 15. The explanation is that 14 days pretty much always elapse between ovulation and the first day of the next menstruation. That's the time the body needs to understand whether it has become pregnant or not. If a cycle is longer or shorter than 28 days, this will primarily influence the length of the period *before* ovulation. If you have a very short cycle, you may ovulate at the same time as you have your period, although you'll never ovulate on the first day of your period. If you have an irregular cycle, the first day of bleeding is the only day you can know for certain that you won't ovulate.

The dance of the hormones

Now that we have an overview, we can start on the really interesting aspect: the dance of the hormones through the cycle. We start at the top of the circle. The period has arrived and you're on the first day of phase 1 – the follicular phase. The action isn't isolated to the uterus, because there are also things going on in the ovaries and the pituitary gland (which we nickname the brain-scrotum). While the uterus is expelling its lining along with all hope of a fertilised egg, the pituitary gland begins to produce FSH. This gland never gives up – even while the period is under way the hormones are already preparing a new egg and the next shot at pregnancy. As you'll recall, all the eggs in the ovaries lie inside what are known as follicles, which begin to mature once they are stimulated by FSH, hence this part of the cycle is known as the follicular phase.

So, the follicles grow because they receive FSH from the pituitary gland. This in turn causes the follicles to start producing oestrogen. As the follicles grow and grow, the oestrogen levels in the blood begin to increase dramatically. The bigger the follicles, the greater the quantity of oestrogen produced.

In turn, the oestrogen influences the uterine lining, causing it to grow. Right after the uterus has finished bleeding, the reconstruction gets under way again. There's no time for a grieving process here. The uterus is a persistent wretch that never passes up an opportunity to receive a fertilised egg, even though it'll be disappointed almost every single month.

While both the follicle and the uterine lining are growing, we approach day 14, the day of ovulation and the transition to phase 2. The follicle changes shape, becoming a bulging, fluid-filled water balloon at bursting point. Now the follicle emits so much oestrogen that it sends the levels in the body sky-high – and this is the signal the pituitary gland has been waiting for.

In response to the powerful oestrogen signal, the pituitary gland begins to produce LH, the ovulation hormone. We're not talking about small doses here: the quantity of LH suddenly sky rockets. If you've ever tried to become pregnant, it's possible you may be familiar with this dramatic rise in LH. Because ovulation tests you can buy are detecting the increase in LH in your urine. When the test is positive, you'll know that the rise in LH has started and ovulation is right around the corner. The immense flow of LH reaches the follicle, which responds by exploding, so that the egg is shot out of its cocoon and out of the ovary. For a little while, the egg floats freely outside the ovary before small tentacles on the Fallopian tubes, known as fimbriae, snap it up and send it on a voyage along the tube towards any sperm cell that may be awaiting it. We are halfway through the menstrual cycle and ovulation is a fact.

Now seems like a good time to take a quick break to comment on a couple of things we didn't learn in science class at secondary school. It's about the egg cell. You probably remember the heroic battle or race between the tough-guy sperm cells, which swim frantically to be the first to fertilise the waiting, passive egg.

Point one: the egg doesn't stand still – there's no hanging around nervously in the bar waiting for the sperm cell. The egg is a diva and, like most divas, she tends to turn up at the party fashionably late. As you can read more about in the section on pregnancy, the best time to have sex if you want to become pregnant is during the days *before* ovulation. The egg isn't passive at all. It's at least as active as the sperm cell. It isn't the sperm cells that swim towards the egg, but rather the egg that comes bobbing down towards the waiting sperm cells. They've often been waiting for her for days...

Point two: an equally heroic battle is waged between the egg cells as between the sperm cells, but for some reason or another, we're not told about that in school. Follicle-stimulating hormones (FSH) don't just affect one egg follicle each month. As you now know, up to 1,000 follicles begin to grow and mature every month, but only one of the very largest ones will have the pleasure of exploding and releasing its egg. The others wither away and die without ever having the chance to meet a sperm cell. Now perhaps you think 1,000 follicles competing isn't as tough as what the sperm cell is exposed to – after all, they have to race against millions! Remember, though, that men produce many millions of sperm cells every single day, whereas we women are born with all the eggs we'll ever have – and they run out.

Why, we ask ourselves, are egg cells (from women) presented as passive and sperm cells (from men) as active when this absolutely doesn't correspond to reality? Just saying...

But back to the menstrual cycle. We're in phase 2, so days 15–28 on the timeline, or the luteal phase. The egg has just been released and the uterine lining has grown nice and thick thanks to all the oestrogen from the follicles. In phase 2, progesterone is the star hormone, whereas in phase 1, oestrogen was in charge. Progesterone is produced from the remains of the punctured follicle in which the egg lived before it was released. The remains of the follicle change shape and colour, becoming a little cluster known as the *corpus luteum*, which is Latin for yellow body, so called because of its colour. Sometimes things are that simple.

As we said earlier, progesterone means 'for pregnancy', so now the body takes the final steps to prepare itself to receive the fused egg and sperm cells. The progesterone prevents the uterus from contracting and expelling the endometrium, at the same time ensuring that the uterine lining is an extra comfy place to live. Meanwhile, the pituitary gland is prevented from producing FSH or LH – those hormones that make new eggs develop and grow – by progesterone released in the corpus luteum. After all, we don't need any more new eggs just now as hopefully we have a fertilised egg on the way!

Unfortunately (for the corpus luteum), phase 2 of the menstrual cycle almost always ends in a tragic tale of suicide, as you will now see. As we've said, the progesterone from the corpus luteum stops the pituitary gland from producing any FSH and LH, but the problem is that the corpus luteum needs both hormones to survive, too. In other words, the corpus luteum prevents production of its own lifebuoy and will only be rescued if fertilisation takes place. Most often, therefore, the corpus luteum falls victim to its own altruistic struggle to keep the potentially fertilised egg alive. Without fertilisation, the corpus luteum fades away and dies, and the progesterone vanishes along with it.

With the corpus luteum out of the way, there's no longer any progesterone blocking the pituitary gland so the levels of FSH and LH in the blood rise again. The follicles in the ovaries get to work once more, ready for a new opportunity to mature, explode and let their eggs fuse with one chosen sperm cell. Without progesterone there's nothing to retain the thick endometrium or prevent the uterus from contracting. We know the outcome: the period. The first day of bleeding. We're back at the top of the circle. The cycle is over, but a new one has already started.

WHEN CAN YOU ACTUALLY BECOME PREGNANT?

It's a given that sex must happen in order for women to get pregnant naturally, but beyond that, there seems to be a great deal of uncertainty. In one episode of the American channel TV3 reality TV show *Paradise Hotel*, a lively discussion started over the breakfast table after two of the participants had had unprotected sex: 'What if she gets pregnant?' Some stubbornly insisted that everything would be fine because the woman in question had just had her period, while others claimed that women were most fertile right after menstruation. The confusion was total and the solution turned out to be emergency contraception funded by the television channel. This pregnancy business isn't simple.

Pregnancy is a watershed in women's lives. We can go from being terrified of it and expending a considerable amount of brainpower on how best to avoid it to wishing for it so much that it can't happen quickly enough. It's the worst and the best that can happen to us, depending on where we are in life and who we are with. It may therefore seem remarkable to write a section about pregnancy that will serve both groups, but it's actually very simple. Knowledge about how we become pregnant is the best medicine whether you want to prevent pregnancy or wish to be pregnant. So, what does it take?

Let's start off by stating the obvious. You can't become pregnant from anal sex, oral sex or from sitting on a toilet seat with sperm on it (yuck). You must have vaginal sex. After that it gets a bit more complicated.

When the man has an orgasm, many millions of sperm cells are squirted up into the woman's vagina. Most of them die after a short time; the majority by running out of the vagina after sex or by swimming off into some dark corner of it. Very few sperm cells manage to find the cervical opening, and even then, it's all a matter of timing. Most of the time, the cervical opening is, in fact, closed by a thick, gelatinous mucus plug that the body produces in response to naturally high levels of progesterone. Only around ovulation does the mucus plug dissolve, opening the passageway into the uterine cavity. In the days before ovulation, you may even notice this since your discharge changes, and contains elastic threads of mucus! This mucus, which is similar to egg white, can be stretched to incredible lengths between your fingers if you fancy trying.

When ovulation approaches, the progesterone level diminishes and the body produces more oestrogen. The oestrogen causes the cervical opening to produce a runny, watery fluid instead of gelatinous slime and this makes it possible for the sperm cells to swim up into the uterine cavity. Again, you can observe this from your discharge, which becomes more runny and milky when you are ovulating and so at your most fertile.

Now let's say you have unprotected sex in that window around ovulation when your cervix is open and a little gang of 200 sperm cells have managed to find their way into your uterus. They will now spend between two and seven hours moving through the uterus and up into one of the Fallopian tubes. They're helped along by small, rhythmic movements in the uterus and Fallopian tubes, which create waves they can surf along on. Their choice of direction is vital, because the eggs almost always comes from only one ovary at a time. Once inside the Fallopian tube, the sperm cells have a rest and wait for the egg that may turn up – because, as you now know, the egg is clearly the diva of the party. She keeps the sperm cells waiting. Sperm cells normally survive in the uterus or Fallopian tubes for around 48 hours, although living cells have been found as many as five to seven days after sexual intercourse. Patient chaps, sperm!

After ovulation, the egg will bob down along the Fallopian tube towards the waiting sperm cells. Fertilisation occurs when one sperm cell fuses with one egg in the Fallopian tube, creating the precursor of a foetus, known as a zygote. Now and then two eggs will be released during ovulation and then you may get two-egg twins. This happens more often as women age, and it's hereditary, so that some families will have several sets of twins. More rarely, a set of one-egg (identical) twins may be born. This happens when the zygote splits into two separate pieces immediately after being fertilised.

One day after fertilisation, the fertilised egg will still be floating around in one of the Fallopian tubes, but now the cells have begun to divide. Even so, this is no guarantee that you will become pregnant. For the pregnancy to be successful, the growing cluster of cells must find its way down into the uterus and attach itself to the mucous membrane on the wall of the uterus at the right time. In addition, the body must receive a signal from the uterus indicating that the cluster of cells is in place via a hormone called hCG (human chorionic gonadotropin) – this is the hormone that pregnancy tests detect in the urine. This is also the hormone that ensures that the corpus luteum we spoke about in the previous section survives and continues to produce progesterone. If this doesn't happen, the fertilised egg will be flushed out with the next menstruation without you noticing a thing.

It takes between seven and ten days from fertilisation for the cluster of cells to attach itself to the lining of the uterus. Only then are you actually pregnant. The next nine months are such an extensive journey that we have opted to skip them. After all, there are plenty of pregnancy books available for you to read.

Back to our *Paradise Hotel* couple. Is the woman likely to have become pregnant if she's just had her period? In a study of couples who were trying for a baby, only those who'd had sex during a six-day window around ovulation achieved pregnancy – that's five days before ovulation plus the day of ovulation itself.[19] Those who had sex the day before ovulation or the day on which it occurred had a 30 per cent chance of becoming pregnant. Five days before ovulation, 10 per cent became pregnant. So, a good many became pregnant even though they had sex long before ovulation. As we said earlier, sperm cells can survive in the woman's body for up to a week before dying, so in theory, you're fertile for a period ranging from seven days before ovulation until one day afterwards, or a total of eight days. In other words, there is an eight-day fertile window. Most of us aren't aware of our ovulation, so the key to knowing whether the *Paradise* participant was in the risk zone would have been to map her cycle to see how long it was.

As we described in the section on the menstrual cycle, ovulation most often occurs 14 days before the next menstruation. If you have a totally consistent cycle of 28 days, ovulation will always occur in the middle of the cycle, on the 14th day, or two weeks after you last had your period. Given the eight-day window, this means it's possible for you to become pregnant between days 8 and 15 of your cycle.

Let's say that the *Paradise* participant has a stable 28-day cycle and a period that lasts seven days – days one to seven in her cycle. That'll mean she has only one day after her period before her chance of becoming pregnant arises. So, five days after she's finished her period, there's a considerable chance of her becoming pregnant. In such a cycle, it definitely won't be safe to have unprotected sex when she's just had her period. But in the week before she's expecting her next period – days 21 to 28 – it will be safe. We can thank emergency contraception or sheer luck for the fact that there was no *Paradise Hotel* baby.

Now it may sound as if it should be pretty simple to work out what your safe time is if you can only get pregnant eight days in every cycle. The problem is that very few women have entirely stable cycles. You've probably noticed this yourself too. Since you never know in advance whether you'll ovulate sooner or later than normal this month, you must operate with a wider window. If ovulation shifts either backwards or forwards by just two days, this will lengthen your unsafe time to 12 days. Many women have greater variation than this. If, in addition, you're the kind of person who doesn't like having sex during her period, you're left with just a few days when you can have sex without using contraception and still be confident that you won't become pregnant. In other words, it's always sensible to use contraception.

SEX

If there's one thing we humans have had in common since the dawn of time, it's sex. Most of us have had or will have sex, both with ourselves and with other people. Without sex, there would be no more humans on Earth, and we think humans would have had much more boring lives. Sex is one of the most natural things we can do. Even the way we have sex – whether homosexual or heterosexual – isn't so different from other animals.

The difference is that the human race is the only species that's ashamed of having sex. We hide away when we screw – or at least that's the norm. This secrecy means sex has always been clouded in uncertainty. We don't know what everybody else is up to, we don't know if our desires are normal and we can never be quite certain that we come up to scratch. Paradoxically enough, even though we do it as a twosome, sex is a pretty lonesome business. This is especially true when you're at the very beginning of your sex life, in puberty.

A great deal is written about sex these days, and many young people spend hours watching porn. Sex videos are shared on social media and teens send snaps of hard penises and erect nipples to people they're involved with. Some might claim we're living in the most openly sexualised society ever.

This has created a remarkable duality. We have unique access to inspiration and insight about horniness, desire and bodies. Knowledge is just a mouse click away. At the same time, this openness doesn't seem to have made us any more confident – in fact, it's probably quite the opposite.

The problem is that what we get shown is a glossy version. Ideals about sex have been raised, but at the same time the uncertainty lives on inside us. We still want to hide away when we're turned on, but our environment tells us that everything should be shared. The contrasts can feel overwhelming. The result, we believe, is that a lot of women feel as if their libidos are too low, they have too little exciting sex and too few orgasms.

There's a need for a new understanding of reality. In this chapter, we want to talk about what we call a normal sex life. And of course when we use the word 'normal', we don't mean to say anything that falls outside this is wrong or something to be ashamed of, it's just not what most people get up to. Sexuality comes in a thousand forms and only you know what's right for you. We hope to add nuance to the way we think about sex and to offer some tips about how to find your way to a satisfying and chilled sex life.

FIRST-TIME SEX

Few experiences in life are so veiled in legend as *doing it*, or having sex for the first time. Your expectations about performance – yours and your partner's – can be sky-high and it's difficult to imagine what lies ahead.

As a result, some people are disappointed in themselves or their partner when they make their sexual debut. Didn't you have an orgasm? Was it difficult to get into the positions you'd read about? Did your boyfriend's penis go soft after ten seconds? Didn't she touch your clitoris?

Courage! Sex is like most other things in life

You don't get good at it without practice and nor does your partner. It's important to bear in mind that the first time won't be perfect, but if you lower your expectations a bit, it can still be a positive experience. There's got to be a first time, after all. We've collected a bit of information that may help make that first time as good as possible.

The Norwegian film *Just Bea* (2004), follows a group of friends in their first year of upper secondary school (sixth form in the UK) in Oslo. Bea is the only one who hasn't 'done it' yet. One of the rituals in her gang of girlfriends is that you get a piece of marzipan cake from the local patisserie once you've been initiated into the ranks of the 'shaggers'. Bea is now 16 years and nine months old, and feels as if everything depends on whether she can get laid. The slice of marzipan cake in the patisserie window is calling out to her. But Bea isn't the only one out there who thinks 'everyone else has done it', and that there's some rush to get it out of the way. When these kinds of thoughts pop up, it's handy to have a few facts on the table.

The average age for women in Europe to make their sexual debut is around 17, but critically that's just an average, not a deadline.[1] Some people start earlier, some later. In Norway, only 20 per cent of all young people start having sex before they're 16. So, four out of five young people haven't had sex when they start in sixth form or college. In other words, there's no need for Bea to be in a hurry for that slice of cake.

Although it may be good to have an average age to relate to, it's important to remember that your first time is about you and your partner. You should start having sex when you're both ready for it. You're ready when you feel desire (desire is in your head), and when you are turned on or horny (this is in your body). Now and then, your head and body might not be on quite the same page, and in that case, it may be a good idea to wait a bit. When we become horny and who makes us feel that way varies from person to person. Some people feel ready before they're 16, others when they're in the sixth form, and yet more wait until they're 20 or 30 – or even older.

Many people have sex for the first time with a partner of their own age, but there are no rules (as long as they are above the age of consent). Some people do it with their girl- or boyfriend, others with a one-night stand, others with a mate or a female friend. For some it happens in a bedroom and for others, it's behind a Portaloo at a festival. None of these things is wrong, as long as everybody involved actually wants to play the game.

Just remember that the Cardamom Law applies:* you and your partner may be horny and keen to have sex NOW, but it may be best to have sex in a place and at a time that isn't going to bother other people. For example, it isn't cool to sit next to a couple having sex on a plane. Ellen can vouch for this, having experienced it on a flight to New York. The fact that these lovebirds pretended to speak neither English nor Norwegian when they were clearly from Kristiansand (a town in southern Norway) was the last straw. Have some respect.

A lot of people think a great deal about what it takes to be able to say that you've had sex, and what it means to be a virgin. For example, is it possible to engage in some sexual activities and still be a virgin? Are you a virgin if you've had anal, but not vaginal sex? What about oral sex or fingering? What counts – what is *real* sex? We haven't got the answer to that, but we believe there's far too much focus on labelling things. There's no wrong or right sex

---

*   The Cardamom Law, from Thorbjørn Egner's children's book *When the Robbers Came to Cardamom Town* translates roughly as: 'don't bother other people, be both good and kind, other than that feel free to do whatever comes to mind.'

– at any rate there's no sex that is 'real' or 'less real'. You're the one who decides the terms of your sex life. First-time sex can be so many things, since sex includes oral sex, fingering, vaginal and anal sex. You can have fantastic sex without having traditional vaginal intercourse. After all, it's totally absurd to claim a lesbian is a virgin until she's had vaginal sex with a man.

Most kids today know a bit about what sex involves. This isn't just down to sex education because most of them have actually seen sex in the form of porn.[2] Despite (or perhaps because of?) this, a lot of them are worried about whether they're good enough before their first time.

The first time you have sex, you can expect it to involve a lot of flailing about. No matter what you do, it's not going to be like it is in a porn movie. Like other films, some porn movies use special effects so that things look different than they do in reality and there's a lot of make-believe doing the rounds. So, it isn't possible to do all the things you see in porn movies in real life, even though porn is inspired by and based on something that is real. It's a bit like the *Hobbit* films – there may be mountains in real life, but that doesn't mean there are dragons living in them. And even if there were, they wouldn't have Benedict Cumberbatch's voice.

It's also important to remember that porn actors should be viewed as extreme athletes. They've done it all before, so to say. The American skier Lindsey Vonn makes downhill look easy, but you'd probably break your neck if you tried to be her the first time you put on a pair of skis.

Don't expect to be able to perform like Stoya, the famous American porn actor. You won't be able to achieve advanced Kama Sutra positions on your first attempt. You'll probably never manage them at all, and that's fine: you don't need to be able to in order to have good sex. It will be pretty clumsy the first time, but that's the way it's supposed to be. That's part of the charm. You'll almost certainly feel as if you have one arm too many or two legs too few, but it'll get easier with practice.

It isn't just important to lower your expectations about your own performance. Remember to cut your partner some slack too. He or she won't know what you like the first time you have sex together and will probably be at least as nervous as you are. In any event, it may be good to talk about it afterwards, have a debriefing. What worked? Will there be a next time? If so, what should you both do differently?

How am I supposed to get anything in there?

Sex is so many things and an exaggerated focus on vaginal intercourse excludes too many people. After all, sex doesn't just have to be between a woman and a man, although it may often seem that way in our heteronormative society. In the UK around 18 per cent of women have had a sexual experience with somebody of their own gender.[3] Nonetheless, we'll give a little extra space here to first-time vaginal sex. Not because it's the only way to have sex, but because it's what we get most questions about.

An incredible number of girls ask themselves the following questions before they have vaginal sex. Will I bleed? Will it hurt? A lot of women are afraid their vaginas will be too tight: how am I supposed to fit anything in there? I can't even get a tampon in!

The idea of getting something as big as a penis into a vagina may seem dramatic, but there's actually plenty of room. Your vagina is incredibly flexible and can expand in all directions when you're turned on. A lot of people think women who haven't had sex have tighter vaginas than those who have. You've probably heard that your vagina gets saggier and saggier the more you screw. That's not true.

The vagina is a powerful muscular tube and you can regulate how tight it will be yourself. And this regulator works regardless of how many penises or dildos you've had in your vagina. If you really relax, it'll be easier for a penis to slip in, but if you clench, it may be difficult to get *anything* in. Even if you've had sex a lot of times, you can still tighten your vagina and make it narrower. If you use your vaginal muscles actively during sex, you can regulate the friction between the vagina and the penis. Just experiment!

A lot of girls are nervous before having sex for the first time and that's hardly surprising, given all the pressure of expectation. It's perfectly fine to be a bit nervous, but if you're too nervous, it can make the experience an unpleasant one. If you're nervous, it's easy to unconsciously tighten the muscles in your vagina and that makes it difficult to get anything in there. It can even hurt a bit.

When women are horny, their genitals often react by producing more moisture. This slick fluid serves as the body's natural lubrication.* If you're

---

* This doesn't apply to all women. It's quite possible to feel horny without getting wet and vice versa. You can be wet without feeling any desire whatsoever. You can read more about that in the section on desire.

very stressed, it's difficult to get turned on and wet. This can happen even if you've decided that you want to have sex. In a way, nervousness can prevent your body from going along with what you want.

If you're dry or are involuntarily tightening your vagina, it's easy to get small tears in the vaginal wall that may bleed a bit. This isn't dangerous, but it can be unpleasant and sting. The key is to take it easy the first time. Spend time on kissing and foreplay, so that it's easier for your muscles to relax. Give yourself time to be really turned on and that way you'll also produce more moisture.

Some girls don't get wet, even if they relax, spend time on foreplay and want to have sex. On the other hand, some women become wet when they don't feel horny. There's not always a link between the brain and the genitals. The great thing is that there are alternatives to the vagina's natural moisture. It's equally good to use spit or lubricant from the supermarket or the chemist. Lubricant may improve a lot of people's experience and it may be a good idea to have some around the first time, when you don't know exactly how your body is going to react.

And then there's the hymen, unfortunately also known as the virginal membrane (see p. 19). We've already dedicated a whole section to this, the narrowest part of the vagina, but we might as well repeat some of the points. Your hymen won't necessarily bleed the first time you have sex. It's roughly as likely that you won't bleed as that you will. And nobody will be able to tell from looking at your genitals afterwards whether you've had sex or not. There is no membrane covering the whole of your vagina, so there's no vaginal membrane to rupture, just a flexible ring of tissue. Don't waste energy worrying about your hymen, it isn't worth losing sleep over. Spend time worrying about serious things instead, like global warming, the refugee situation and deficient sex education in schools.

Tips and tricks

You now know a lot about what happens in the vagina when you have sex, but how are you supposed to go about doing it from a practical point of view? We have two suggestions for how you can sleep with a man (or boy) for the first time, from a strictly technical standpoint, but you may well opt for a third alternative. It's your vagina, after all. The alternatives are different, but equally good.

The first is super traditional, but definitely worth considering. The missionary position isn't often used in porn because you see so little of the sex organs (and what would porn be without exposed sex organs?), but in the real world, missionary is a winner when you're having sex for the first time. It involves you (the girl) lying on your back, while the boy lies between your legs, so that your chests and stomachs are facing each other. The penis goes into your vagina when the boy moves back and forth on top of you. It's not an active position from your point of view, but there are several reasons why this is a good place to start. You have full access to and oversight of each other's bodies; you can snog as you go along; and, last but not least, it's possible for you to observe each other's reactions, so you always know that the other person's having a good time. This is especially important the first time, when both of you are nervous. If there's too much eye contact, you can just shut your eyes.

Some find it scarier to give up control than to take charge themselves. A lot of people are scared witless of being driven along the motorway by other people and feel the need to be backseat drivers. Are you like that? If so, it's much better for you to take control yourself. *We'll put you on top.* A good starting point is for the boy to lie on his back and you to lie on top of him. It's a bit like a reverse missionary position. Place your knees on either side of his hips and sit on his penis. If you like, you can give yourself extra support by resting your lower arms or hands on the bed. You absolutely don't have to sit as if you were on a horse even though people often talk about this position as the girl riding the boy, or cowgirl position. If you feel too exposed sitting upright, you can lean forward. If you like it that way, you can ride on. Now you're the one who's going to do most of the moving. You can control how and how deeply the penis slides into your vagina and how quickly things will go. That's the advantage of sitting on top!

As with the missionary position, you'll still have a good view of each other's faces. Yes, it can be a bit scary, but it's easier to communicate if something's good or bad.

Not all sex ends in orgasm – although that may be the impression you get from porn or Hollywood films. This applies to both boys and girls. Orgasm is something that comes with practice and not something you should expect of yourself or your partner the first time you have sex. To have an orgasm, it's important to know your own body well and to feel safe.

For just those reasons, some women seem to find it easier to have an orgasm with a person they're in a steady relationship with.

Another important way to get to know your own body is to masturbate. For a lot of people, it takes several years to manage to have an orgasm with their sex partners. It's often easier to come when you do it all by yourself, but practice makes perfect! We'll come back to that later.

Communication with your partner is also important. By all means say what you want, but don't expect him or her to be able to sort out your orgasm for you. It's perfectly fine and normal to take things into your own hands. Having sex with a partner doesn't mean you can't devote attention to yourself at the same time. After all, you can show your partner what you're doing and then your partner can show you what he or she likes, too.

Don't forget about contraception

Sex is fun, but like other fun things, there's a risk attached. In the same way as seat belts and cycle helmets reduce the risk of serious injury, contraception reduces the risk of sexually transmitted infections and pregnancy.

Contraception is definitely a shared responsibility. If it takes two to have sex, it takes two to sort out contraception. Even so, it isn't always sensible to assume that your partner will come prepared. Our advice to you is always to take matters into your own hands. That's also our advice to any boys who might be reading this. If your partner is prepared too, that's a good sign. It may mean this is a person with a good head on their shoulders.

Contraception requires planning, so find out how to use it well before having sex for the first time. Go and seek guidance from a doctor or nurse and read the chapter on contraception too. You'll find everything you need to know in there. We recommend combining condoms with a contraceptive method that gives high protection against pregnancy. For now, the contraceptive alternatives on offer are almost exclusively for women, but luckily, good options for men are also in the pipeline. The condom is the only form of contraception that offers protection against sexually transmitted infections. By all means use a condom on its own, but make sure it doesn't become damaged when you're in the middle of the act by following our condom course (see p. 122). It may also be a good idea to have a morning-after pill to hand in case anything goes wrong. You'll learn more about that soon too.

If you feel like having sex and you have the contraception under control, go right ahead. You're the only person who knows whether you're ready or not. Nonetheless, our most important advice is to take the first time for what it is: *the first time*. There'll be plenty of others; you'll become more skilful and it will get better.

ANAL SEX

We closed the section called 'The other hole' in chapter 1 with a real cliff-hanger: the area around and right inside your anus is full of nerve endings just waiting to be stimulated. Some people find that it expands the dimensions of their sex life if they invite it to the party (see p. 23).

Great – we have masses of anal nerve endings, but how are we supposed to go about stimulating them? Perhaps you think it sounds a bit over-optimistic to 'invite the other hole to the party'. Lots of people think anal sex sounds scary and a bit dirty, in the same category as whips and blind-folds. 'What? Are we supposed to have sex with the same hole we poo out of?'

Anal sex is undoubtedly 'sex 201', or advanced sex. It's not something you have to do if you don't particularly feel like it. Nonetheless, it's becoming steadily more common among heterosexual couples. Nearly one in five of all young Britons aged 16 to 24 has had anal sex in the past year.[4] There's no reason to think young people elsewhere are any different.

So, people have anal sex, but they often have it for the wrong reasons. Unfortunately, it's been observed that anal sex is all too often an activity that girls are pushed into having and something that they experience as unpleasant or painful.[5] There's a widespread perception that girls must 'learn to enjoy' anal sex. That's not the way it should be. Anal sex should be voluntary and it should be good. If you're not interested, don't pursue it. Set your own boundaries.

A section for the curious

If you are curious this section is for you. Many women like anal sex, which can be so many things. The term includes all types of stimulation of the anus. It may entail penetrative sex with a penis or a dildo, it may involve fingering or oral sex, licking on and around the anus, which is also known as rimming. The fact that you don't fancy a penis in your anus doesn't mean you can't find other ways to get pleasure from it.

The advice in this section deals with penetrative anal sex, with fingers, penis or other objects. Since having anal sex is a bit different from having vaginal sex, there are a few things you need to know before you get started.

As you may remember from earlier, the anus has two strong, adjoining sphincters: one that works automatically without you doing anything at all, and another one that's a voluntary muscle. This is practical because it means we aren't constantly having to dash to the loo for a number two. The sphincter keeps the anus tight, making it as wrinkled as a pleated skirt and concealing the actual size of the ring.

A lot of people think the anal canal and rectum are very narrow, much tighter than the vagina. This may be one of the reasons for its apparently magical power of attraction for men, but it's only a partial truth. The rectum is actually like a balloon, just tied shut at one end with a knot. The sphincters are at the very end, and press the last section of the gut together with immense force. This means that it is extremely narrow at the sphincters, but once you get past them there's plenty of room. The vagina, on the other hand, is a tube full of muscles all the way from its opening up to the cervix. So, the vagina can be narrow all the way up, whereas the rectum is mostly narrow right at the end. What's more, it isn't as if the sphincters are narrow all the time. After you've been going at it for a little while, they relax so that the rectum isn't especially narrow at any point.

The balloon knot means that anal sex involves some very particular challenges. When you're going to have vaginal sex, we talk about *relaxing* so the pelvic muscles won't contract and make it difficult to have sex. The sphincters in the anus don't work in the same way. As you know, your anus remains closed when you are totally relaxed, and stays like that even when you're sleeping or in deep meditation; this is the involuntary ring muscle at work. You can't actively make the opening larger by relaxing. What you can do is prevent the *voluntary* sphincter from contracting as well. You have no control over the involuntary sphincter but, as we've said, it will gradually become looser with stimulation.

The most important advice, therefore, is to take it easy to start off with.

Don't launch yourself at a hard penis or a massive dildo if you've never had anything up your back passage before. It takes time for the sphincters to relax. First you need to get the muscles that you can control to relax and after that, the involuntary sphincter has to take the hint. Start out trying smaller things, fingers or smaller sex toys, and get used to the feeling. Most people need to warm up for a considerable amount of time before they're ready.

If you take it too fast, the anus is prone to small tears that can be horribly painful over the next days. Anybody who's ever aimed for the vagina, but ended up with the full length of their partner in the wrong hole instead knows all about that. It hurts. If you're going to have anal sex, you must be ready for it. This also means that your partner must be prepared to be incredibly patient. Just going for it won't work.

Once you're under way, things get easier. Your anus becomes more and more slack – and that brings us to something a lot of people find scary. The balloon knot doesn't close up again straightaway once you're finished. 'Oh no! Is my ring going to be saggy for ever?' Far from it – relax. The muscles do slowly tighten again, it just takes a bit of time.

True enough, it is possible to permanently injure the sphincters, in the same way as it's possible to injure any part of your body. But you'd have to give them a real pummelling. Remember that the anus is designed to allow larger things out than your average penis. Start off calmly, proceed carefully, and stop if anything feels wrong; that way everything will be fine.

Another important aspect of anal sex is moisture. While the vagina usually becomes wet of its own accord when you're aroused, you have to use lubricant or some equivalent type of artificial moisture to have anal sex. Without it, it'll be difficult to get anything in and if it's too dry, there'll be a lot of friction – and friction increases the risk of tears and light bleeding.

It's true that a little moisture is also produced by the glands in the rectum, but that happens regardless of whether you're turned on. The inside of your gut has a mucous membrane, just like the inside of your vagina and mouth. Mucous membranes produce moisture: spit in the mouth and vaginal secretions in the vagina. When the mucous membrane in the rectum is irritated by, say, a penis, it produces mucus to protect itself. So, sex in itself will trigger the production of a bit of moisture, but it isn't enough. You need lubricant as well.

And so on to the big question: poo. We've all heard urban legends about women who've accidentally pooed on their partners during anal sex. It's hardly a tempting prospect for most of us, but there's no getting away from the fact that there are faeces in the rectum – after all, that's what the gut is designed for. Even if you don't feel as if you need to go to the loo, faeces accumulates in the gut until it is full. The rectum is a storage place for the poo before it escapes into the outside world. This means faeces can end up on a penis, sex toy or finger and if you haven't thought about it in advance, it may come as a bit of a shock. If it does happen, there's nothing wrong with it and no reason for you to feel embarrassed. If you're going to have sex involving your gut, that's part of the game.

It is, however, possible to reduce the risk of poo. Some people choose to solve the problem by flushing out their gut first with a little enema bought at the chemists. Doctors don't recommend this, however, because the irritation of the mucous membranes can make you more susceptible to sexually transmitted infections. Others take care to go to the loo before they get going.

You cannot, of course, become pregnant from having butt sex, but you absolutely can get sexually transmitted infections. Many people forget this, or believe they're less likely to be infected in the anus. In fact, it's quite the opposite. Some sexually transmitted infections are more easily transmitted through anal sex. If you have sex with new partners, it's important to use a condom until you and your partner have been tested. This applies regardless of what kind of sex you have.

Be safe too

As you know, it's fine to have vaginal sex without a condom after you and your partner have been tested for STIs, but your anus contains gut bacteria, so hygiene is important! You don't want to get gut bacteria into your vagina or your urethra where they don't belong, because that may lead to infections. This also applies to men, too. So be careful when you're switching straight from anal to vaginal sex, with either finger or penis. It's a good idea to use a condom during anal sex and take it off if you want to continue with vaginal sex. Remember to clean the sex toys you use anally as well.

Incidentally, there are toys designed specially for anal use. They often have a plug at one end to prevent them from disappearing right up into your rectum. Nothing can disappear in the vagina, because it is no more than 7 to 10 centimetres long and is closed at the top. However, the gut is endless, practically speaking. It's pretty crappy to have to go to your local hospital A&E to remove objects that have got stuck, but it does happen. Doctors get a tremendous amount of enjoyment out of exchanging stories about all the strange things they've had to fish out of people's backsides: chunky candles, toy cars, iPods or bottles – they must be allowed their fun too.

This was a to-do list for those of you who want to try anal sex. Done properly, it can be wonderful for women and men alike, but for that to happen, girls must stop doing it for the man's sake. Anal sex, like all other sex, must happen because you both want to do it.

A TOTALLY NORMAL SEX LIFE

When the American TV series *Girls* (2015) first took our screens by storm, many people described it as revolutionary to finally see normal women having normal sex – whatever that is. Instead of multiple orgasms and steamy sex on the kitchen counter, we got to see clumsiness, awkward pauses and failed attempts to turn up at boyfriends' houses wearing sexy underwear. It's striking how hard the girls in the series try to live up to the sexual ideals of popular culture, with wildly varying degrees of success. Dirty talk and spanking seemed sexy in the latest *Elle* article, but when Adam and Lena try it in real life, it turns into the very best kind of cringe TV. However, *Girls* is the clash between the ideal and the reality.

Girls is a reaction to the fact that sex has become public property. People talk loud and long over bottles of red wine about the most intimate details of their friends' sex lives. Women have taken ownership of sex. It's cool to be horny, cool to know what you want. And that's great, for those who achieve it.

Unfortunately, expectations about how your sex life ought to be come along as part of the baggage. Our sex life has become yet another arena where we are supposed to perform. Only in a tete-à-tete with a good female friend do the more shameful questions come out: 'Is it normal only to have sex every other week?' 'Do you normally suck your guy off every time you have sex?' 'Am I abnormal if I can only come by touching myself during sex?'

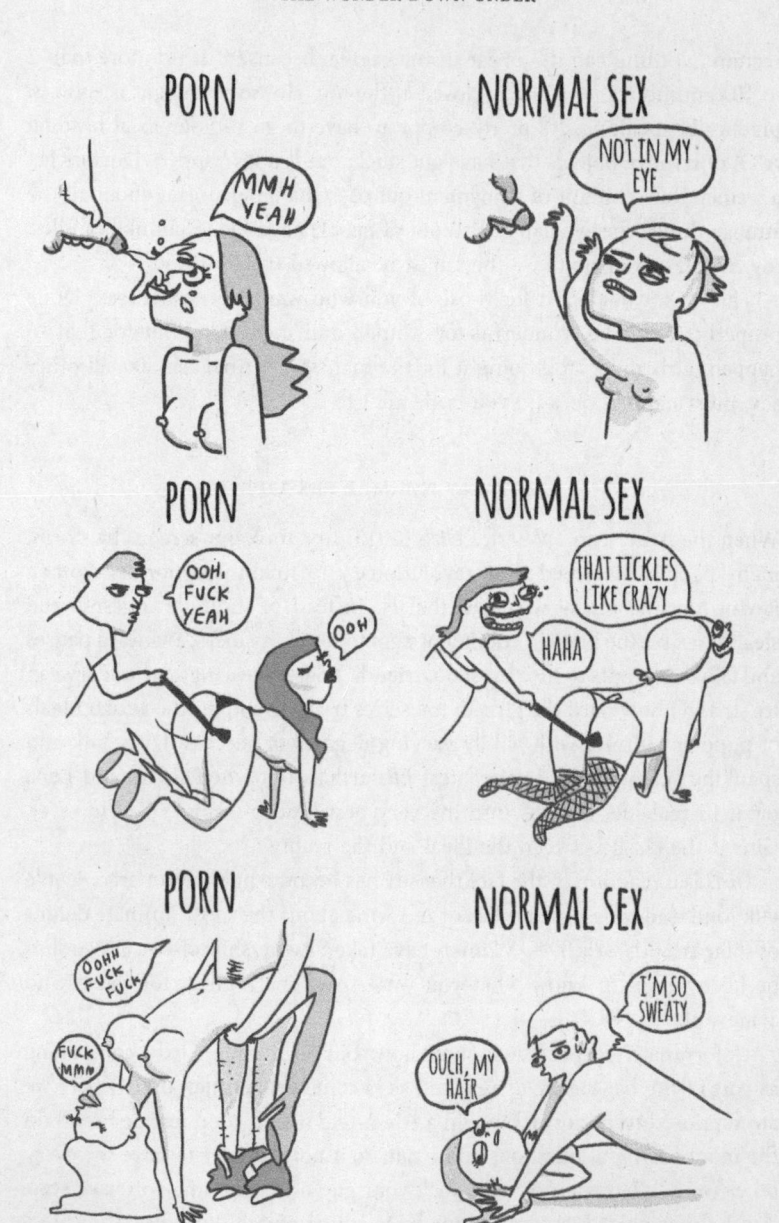

What actually constitutes a normal sex life?

We went on a quest to discover standard sex. When people are assessing their sex lives, the *amount* of sex is generally the easiest aspect to compare with others. Quality is so subjective, after all, but it's easy to count. If you ask heterosexual people how often they have sex, you get the same answer in large parts of the Western world. Heterosexual couples have sex once or twice a week. Co-habiting couples have more sex than married couples. Single people have the least sex.[6] We know less about homosexual men and lesbians, but some data suggest that lesbian couples have around as much sex as heterosexual couples.[7] In a Norwegian study involving couples aged between 23 and 67, around 40 per cent had had sex once or twice a week in the previous month.[8] Only one eager group, 10 per cent of the total, had had sex three, four or more times a week, but just as many hadn't had sex at all in the previous month. The rest had had sex once every other week or less.

In the latter study there was, perhaps surprisingly, not such a great difference between how often the different age groups had sex. Only when the couples hit 50 did they begin to have sex a little less often, but even then, more than 40 per cent had sex once or twice a week or more. Even so, we know from a long series of studies that age is one of the most important factors when it comes to how often people in relationships have sex. Among other reasons, this is because the body's sexual functioning deteriorates with age. The libido falls, men can have erectile problems and women may find the mucous membrane in their vaginas becomes fragile and thin owing to low oestrogen levels, leading to more discomfort during sex. However, there are other factors apart from age that explain how often we have sex. One of them is being in love.

The first stage of a new relationship can feel like being in a bubble. The brain is overflowing with neurotransmitters that convey pleasure, satisfaction and desire. Absorbed in the feeling of being in love, you forget that anything exists apart from the two of you. Sex becomes more important than sleep, food and friends. It becomes a shared language through which you can convey everything you don't yet dare say with words – it's you and me now, we're the only thing that matters.

Everyday life has a way of sneaking up on you in the end. One evening, you catch yourself looking at the clock as an eager hand creeps under your knicker elastic. 'Can't we just spoon a bit? I have to get up so early,' you say with an apologetic smile. Is there something wrong with your relationship if you're suddenly not so keen on having sex 24/7? Or is it just a natural progression?

A German study examined the sex lives of 1,900 students in their 20s who were in steady relationships.[9] It found a clear connection between how long the couples had been together and how often they had sex. On average, the newly enamoured couples had sex ten times a month, or two and a half times a week, but 70 per cent had sex more than seven times a month. After the first year, the number of times people had sex began to decrease. When the relationship had lasted between one and three years, fewer than half of the respondents had sex two or more times a week. After five years, shagging hit rock bottom. By then, the frequency of sex was halved, from ten to five times a month. These findings have also been seen in other studies[10] and among lesbian couples.[11]

In other words, you're not alone if you feel you're having less sex than before, so what's going on? The German study made some interesting observations. At the beginning of the relationship, women and men experienced similar levels of sexual desire, and had the same desire for intimacy and nearness. Then something odd happened. While the men were still just as horny three years on, the study found a dramatic reduction in sexual desire among the women after the first year of the relationship. During the first year, three out of four women agreed that they wanted to have sex often. After three years, the number had fallen to just one in four, and twice as many, up from 9 per cent (at the beginning) to 17 per cent, said they often experienced a lack of sexual desire.

One illustration of this is how often men and women in a relationship find themselves being rejected when they fancy having sex. In the Norwegian study we spoke about earlier, half the men said they were sexually rejected now and then, while one in ten felt they were often rejected. The number was reversed for women; 90 per cent said they'd never, or rarely, been sexually rejected by their man.[12]

One aspect that didn't decrease, but rather increased over the course of the relationship was the women's need for intimacy and closeness. For men, however, the desire for cuddling actually *decreased* over time. Perhaps the cliché is truer than we'd like to believe: women want to cuddle, men want to screw. Why, we don't know. The researchers behind the German study thought the best explanation was evolutionary. Women unconsciously use sex as a means of binding the man to them and then lose interest in sex once their goal is achieved and the man is stuck. Others believe the answer lies in different degrees of biological sex drive (how far sex is a drive at all is something we'll come back to). Others again point out that society has so-called sexual 'scripts' for how men and women should behave. People think of being horny as manly, whereas it's considered unfeminine for women to express the same degree of horniness. This may make it easier for women to settle into asexual patterns than men, but it can also increase the experience of shame in the men who have little interest in sex.

So far, we've seen that the longer a couple is together, the less sex they have. At the same time, we know that the happiest couples are the ones who have the most sex. One consolation is that there seems to be a happiness ceiling. A Canadian study of 30,000 people found that the level of happiness didn't increase among the people who had sex more than once a week.[13] So it seems that human beings may have found their way to a golden mean of once or twice a week all by themselves!

So, which aspects other than frequency are involved in determining how satisfied we are with our sex lives? Again, the answer may seem obvious: the quality of the relationship.[14] There is a close connection between how satisfied we are with our relationship and the quality of our sex life. Put simply, a good sex life is a good relationship. We don't know whether it's the good sex that makes us satisfied with the relationship or the good relationship that produces good sex. It's probably a combination.

It's good to talk
A good relationship has a lot to do with communication. You need to talk to each other about sex and feelings. Oh God – how lame! Why on earth do we have to talk about sex? Isn't that just the ultimate proof that your relationship is sexually dead? The sexiest thing about one-night stands and new relationships is precisely the lack of talk. Some people are so afraid of talking that they'd rather forget the condom than risk killing the

atmosphere. This little chat is a threat to the fragile state of mystery and excitement.

Even so, it is simply a fact that the couples who can achieve emotional intimacy by talking about their feelings, needs and expectations are more satisfied with both their relationship and their sex life in the long run.[15] By speaking openly about what you want and need sexually, you create security and, in turn, satisfaction. As a bonus, couples who talk about sex aren't just more satisfied, they also have more sex.[16]

There are many things in a relationship that can kill sexual desire: stress, lack of shared quality time, the feeling of not coming up to scratch sexually, a negative self-image and poor body awareness. If you feel that you and your partner have different sexual needs, you can quickly find yourself in a vicious circle in which one of you is always taking the initiative and the other is often rejecting the advances. It's no fun rejecting somebody. You feel guilty because you can't live up to the other person's expectations and you may start to become anxious that the other person will eventually get tired of it and leave you. The more you worry about these things, the less desire for sex you have. In the end, you avoid even innocent cuddling or kissing for fear it might lead the other person to expect something more.

This is often the underlying dynamic when couples stop having regular sex. It's naïve to think that you can get over this without talking to each other. If more couples dared to have a talk as soon as they noticed something wasn't right, a lot of problems could be avoided. So, sit down with your partner, put away your mobile and have a proper chat. Perhaps you'll get more and better sex in exchange.

Now perhaps you think that quantity isn't everything and we absolutely agree. It's all very well having sex twice a week, but it's the *content* that matters. What kind of sex do people actually have? Sex can mean so many things, after all. It may involve sucking and licking, vagina or anus. People may come or not come, screw in a double bed, on the sofa or in a hotel lift. For some people, routine sex is their mortal enemy: they miss the excitement and unpredictability of their single life, or the beginning of their relationship.

An Australian study from 2006 involving 19,000 people looked at which combinations of sex people had last had.[17] The answer they got was that 12 per cent had had only vaginal sex. Half had vaginal sex as well as stimulating each other's sex organs with their hands. A third had also had oral sex. Hardly surprisingly, the study found that the more hands and tongue were involved, the more likely the woman was to have achieved orgasm.

There are a lot of expectations attached to the idea of a good sex life. The reality is that a normal sex life is, well, pretty normal. Very few people are at it like rabbits. People get a bit bored as the first crush dissipates and everyday life catches up with their sex lives. A minority go down on their partner every time they have sex. Even so, most are very satisfied. And if you want things to be better, there's only one thing to do: talk to each other.

THE DISAPPEARANCE OF DESIRE

Being horny is no longer taboo. It's almost become an ideal among young women. The notion of perfection involves enjoying sex, initiating sex and experimenting with sex. But what are we supposed to do if desire vanishes, or never arrives in the first place. That can leave people feeling horribly excluded.

In winter 2015, Nina had the pleasure of meeting an unusually fascinating woman. The American sex therapist Dr Shirley Zussman (then 100 years old) is a little hunch-backed lady with full lips and sparkling eyes. She might be said to have had a front-row seat in the sexual revolution. She studied with William Masters and Virginia E. Johnson – renowned for their 'discovery' of the female orgasm and the inspiration for the SHO series, *Masters of Sex*. Dr Zussman has practised as a sex therapist in New York since the 1960s and 50 years later, she's still treating patients in her office in New York's Upper East Side, with its floral décor and its book-shelves decked with wooden figures in different sexual positions. This gives her a unique overview of the development of sexual problems over time: 'Before, my patients used to come to me with orgasm problems – premature ejaculation or the absence of climax – but now it's simply the spark that's missing,' she says. People definitely have better sex nowadays, according to Zussman, but that's no help when they just can't bring themselves to do it. She blames it on technology and high pressure at work. 'The women who come to me are so tired that they'd rather look at those darn iPhones than set aside time for intimacy. We forget to touch each other and look each other in the eyes.'

Dr Zussman may well be right. It can seem as if lack of desire is the new female ailment. A major study from 2013 showed that one in three British women had suffered from an absence of sexual desire in the previous year.[18] Among women in the 16–24 age group, one in four reported that they lacked any interest in sex. It makes for sad reading.

What yardstick are women who suffer a lack of desire measuring themselves against?

Since the 1960s, a kind of domino model has been used, involving four stages of sexual response: Desire–Excitement–Orgasm–Resolution. Desire is defined as a wish for sexual activity, including fantasies and thoughts. Desire is a purely mental process: I'm keen on sex NOW! Excitement, however, is both a feeling of pleasure and a purely physical reaction that involves, among other things, an increased supply of blood to the genitals, moistening and expansion of the vagina, a higher pulse rate, higher blood pressure and more rapid breathing.

Only lately have researchers begun to question this model. Surveys have, in fact, shown that up to one in three women rarely, if ever, experience sexual desire – they do not feel 'spontaneous desire' as it's called technically. Even so, most of them experience physical excitement and enjoyment of sex. Perhaps that sounds peculiar. Can it really be true that there's something seriously wrong with so many women out there?[19]

DESIRE

EXCITEMENT

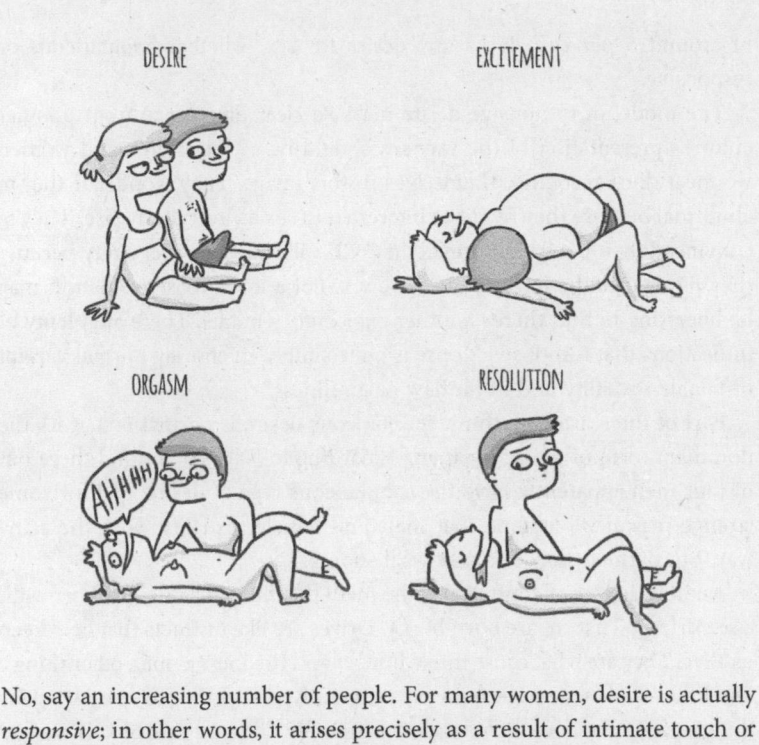

ORGASM

RESOLUTION

No, say an increasing number of people. For many women, desire is actually *responsive*; in other words, it arises precisely as a result of intimate touch or a sexual situation.[20] Physical excitement precedes desire, you might say, and so these women are more dependent on foreplay and nearness to flip the switch. Women with responsive desire have low interest in sex and take little initiative in bed, but they still have the capacity to have marvellous sex once they get going. Desire just needs to be nursed along a little more carefully.

The American sex researcher Emily Nagoski has taken up the banner of educating women about responsive desire. In her book *Come As You Are*, she claims that nearly one in three women have a responsive form of sexual desire. At the opposite end of the scale, there are the 15 per cent who have the 'classic', spontaneous form of sexual desire, in which you feel a desire for sex out of the blue. All the other women are somewhere in between the two.[21] Now and then, they fancy having sex without quite understanding why, whereas other times, sex sounds like a bit of a drag until they feel their body responding and their head slowly joins the party. Only a small group of around 5 per cent lacks any desire for sex, whether spontaneous or responsive.

The model of responsive desire marks a clear divergence from popular culture's presentation of the way sex should be. A lot of girls and women we meet don't recognise themselves in this image. They wonder if they're abnormal because they're not as interested in sex as 'everybody else'. They're convinced their boyfriend thinks they're boring and they feel guilty because they never take the initiative to have sex. For a lot of these women, it may be liberating to find there's another explanatory model. There are plenty of indications that responsive desire is quite simply an entirely normal variant of female sexuality and not a flaw or an illness.*

Part of the reason we think spontaneous desire is normal is that it's the dominant form of desire for men. According to Nagoski, around three out of four men apparently have the spontaneous type of desire, and for some strange reason we assume that male and female sexuality work the same way. But perhaps they don't, as we'll soon see.

Another source of confusion is the myth that human beings are born with a sex drive.[22] That we are born horny. Drives are like instincts that help keep us alive. They are what cause thirst, hunger and tiredness among other things. Our brain sends a message, quite unconsciously, that it's time to do a particular thing to keep the body in balance, for example sleep, eat or drink. If we had a sex drive, it would tell us that we have a need for sex along the same lines as our need for food, sleep and warm clothes. In that case, it would be a need fundamental to our survival. When sex is defined in that way, it's hardly surprising we think something's seriously wrong if we don't experience sexual desire.** And just in case any of you are in any doubt about it: nobody ever died from lack of sex. Sex isn't a drive but a reward.[23]

---

* This distinction in types of desire obviously also applies to men. Men may also experience responsive desire. It's just a little bit rarer for this to be a man's primary form of desire. According to Nagoski, around 75 per cent of all men primarily experience spontaneous desire, versus 15 per cent of all women. Five per cent of men have responsive desire as their main form, versus 30 per cent of women.

** Absence or loss of sexual desire is actually a diagnosis in the international classification of mental and behavioural disorders (ICD-10). It is possible to be assigned this diagnosis even if you experience sexual pleasure and arousal.

As long as sex gives enjoyment and is pleasurable, it's like dope for the brain: we want to have more. Desire is stimulated and we begin to seek out situations in which we can get sex. And that's where we come to Nagoski's important point: if sex doesn't serve as a reward for you, for example, because it's painful, carries associations with earlier assaults or is quite simply boring, your desire diminishes. The system only works as long as sex serves as a reward for the brain. In other words, we're not born horny, we *become* horny.

There are two lessons to learn from this
First of all, it means that women (and men) who have little desire for sex – either generally or because they only experience responsive desire – are not abnormal or sick. Some people love chocolate, others don't. We don't think there's anything wrong with people who don't like chocolate, even though *most* brains react positively to this delightful combination of cocoa, fat and sugar. And does it matter whether we label people as sick? The answer is yes, as the tiny remnant of sexual desire that's left inside is killed stone dead if you're made to feel like a walking deviant.

Secondly, it implies that sexual desire is not a constant. We are born with the *potential* to become horny, but the extent to which we do so varies over time according to how much pleasure and satisfaction sex gives us and what our general life situation is like. In addition, our sexual history – the experiences we have in our baggage – helps shape our sexual desire.

This explains why sexual desire rises and falls in waves over the course of our lives and the relationships we are involved in. It also gives us a fantastic means of influencing desire. The brain's system of reward can be manipulated if we understand how it works. And that brings us to the biggest difference between men and women.

Sex researchers come up with some very strange ideas
In a raft of experiments, men and women have been equipped with measuring apparatus on their penises and in their vaginas to measure the blood flow to their sex organs. This makes it possible to obtain a measure of how *physically* excited a person is. These are automatic responses that people don't consciously control. In the experiments, the subject may watch porn: hetero sex, homo sex, cuddly sex, violent sex, yes, even sex between apes.

Something for every taste, in other words. Then they're supposed to report how horny they feel as they watch the different clips. And that's when a very interesting discovery is made.[24]

Among men, there's around a 65 per cent correspondence between how hard their penis becomes and how horny they feel.[25] So the head is mostly on the same page as the automatic responses of the male sex organ. *Aha, I'm hard so I must want sex*, thinks the man. (Of course, this is a simplification. Men can also become hard without having any desire whatsoever for sex, as with the well-known phenomenon of morning glory, or teenage boys getting a boner when they have to go up to the blackboard and show the workings of a calculation.) Men's desire is pretty closely connected to the shenanigans of the penis, so pills like Viagra work incredibly well when men are struggling to 'get it up'. Viagra doesn't work on the brain, but simply ensures that the veins carrying blood back *out* of the penis become constricted, making the penis grow harder and more engorged with blood. This is more than enough – if you get the penis onside, the job's mostly done.

In women, however, it's been found there's only a 25 per cent overlap between the head and the workings of the sex organs.[26] The connection is so minor that it's simply impossible to say anything at all about how far a woman feels sexual desire based on how wet or engorged her sex organs are. A woman's genitals swell and grow wet from seeing men having sex with men and apes in full swing, but she won't necessarily feel turned on as a result. The woman's genitals also respond strongly to lesbian sex, often more than to hetero sex. More disturbingly, it has been observed that women can become physically excited and experience orgasm during assaults.[27] What does this mean? That women actually dig ape sex, or that some girls like to be raped?

No, no and no again! It means that women, unlike men, have a much higher degree of what sex researchers call 'arousal non-concordance' or 'subjective-genital (dis)agreement'. These complicated words actually just mean that there isn't any correspondence between the brain and the nether regions when it comes to desire. The two body parts evidently don't speak the same language and women with a very low degree of desire score highest of all; their brains are almost incapable of picking up the signals from their genitals.[28]

Women's desire is first and foremost located in their heads. It simply isn't enough for an attractive person to be lying in our bed, or for us to become wet and erect, the way men often do. We need more – it's our brain that needs stimulating, not our genitals. That's why Viagra only works on vanishingly few women, even though a lot of effort has been put in.[29] For women's sexual desire to be affected by pills, you have to fiddle with the intricate pathways in the brain and *that's* medicine at a whole new level.

Could a pill make a difference?
Many efforts have been made to develop a 'pink pill' for women's sexual desire. One attempt involved giving women testosterone, since this sex hormone is believed to be central to sexual desire. The problem is that it's not a good idea to give testosterone to fertile women as it could have potentially damaging effects on the foetus if the woman becomes pregnant. So, most of the studies were carried out on women who were almost entirely lacking in testosterone either because of cancer surgery or because they'd reached menopause. In such cases, the testosterone boost has mostly been seen to have a moderately positive effect on sexual desire.[30] In the best study, carried out on slightly younger women aged 35 to 46, no rise in levels of desire was found.[31] However, the women who received a medium-sized dose of testosterone experienced a 0.8 increase in 'satisfactory sexual events' in the course of a month compared with those who received a placebo.

The findings indicate that more testosterone has little effect once a very low minimum level has been exceeded. In fact, studies looking at the effect of testosterone on sexual desire cannot boast any major findings. Whether you're high or low, this doesn't appear to predict where you are on the desire scale.[32] It seems as if sex hormones simply don't have such a strong influence on women's sexual desire as had been believed.[33]

Other medication has also been tested, although this isn't legal in the UK: Melanotan II, popularly known as the 'Barbie drug', attracted a lot of attention in the media at one point because teenage girls, led by Norwegian celebrity blogger Sophie Elise Isachsen, were buying it on the internet. Melanotan is a synthetic hormone that imitates one of the body's hormones (melatonin) that tans our skin and gives us freckles. To start off with, Melanotan was developed to help us tan without sun – in other words, as self-tanning in pill form. Then it was discovered Melanotan's side-effects included reduced appetite and, possibly, increased sexual desire. Thus was the dream of the perfect woman born: golden brown skin, thin and horny. Understandably enough, the pharma companies saw dollar signs.

The problem was that Melanotan use eventually turned out to have potentially life-threatening side-effects. All experiments with the medicine were halted. Then the pharmaceutical company found that it could produce a less dangerous variant called *bremelanotide*. After years of experiments, this medicine is now undergoing a final round of studies and it looks as if it'll be approved. The problem is that this expensive medicine has to be self-administered with an autoinjector before sex and even then the effect isn't especially great. On average, the users reported half an extra 'satisfying sexual event' *per month* compared with those using a placebo injection.[34] Nothing to write home about, then.

Another medication, *flibanserin*, was originally developed as an anti-depressant, but was approved in August 2015 for use on people diagnosed with low sexual desire. This medication is also incredibly expensive – costing several hundred pounds a month – and must be used daily. You can't drink alcohol while you're taking it either, owing to the risk of life-threatening drops in blood pressure. Side-effects such as nausea, dizziness and fatigue are relatively common. Here, too, the effects are not dramatic. The users have between 0.4 and one extra 'satisfying sexual event' per month.[35]

In other words, pills do not so far appear to be the miracle cure people had been hoping for. None of the medicines mentioned above amounts to much once you take into account the side-effects, price and result. However, these kinds of studies have emphasised how much of an impact our feelings have on sexual desire and satisfaction. Indeed in some of the studies, an incredibly high placebo effect was observed – higher than has been seen for almost any other 'medicine'. In a Viagra study, 40 per cent of the women who were given sugar pills were seen to have experienced an improvement in sexual desire.[36] By taking a pill, they entered into a new mode and a new role – they managed to break out of old, ingrained patterns in which they identified themselves as people who didn't want sex.

The placebo effect shows us this: our sexual desire sits in our head and it can be manipulated. But how? Emily Nagoski explains it very well.[37]

Imagine the brain, holding sway at the top of the body like a sensitive conductor. The body's conductor is constantly receiving signals from the body and its environment, which it interprets, fitting them together to form a finely tuned image. Our nervous system and the signals it sends to the brain are very simply structured, a bit like the codes in a computer, where everything is either 0 or 1. We have one signal that tells us to 'drive', known as *excitation*, and another that tells us to 'brake', or *inhibition*. The balance between the signals indicating excitation and those indicating inhibition determines what the brain will decide to do with the body at any given time. If you're pushing the brake to the floor, it doesn't make any difference if you accelerate a bit at the same time. The sum effect is what counts.

Imagine that each of the reasons preventing you from wanting sex – consciously or unconsciously – puts a little pressure on the brake. Examples could include stress, depression, poor body image, feelings of guilt and fear of not achieving orgasm. All these slight pressures on the brake can build up so that the brake ends up pressed to the floor, bringing things to a complete halt. To relieve this heavy pressure on the brake, our brains need to receive an even more powerful signal telling us to 'drive' – for example love and pleasure. The reward must be greater than the effort. Now and then, this happens by itself, for example when we're in love; but otherwise, our task is to ensure that the 'drive' signals dominate and that the brake is as weak as possible. This sounds pretty vague, but there's actually no mystery about it. The first step is acknowledging that sexual desire is not something that arises of its own accord, or a constant character trait you were born with. After that, you must sit down and think through what turns you off and on. Do what Nagoski suggests: make a list – here are some ideas.

What turns me off? *Having sex right before I go to sleep because then I worry I won't be properly rested the next day. Feeling down or sad. Fear that my partner will try to have sex when I don't feel like it and then I'll have to reject him/her again. Uncertainty about the relationship. Jealousy. Routine sex when I know exactly what's going to happen. The expectation that I must come for my partner to feel like a good lover. Stress or worry about things I should have done, but didn't get round to during the day. Feeling ugly. Feeling dirty as I haven't showered. When we check our mobiles in bed.*

What turns me on? *Knowing that we have masses of time and there's no hurry to get things finished. A quickie, no talking. The thought of an orgasm. Feeling good in my own body. An erotic book or film, or just porn. Sex after exercise, when the endorphins are flowing and the blood's still pumping. Sex in the middle of the day in broad daylight. Pitch-black, sheltering darkness. Clean bedclothes. Feeling loved. Compliments. New surroundings. Safe surroundings. Seeing my partner in his or her element. Being in my element. Having my back tickled. Daring to try new things in bed. When I'm sure that what I always do in bed is absolutely the best thing my partner can imagine.*

When you've made your own list, the real work begins. You have to arrange things so that the balance tips in favour of 'drive'. That means eliminating as many of the brakes as possible, while simultaneously creating a setting in which as many of your drive switches as possible are flipped.

It's pretty much impossible to do this alone if you're in a relationship. You must involve your partner and tell her or him what turns you on and what you need. In relationships that have really got stuck in a rut, sex therapists often recommend you stop having sex at all for a while, or establish guidelines for sex – for example deciding on a particular day and time when you'll have sex and clearing your schedule accordingly. It sounds pretty unsexy, but there's a logic to it. If you decide on a sex hiatus, you remove all expectations of sex and by doing so, you get to have a break until the desire returns of its own accord. You can't force desire. The sense that you *ought* to be feeling desire is just another brake.

This doesn't mean that you should stop being close to each other. For a lot of people, in fact, it works the opposite way, because they have space to cuddle and be intimate without feeling any pressure for anything they're not ready for. You should be kind to yourself; be patient. If your partner doesn't think this is important, perhaps you've got to the root of the problem.

Grandma Zussman, with her 100 years of experience, grasped something vital. Sexual desire doesn't occur in a vacuum. Desire is tightly interwoven with the relationships we live in, and not least our relationship with ourselves. There are no quick fixes out there. But most of us are capable of feeling desire.

THE BIG O

The orgasm is a wonderful, fabulous phenomenon. It stands apart from all the tedious routine work the body does to keep us alive. While the heart beats to pump blood around our bodies, the gut rumbles and churns to give us nourishment and the brain quivers with nerve signals to move our body and make plans, the orgasm has an entirely special function. The orgasm is quite simply toe-curling, hair-raising, moaning bliss. The orgasm is our little reward.

People have tried to come up with many different definitions of what an orgasm actually is and the researchers aren't entirely in agreement about it. The traditional medical understanding of it is that it's a transient peak sensation of intense sexual pleasure, associated with rhythmic contractions of the musculature in the pelvic region.[38]

Modern sex researchers think this definition is too narrow. One woman's experience will be different to another's and what's more, it's physically possible to have unpleasant orgasms or asexual orgasms – for example, during an assault or while asleep. In fact, as many as one in three women experiences orgasms in their sleep.[39] They therefore think it's better to say that orgasms are a sudden, involuntary release of sexual tension, like the release of a tensed bow.[40]

So, people can have orgasms without pleasure, orgasms without physical contact with the genitals and orgasms without circumvaginal contractions. Some describe just having a warm, tingling feeling that spreads throughout their whole body, and then getting an unmistakable feeling of being 'finished'. Common to all is that you know it when you've had an orgasm. If you don't know whether you've had an orgasm, you haven't had one. So, vague and yet so simple.

If, that is, we stick to the classic concept of the orgasm, which is the most normal one, after all, that the orgasm is the peak of sexual response. When women are physically excited, their inner labia and the inner parts of their clitoris fill with blood, in the same way as the man's penis becomes hard. In fact, the clitoral complex doubles in size when you're horny! Just 10–30 seconds after stimulation of the genitals has begun, the vagina will, often as not, start to become wet. It will also become at least 1 centimetre broader and longer. The closer you come to climax, the more your pulse quickens, your respiration speeds up and your blood pressure climbs. Many people also feel the muscles in the rest of their body tensing, and their fingers and toes curling against the sheet. There's a wonderful name for this: *carpopedal spasms.*

In the end, the orgasm arrives. A feeling of wellbeing spreads through you from head to toe. It feels as if your genitals are exploding and the muscles in your pelvic region will often tighten in rhythmic contractions. The contractions start in the lower part of the vagina and spread upwards to embrace the whole of the vagina and the uterus. The muscles around your urethra and anus are often involved too. On average, women's orgasms last around 17 seconds.[41] When you're finished, however, the blood will begin to withdraw from the genitals, in the same way as the man's penis becomes flaccid after orgasm. At that point, the body has completed the resolution phase – where everything slowly returns to its normal state.

Unlike men, women may have several orgasms in a row if they continue to stimulate themselves. The world record for the number of female orgasms is unknown. For some reason or another, the *Guinness Book of Records* hasn't published it. It does list other wickedly exciting sex records such as 'most frequent sex' on its website. If you were wondering, an Australian cricket, *Ornebius aperta*, is the record-holder, having completed 50 sex acts in the course of three to four hours. The little rascal.

The highest unofficial figure we know of for the number of orgasms is from a so-called Masturbate-a-Thon – which is, marvellously, a self-pleasuring competition to raise money for charity.[42] The record came from the Danish Masturbate-a-thon in 2009, in which the winner is supposed to have had a total of 222 orgasms in the course of one, presumably pretty long, masturbation session. That leaves most of us with something to aim for...

Now, perhaps you're surprised we're talking about orgasms in general, because, after all, there are clitoral orgasms, vaginal orgasms, G-spot orgasms, tantric orgasms, squirting orgasms and orgasms from having your tootsies sucked. Aren't there?

Actually all orgasms are the same: an orgasm. The physical and mental response is the same. The only difference is what releases it. Our entire body is an erogenous zone. There are nerve endings everywhere that can be stimulated and give pleasure. Just think how delicious it can be to have someone kiss your neck, tickle your hair or stroke the inside of your thigh.

We've also met women who have spontaneous orgasms throughout the day, every single day, without any kind of physical stimulation, as well as women who can breathe their way to orgasm.

The terms vaginal orgasm and clitoral orgasm are especially widespread, although there isn't any difference between them.[43] We now know that the clitoris is a large organ and not just a little nub at the front of the vulva. The inner parts of the clitoris surround both the urethra and the vagina, and can be indirectly aroused through most forms of stimulation of the vulva and vagina. To talk of 'clitoral orgasm' and 'vaginal orgasm' is imprecise, since the clitoris is thoroughly involved in vaginal sex. The vagina itself is pretty insensitive. As you'll see later, the head of the clitoris is also placed differently for different women. Some people claim that this placement can make it harder or easier for women to achieve orgasm during vaginal intercourse.[44]

Squirting orgasm, female ejaculation or squirting, is shrouded in legend and has been described in literature for more than 2,000 years, ever since the times of the Ancient Greek philosopher Aristotle.[45] For most women, however, the urethra isn't especially involved in their sex life, despite being positioned between the head of the clitoris and the vagina. That said, some women find something special happens with their urethra when they orgasm – a cause of much head-scratching among the women as well as researchers. When the women come, clear or milk-white fluid squirts out of their urinary opening. Some women report several millilitres, while others talk about an amount equivalent to a glass of milk. What kind of orgasm is *that*?

We don't know how many women have squirting orgasms, but we do know that it happens, and lots of us have seen it on the internet. Porn depicting ejaculating women was banned in the UK in 2014.[46] We don't know why female ejaculation is worse than any other porn – for example, porn involving male ejaculation – but it seems that some people find female ejaculation especially offensive, perhaps because they think the ejaculate is wee? But is it?

It's still unclear what the fluid consists of. Some studies take the view that the ejaculate comes from some small glands known as *Skene's glands*. These glands are in the anterior wall of the vagina, around the lower part of the urethra. Apparently not all women have them, and they can vary in size from one woman to the next – which could, at any rate, explain why only some women have squirting orgasms. The glands are supposed to be the equivalent of the man's prostate, which is involved in producing the fluid in sperm, and they empty their secretions into the urethra during orgasm.[47] This theory is supported by the fact that prostate substances have been found in the fluid from some ejaculating women.[48] However, one study from 2015, which used ultrasound examinations on seven masturbating women, concluded that the ejaculate mostly consisted of urine, although small amounts of prostate substances were also found in the liquid.[49] Some researchers think we're dealing with two different phenomena: some women ejaculate small amounts of white fluid from their Skene's glands, while others squirt larger amounts of clear liquid from their bladder.[50] In any case, perhaps it doesn't really matter what the secretion consists of. It's a natural part of the orgasm for a number of women.

Let's go back to the story of clitoral and vaginal orgasms

Women have long struggled with a sense that there's a hierarchy of orgasms, with the so-called vaginal orgasm, triggered solely by vaginal penetration, at the top. They feel as if there's something wrong with them if they don't get orgasms from nothing but 'the old in-out', as Alex DeLarge in *A Clockwork Orange* (1962) liked to call it. They feel as if they're cheating if they have to help things along with a finger or need to be licked.

This is peculiar. Not just because an orgasm is an orgasm whichever way you look at it. But also because this way of reaching orgasm is actually unusual for women. How has this strange ranking of female orgasms come about?* It is, in any event, not a leftover from the really olden days. Before The Enlightenment of the 18th century people believed a woman had to have an orgasm to become pregnant and if she really wanted to be certain of pregnancy, the man and woman supposedly had to come *simultaneously*.[51] At the time infant mortality rates were incredibly high, so having plenty of children was an important goal. Giving women orgasms therefore became an art men had to perfect if they wanted to ensure they had heirs. The key to the woman's orgasm lay in direct stimulation of the head of the clitoris.

---

* The following historical account is inspired by Liv Strömquist's fantastic graphic novel, *Kunskapens frukt* (Galago, 2014).

Thus it was that the physician to the princess of Austria recommended in 1740 that 'the vulva of Her Most Holy Majesty should be titillated before intercourse.'[52] Doctors these days could draw some inspiration from this. Imagine if instead of being told to live healthier, you were told you ought to get your lady parts titillated more often. Now that's what we call popular health! So, the men of the 1700s knew the lie of the land even though they'd misunderstood a lot of other things here on Earth. The source of the inferiority complex surrounding the so-called clitoral orgasm lies a lot nearer to our own times. We need to take a trip to the 1900s.

The distinction between vaginal and clitoral orgasms and the elevation of the vaginal as the *true* orgasm is quite simply a pretty modern, male invention. Sigmund Freud, the father of psychoanalysis, proposed a new theory in 1905 that viewed the clitoral orgasm as the immature, young woman's form of orgasm.[53] It was the kind of thing that should only happen in a little girl's bedroom. As soon as the girl got a sniff of a male member, her interest in the clitoris should vanish and be replaced by a burning desire for penetration. The fusion of man and woman was the only healthy form of sex, and the only form that should give women pleasure. Real women, according to Freud, had vaginal orgasms.[54]

Where did Freud get this from? His own head of course! It didn't matter that there were masses of women out there who profoundly disagreed with him – they were ill. They were suffering from a vague condition known as *frigidity*, characterised first and foremost by the fact that they were unable to take pleasure from a man's noble part the way they ought to. It was the ultimate manipulation technique: either you agreed with Freud or you were mad.[55]

According to Freud, women should seek immediate help from a psychologist if they thought it was wonderful to touch their clitoris or – heaven forbid – failed to have orgasms during vaginal intercourse with their husband. Of course this was great for the man. If the woman didn't come, it wasn't his qualities as a lover that were in question, but the woman who needed to do a bit of work on herself. The man had now been given an official blessing to go for it, come, then happily turn his back as he switched off the light. The woman's pleasure was her own responsibility.

Freud was hardly a nobody and his theory gained plenty of support. So it came about that thousands of years of female experience were suddenly written off as maidenly neuroses. The clitoris, known for centuries as the core of female sexual pleasure, was consigned to oblivion and vanished from the anatomy books. It would be nearly 60 years before anybody dared contradict his theory.

In the 1960s, a quiet revolution began to take shape at Washington University Hospital in the USA. The gynaecologist William Masters and his research partner Virginia E. Johnson began to develop an interest in female sexuality and set up a series of experiments that were quite insane by today's standards. They recruited couples to have sex in the laboratory, hooking them up to measuring equipment, with the researchers as eager observers. They even made a vibrating plastic penis with a camera in its tip, so that they could observe what was happening inside the women's vaginas when they came. The result of their studies was seen as a shocking medical discovery: that the clitoris was absolutely central to female orgasm. A bombshell? Obviously.

Today, we know that fewer than a third of women regularly come from vaginal intercourse alone, and even then, there's much to suggest that the clitoris is central. Some researchers think these women drew the golden ticket in the anatomical lottery. Because it seems they also have an advantage when it comes to the size and placement of their clitoris. The first person to conduct scientific research in this area was psychoanalyst and author Princess Marie Bonaparte of France (1882–1962), who – despite her great appetite for sex and lovers – was never satisfied because she couldn't come vaginally.[56] Bonaparte and modern researchers both agree on one thing: a larger clitoris head combined with a short distance between the clitoris and vagina make it easier to have orgasms,[57] because the clitoris enjoys a greater degree of indirect stimulation during penetration, both externally and towards its inner parts. Bonaparte took the drastic step of opting to have her clitoris moved further down by surgery – unfortunately with poor results.[58]

We wish Bonaparte had known that not having an orgasm during ordinary intercourse with a man is not abnormal. It is the norm. But because men have dominated the research into female sexuality, and men have dominated the public discourse about sex, this is a message that has passed many people by. Sex has become synonymous with precisely the activity that almost solely ensures that the man comes: the penis in the vagina. Indeed, people say that intercourse isn't 'consummated' unless the man has had an orgasm. If only the woman comes, intercourse is theoretically incomplete – it is interrupted intercourse. The woman has vanished from the picture.

To be fair, everyday sex should be all about pleasure and orgasms for both partners, so couldn't having sex in a hetero relationship just as well mean, for example, 50/50 licking and penetration? Lesbian women report having orgasms more frequently during sex than their heterosexual sisters, so there's clearly something to be said for broadening one's repertoire.[59] It's wrong to write off the female orgasm as a pure bonus. Orgasm should be the rule, for women as well.

It's more difficult for women to have orgasms than men

Still, there's no getting away from the fact that between 5 and 10 per cent of women are *anorgasmic* – in other words, they've *never* had an orgasm, either alone or with another person.[60] For men, the opposite most often applies – they struggle with coming too quickly. A major British study found that 21 per cent of women aged 16–24 found it difficult to have orgasms during sex.[61] Most women find themselves in the 'comes now and then' category.

Some fortunate women don't know what we're talking about. We all have one of those irritating friends who tells us that she *always* comes, and generally three or four times every time she has sex. What's the magic trick, you might ask? Unfortunately, the chances are she won't be able to help you. Although of course magic tricks may make a small contribution, there are also real differences between us in terms of how easily we come, and there's nothing we can do about it. These differences are determined by, among other things, our genes. Very few of us like to think about our parents having sex, but it's not unlikely that their sex life is a bit reminiscent of your own. If you're an orgasm queen, perhaps you should thank your mum and dad.

Researchers who have studied twins have found that our genes can explain up to a third of the variation in how often people have orgasms during sex.[62] Perhaps that doesn't sound like so much, but in the context of genetics, it's not to be sniffed at. Researchers have also looked at the frequency of orgasm during masturbation, and here heredity plays an even more important role. In fact, their studies show that our genes explain half of the variation in masturbatory orgasms. At first it may seem peculiar that there's a difference between how much genes influence sex and masturbation, respectively.

However, masturbation can be thought of as a more genuine reflection of your physical capacity for orgasm, since you're eliminating a greater degree of psychological uncertainty and sexual interplay with a partner.

Another thing that has a major influence on women's capacity to have orgasms is the context in which they have sex. Nearly all women have little chance of reaching orgasm during a one-night stand. American college students responded that only one in ten had an orgasm the first time they slept with a new partner, whereas almost 70 per cent of the girls had an orgasm when they'd been in a relationship for more than six months.[63]

So, there are hereditary differences when it comes to how easily we have orgasms, but the encouraging news is that most women can have orgasms if they want to. The challenge is taking the step from having orgasms alone, and now and then, to having them almost always. We're not saying that it's easy, or that it's particularly important to stress about having orgasms, but it is possible if you're willing to put in a good deal of hard work. Here is our orgasm bible, inspired by the advice women who can't achieve orgasm are given in therapy.

ORGASM BIBLE

1. Practice makes perfect. If you've never masturbated before, it's time to clear some time in your diary, literally – masturbation works.[64] In studies of women who have never had orgasms, between 60 and 90 per cent managed to achieve one, both alone and with a partner, after five or six weeks of regular *training*.[65] We promise that it's the most fun form of exercise a doctor can recommend. Use your fingers or buy yourself a vibrator. Do whatever turns you on and gets you into the right mood. Do you prefer erotic literature, do you like porn or do you want to fantasise? The most important thing is that you must NOT start out thinking about the orgasm as a goal, but rather focus on finding techniques you like. Practise feeling your way towards pleasure and opening yourself up to it. Practise emptying your head of all disturbing thoughts, whether it's the extra rolls of fat on your belly or that looming exam. The better you get at giving yourself orgasms, the greater the likelihood that you'll have them when you're with a partner. Remember, too, that it's never wrong to take matters into your own hands when you're with a partner. Who does what isn't so important, as long as you're having a steamy time together.

2. Demand your rights. Your partner must be included in *Project Orgasm*. It's important here not to step on anybody's toes – make it a pleasurable joint project. It isn't your partner's fault that you're not coming, unless he or she downright refuses to make any effort to satisfy you. In fact, you need to do the spadework. Your genitals don't come with a user manual, so without your guidance, your partner could spend a year and a day finding out how you come. The simplest thing is to do the job yourself at the outset, by touching yourself while you have intercourse or by masturbating together. After a while you can teach your partner your tricks. A lot of people find this embarrassing, but it's the best way to do it. Don't expect to get it right at once. Be patient and praise your partner every time he or she does something that works; that way you'll gradually train up a super lover.

3. Teach yourself the CAT position. There are masses of sexual positions and, as you've now learnt, few of them are especially suited to giving women orgasms. However, one sexual position has a special status: the CAT position. Because it has been shown that a variant of the missionary position known as coital alignment technique, or CAT, is especially good for giving women orgasms.[66] This is a position that requires a little practice and coordination, but it repays all your patience, in all respects.

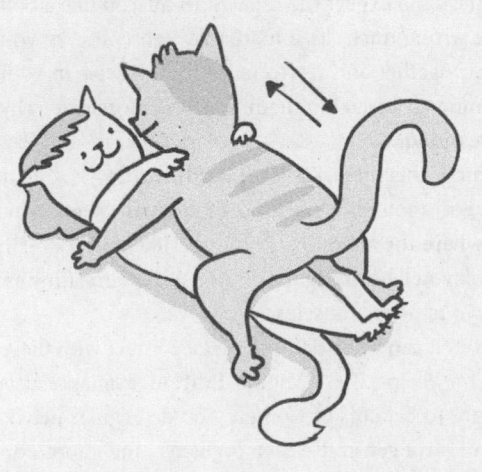

In the CAT position, instead of resting on his hands, your partner must rest on his lower arms and keep as much of his body as possible in contact with yours. Instead of the usual in-and-out thrusting, he should slide his body up along yours horizontally until his genitals are lying right on top of yours. At the same time, you should press your crotches together, like a wave crashing against the shore (clichéd, but true). His hips should tip downwards so that his pubic bone and the root of his penis rub against your clitoris. You'll be able to tell when he's doing it right. You should keep your legs as straight and closed as possible, perhaps by wrapping your legs around his so that your ankles are resting on the top of his calves. Whereas the regular missionary position involves humping, the CAT position is based on good old-fashioned rubbing. The penis won't go very deep into your vagina, but will instead give maximum stimulation to the outer couple of centimetres where most of the nerve endings are located and your clitoris will receive constant contact at the same time.

Once you've got the hang of it, you can try reverse CAT, where you lie on top. Then you have full control and can direct the clitoral stimulation with exactly the tempo and pressure you want.

4. Don't relax! Relax, relax, you're often told. This may be the world's best and worst advice. Yes, you should try to relax in your head, but if you lie there motionless and expect the orgasm to hit you like a bolt from the blue, you're on the wrong track. It's a matter of tightening up your body. Clench your buttocks together and try to tense the muscles in your genitals, preferably tightening and relaxing them, as if in an orgasmic rhythm or in time with your breathing.

For one thing, this increases the blood flow to your genitals – you turn yourself on. For another, it's a kind of mental exercise in directing your attention to where the action is. Try if you like, but it's really hard to think about the steak you'll be eating for dinner at the same time as you're working to clench all your pelvic muscles.

At the outset, it can be difficult to make contact with these muscles. After all, there isn't a 'Shape Up – Vagina Edition' available at your local gym. But there ought to be. Lots of women who do regular pelvic-floor exercises find they have stronger and easier orgasms, and more contact with their genital area. In addition, this prevents urine leaks and pelvic-organ prolapse, and may help combat pain during sex.[67] You can do your pelvic-floor exercises anywhere – on the bus or before going to bed. You can also use vaginal balls, although that's absolutely not necessary.

6. Go for a run. Exercise, especially right before sex, makes it easier for you to get aroused and increases many people's capacity to reach orgasm.[68]

7. Put on some socks. This advice is both jokey and serious. The point is that our brain is continually getting signals from the body about how we're feeling. These signals, and the thoughts they provoke, compete for our attention. It's difficult to have an orgasm when your mind's on anything other than what's going on in your genitals – for example, the fact that you've got cold feet. We women are especially prone to these kinds of distractions, and those from our surroundings too. The sex researcher Alfred Kinsey observed that female rats, unlike male rats, were easily distracted by tempting crumbs of cheese during the sex act.[69]

The lesson here is that you must do everything you can to create the conditions in which it's possible to focus all your attention on having a sizzling time. If that means all the lights need to be switched off, that you want to have sex with your T-shirt on or, yes, that you need to put on a pair of socks, listen to that inner voice. Be kind to yourself. Orgasms only come when you feel so comfortable, both physically and mentally, that you can shut everything else out. This is probably the most difficult lesson and most people forget it along the way.

CONTRACEPTION

When a woman and a man have sex, it can result in a baby. This shouldn't come as a shock because that's the way it's always been – children have never been delivered by the stork. Sex is fab, and most people want to have sex more times than the number of children they plan to have. If you're heterosexual and want to have vaginal sex without having babies, you're going to have to use some form of contraception.

By *contraception*, we mean all methods that can reduce the risk of sexual intercourse leading to pregnancy. In other words, for example coitus interruptus, also known as withdrawal, is a method of contraception – although not one we'd recommend.

Contraception is hardly new, but as medicine has developed, more sophisticated methods have come onto the market. All the same, many of the current forms have a long history. There's nothing new about condoms, but they used to be made of animal hide rather than latex. Four thousand years ago in Ancient Greece, women are said to have put a mixture of honey and leaves in their vaginas to keep sperm cells out of the uterus. This is reminiscent of the modern-day diaphragm, a silicone disc that's placed over the cervix to bar the way to sperm cells. Contraception is also a matter of fashion. Withdrawal is hardly a new discovery at any rate. There's even a story about it in the Bible's *Book of Genesis* (about a guy called Onan) and you can be sure that some couple somewhere will be doing just that this evening – or right now.

We humans have given most things a try, but the advantage you have today is that you can choose. We have plenty of tried-and-tested alternatives that we know work well. You can find a reliable method that suits you, your health and your lifestyle.

Perhaps you take it for granted, but contraception really is incredible. It gives you the option to choose whether you want to have children at all without this choice affecting your sex life. If you want to have children, you can choose when, with whom and how many children there will be. Withdrawal, the diaphragm and a combination of plants and honey in the vagina probably had a certain effect, but the big difference came with the introduction of the contraceptive Pill in the 1950s.

It was a revolution. The Pill was an effective means of contraception then, and it is even better today as it's been tried and tested for years. The Pill changed women's ability to choose what kind of relationship to be in. They could control their own sex lives and plan their family to suit their own career and economic situation. Since then, many new forms of contraception have been developed, including long-acting methods such as the contraceptive implant and the hormonal intrauterine device (IUD).

The facts about contraception are dry, very dry
Now that you have a bit of historical background, it's time to talk about the situation today; and here we must allow ourselves to be completely honest. In this part of the book, we've done our best to explain the difference between the various methods of contraception. We've written a bit about how to use them, and have provided some tips and tricks as a bonus. But it's all very technical. We're sorry to have to say that the first section of the chapter on contraception will most likely be the most boring part of the book for some of you. Even so, we've decided to include it as it's probably the most important thing we have to tell you about.

After all, we know what young women are wondering about and many of them have complex questions about contraception. That's hardly surprising because it's a complicated business that, for some reason, all women are expected to understand intuitively, almost without guidance. We also know that there are an incredible number of myths about contraception alive and kicking, and many people suffer unnecessary side-effects owing to incorrect use, or feel uncertain about using it because they don't have enough information. We don't know whether this is because health professionals who prescribe it are providing bad or too little information or because it's all too much to take in at one go. The chart below sets out the main variants of hormonal, hormone-free and emergency contraception.

Combined contraceptives with oestrogen and progestin	Progestin contraception with progestin, without oestrogen	Hormone-free contraception	Emergency contraception
PILL	CONTRACEPTIVE INJECTION	CONDOM	COPPER IUD
CONTRACEPTIVE PATCH	CONTRACEPTIVE IMPLANT	COPPER INTRA-UTERINE DEVICE	PILL 1: LEVONORGESTREL (LEVONELLE™)
VAGINAL RING	HORMONAL INTRA-UTERINE DEVICE (IUD)	FERTILITY AWARENESS	PILL 2: ULIPRISTAL ACETATE (ELLAONE™)
	MINI PILL		
	OESTROGEN-FREE PILL		

Our aim here is to give you a basic introduction to contraception so that you have the means to choose for yourself. Contraception is in a constant process of development and we recommend that you listen to advice from health professionals, who may have newer and more detailed knowledge of the contraceptive methods you're interested in.

HORMONAL CONTRACEPTION

What is it about hormonal contraception that prevents pregnancy? What is actually going into your system when you swallow your contraceptive Pill every morning, insert your vaginal ring every third week or get a contraceptive implant put in your arm?

Hormonal contraception contains an extremely low dose of the same hormones that are produced in the ovaries and that are involved in controlling the menstrual cycle. All hormonal contraception contains something called progestin, which is a synthetic version of the progesterone produced by your body. Some types also include another hormone, oestrogen. The latter are known as combined contraceptives, while those that only contain progestin are called progestin-only products.

Hormonal contraception with oestrogen

There are three types of combined contraceptives: the combined Pill, the vaginal ring and the contraceptive patch. The advantage of combined contraceptives is that the oestrogen they contain gives you the option to control your bleeding. The disadvantage is that not everybody can tolerate the oestrogen, which you'll be able to read more about later.

The combined pill is the most commonly used combined contraceptive and there are many types, all of which vary slightly. Firstly, different types of oestrogen and progestin are used. Secondly, each one contains different combinations and dosages of progestin and oestrogen. Both aspects can vary the side-effects you'll experience, both positively and negatively, but you can't know in advance how a particular type will work for you. It's a matter of trial and error until you find the brand that suits you best.

There are two main categories of combined pill: multiphasic and mono-phasic. But what on earth do these terms mean?

Most pills are *monophasic*. If you use this type, it doesn't matter where you start in the blister pack, because the hormone dose is exactly the same in every hormone pill. Most monophasic pills are designed so that you can, in a way, create an artificial menstrual cycle consisting of a given number of days. Most types involve a 28-day cycle. So, you take hormone pills for 21 days of the cycle and during these days, you won't have any bleeding. The last seven days are the so-called pill-free week. Then you can either take the sugar pills included in some packs or take a break from the pills altogether. During these hormone-free days, the endometrium is usually expelled by the uterus, so you'll have bleeding. Examples of monophasic pills that use the 21 + 7 days design are Microgynon and Yasmin. Some monophasic pills are organised so that you take 24 pills in a row, and then take a break from the hormone pills for four days. Examples of combined pills that use the 24 + 4 days design are Eloine and Zoely. If you don't want any bleeding at all, you can go directly on to a new pack of hormone pills without taking a break. More about that later.

Multiphasic pills don't have the same dose of hormones in every pill, and each brand has its own cycle design when it comes to the number of days of hormone pills and the number of days of bleeding. So, you can't start at any point in the pack with multiphasic pills, you must follow the instructions carefully. If you use this type, it's particularly important to read the patient information leaflet and to use them correctly, especially if you're planning to skip your periods. In the UK there are several types of multiphasic pills. For example, Synfase, Logynon and Qlaira – but they are not very popular as there is no particular benefit in taking them.

When you use combined pills, you're protected against pregnancy the whole time, even on the designated hormone-free days. So, you can have sex when you like without having to use additional contraception to prevent pregnancy. But if you accidentally miss your pill, you may lose that protection. How many pills you can miss before there's a chance of becoming pregnant depends on the brand, so refer to the patient information leaflet and instructions from your doctor, nurse or midwife. When missed pills lead to poor protection against pregnancy, we call it contraceptive failure.[1]

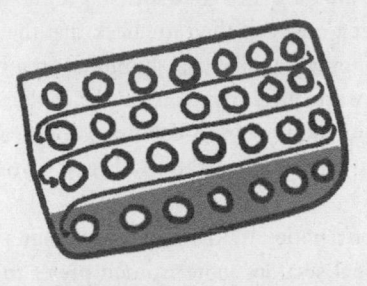

The vaginal ring is a soft plastic ring you insert into your vagina. It looks like a soft, spaghetti-thin ring doughnut. To insert it into your vagina, you simply press it together with two fingers and push it well in. When you release your grip the ring will spring back into its original shape, adjusting to the inner walls of the vagina to stay in place. To remove it, just fish it out gently with your middle finger.

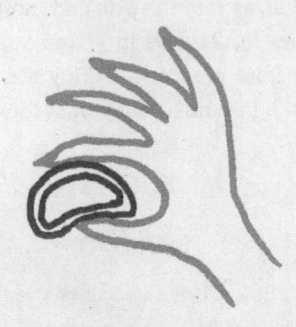

The vaginal ring contains a combination of oestrogen and progestin, which pass through the mucous membranes in the vagina and end up in the bloodstream. A lot of people think it sounds unpleasant to walk around with something in their vagina. They also wonder if the ring can get lost inside them. However, once you've inserted it, you shouldn't notice it's there – just the same as with a tampon. But watch out! Although it isn't common, there have been cases of vaginal rings falling out and ending up in the loo. This happened to one of our female friends when she was out on the town late one night. She told us she didn't notice a thing until the next afternoon. When you're drinking alcohol, it's easy to become a bit less alert than usual and then you may be unlucky. It's a good idea to get into the habit of sticking a finger in your vagina now and then to check that the ring's in place.

As with most monophasic pills, you should use the ring for 21 consecutive days, or three weeks in a row. You can leave the same ring in place for three weeks before taking a seven-day break for bleeding. You can also put a new ring in straight away, without a break if you want to skip the bleeding.

Although you won't notice the ring is there, your partner may feel it when you have vaginal sex. So, some women prefer to take it out before sex. It's perfectly safe to do this for up to three hours at a time, but it's important to remember to put it back in again before the time is up, otherwise you'll lose your protection against pregnancy.[2]

The hormonal patch (Evra) is simply placed directly on the skin, and the hormones pass through your skin and into your bloodstream. You can use each patch for a week and, as with the ring and most monophasic pills, you should receive hormones for 21 days in a row. So, you have to use three patches, one a week, before eventually taking a seven-day break. If you forget to change the patch in time or if it comes loose, contraceptive failure may occur.[3]

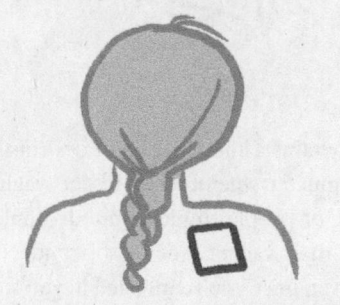

How do combined contraceptives prevent pregnancy?

It may seem a bit odd that hormones we already have in our body can prevent pregnancy, but the progestin and oestrogen in the combined products work extremely well. Combined contraceptives prevent the ovulation that occurs once in every menstrual cycle – roughly once a month. As we've said, if you have unprotected sex from around five days before ovulation, including the day you ovulate, you may become pregnant. This phase is called the fertile window.

Hormonal contraception works a little like pregnancy. When you're pregnant, your menstrual cycle comes to a halt, as if somebody pressed the pause button. If your menstrual cycle stops, there's no ovulation and without ovulation there's no fertile window or possibility of fertilisation.

The progesterone that is naturally produced in the body is responsible for this pause when you become pregnant. Progesterone tells the pituitary gland under the brain (the one that looks like a scrotum) not to produce the follicle-stimulating hormone (FSH) and luteinising hormone (LH) any more. As you may recall, these hormones are necessary to keep the menstrual cycle going. There's no follicular phase without FSH and no ovulation without LH. The progestin in hormonal contraception does the same thing as progesterone when you become pregnant. Progestin tells the pituitary gland it's time to stop the menstrual cycle for a while. In a way, you could say that the combined contraceptives trick the body into thinking it's already pregnant.

Combined contraceptives prevent pregnancy in several ways – they don't just stop ovulation. After sexual intercourse, the sperm cells must swim up through the cervix and into the uterus. There's mucus in the cervix. The progestin in combined contraceptives makes the mucus thicker so that it's more difficult for the sperm cells to swim into the uterus. In addition, the endometrium becomes thinner than usual, which makes it difficult for fertilised eggs to fasten themselves onto the uterine lining.

Oestrogen is usually responsible for growth in the uterine lining or *endometrium*, the lining that later becomes your period (see p. 49). The oestrogen in combined contraceptives makes the endometrium grow a little each month, so most women using combined contraceptives will also have menstruation-like bleeding when they take a short break from hormones, of seven days or fewer.

Oestrogen-free contraception

The advantage of oestrogen-free contraception is that it can be used by anybody, even women who can't take oestrogen for one reason or another.

Long-acting contraceptive methods, such as the hormonal intrauterine device (IUD) and the contraceptive implant, are both oestrogen-free and are the methods that offer most effective protection against pregnancy. The disadvantage with oestrogen-free contraception is that you may not have such good control over the bleeding as with combined contraceptives. In other words, you can't decide when you'll have your period. Usually, though, the bleeding is much less heavy than normal when using all forms of hormonal contraception. Our impression is that some women who use the contraceptive implant have problems with persistent bleeding abnormalities, and that this is less of a problem for women using the hormonal IUD. Again, this is a matter of trial and error.

The contraceptive implant is a bit of plastic containing progestin. It is placed under the skin on the upper arm using a kind of syringe and can remain there for up to three years. It continuously releases a little hormone so that the amount in the blood is constant and low. The contraceptive implant is the safest contraceptive method on the market today. Once it's in place, you can't go wrong. The progestin in the implant will stop your menstrual cycle, allowing you to avoid ovulation for as long as it stays there.[4]

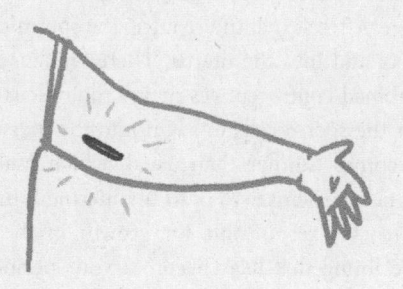

The hormonal IUD is a small, T-shaped object that is inserted in the uterus by a trained health professional. It releases a low dose of progestin that primarily works locally, in the genital area, although small quantities also pass through the mucous membrane in the uterus and are absorbed into the bloodstream. The dosage of hormone circulating in the bloodstream will be extremely low, and a lot of women who've experienced side-effects with other contraceptive methods suffer fewer problems if they switch to the hormonal IUD. You can keep the hormonal IUD in for between three and five years, depending on which type you choose. At present, there are three types on the market in the UK. One of them, which can be left in place for five years, is called the Mirena. This is the hormonal IUD with the highest dose of hormones and is therefore particularly suitable for women who are interested in having light bleeding. A lot of women find that their periods stop entirely with the Mirena. Next comes the Kyleena, which also lasts five years, but is specially designed for women who haven't given birth. It's smaller than the Mirena and has a lower dose of hormones. Finally, there's the Jaydess, which lasts three years, also has a very low hormone dose and is small. Although the Jaydess and Kyleena are particularly marketed at women who haven't give birth, it's perfectly fine for younger women to use the Mirena. It is a bit larger and some women may find having it inserted a bit more unpleasant, but on the other hand, you get better control over the bleeding than with the other two, and it still contains much lower doses of hormones than other methods of hormone contraception. It's a myth that the hormonal IUD is only suitable for women who've given birth!

Some women find they stop ovulating when they have a hormonal IUD, but not all. This is temporary of course, and depends on the hormone dose in the IUD. It is more usual to stop ovulating when you use the Mirena, since it has a slightly higher hormone dose. The Jaydess and the Kyleena often contain doses of progestin that are too low to influence the pituitary gland in the brain, but that doesn't mean they don't work well. The most important effect of the hormonal IUD is, in fact, local – the progestin makes the mucus in the cervix impenetrable to sperm cells. At the same time, the uterine lining becomes thin, making it difficult for any fertilised eggs to survive there.[5]

All three hormonal IUDs provide long-acting, reliable protection against pregnancy. Most women will experience lighter bleeding and less severe menstrual pain than before, and many will also find that they have fewer or less dramatic side-effects than with other hormonal contraceptive methods owing to the low hormone dose. The most normal side-effect, particularly with the Jaydess and Kyleena, is spotting and irregular bleeding.

If you're worried that it will be painful to have the hormonal IUD inserted, it may be a good idea to take painkillers an hour before you're due to have it put in. Some women will experience menstruation-like pains for a little while after insertion, but they quickly pass. After that, you won't notice it's there, except for the fact that you can feel two small strands of thread sticking out of your cervix in the deepest part of your vagina. This is what the doctor uses to remove the hormonal IUD when it's time to change it.

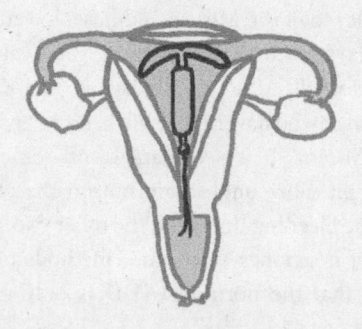

Oestrogen-free contraceptive pills (for example Cerazette) are a type of contraceptive pill that must be taken every day. You never take a break to have bleeding. Nor is there any need to take them at the same time every day. You are only at risk of pregnancy once it has been 36 hours since you took your last pill. The progestin in the oestrogen-free hormonal pills works in the same way as in the contraceptive implant: it influences the pituitary gland to prevent ovulation. In addition, the mucus in the cervix becomes impenetrable and the uterine lining becomes thin.[6]

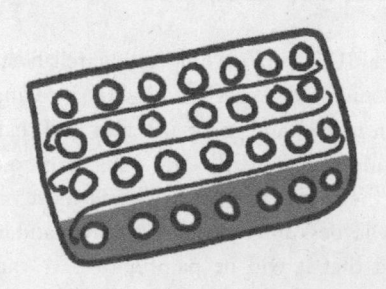

Mini pills (for example Noriday and Micronor) are another pill you take every day without having a break for bleeding. The progestin dose in the mini pills is lower than in the oestrogen-free contraceptive pills above, so you need to be much better at taking it at the same time every day. You only have a window of about three hours, which makes it easier to use the pills incorrectly and risk pregnancy.[7]

The contraceptive injection (for example Implanon) must be administered by a doctor or other health professional no more than 12 weeks after the preceding dose. So, you must visit a health professional for a repeat injection every three months. The hormonal injection contains a great deal of progestin, enough to prevent ovulation. It also works on the mucus in the cervix and on the uterine lining, which becomes thin. As a rule, it isn't recommended for women below the age of 25 because the hormone dosage is so high that it may affect the build-up of bone in the body.[8]

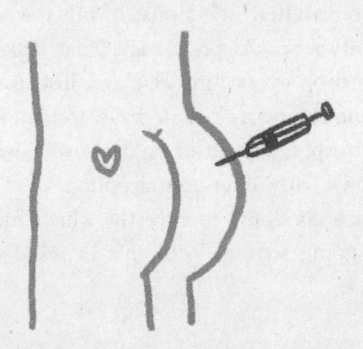

NON-HORMONAL CONTRACEPTION

Are you one of those people who wants a hormone-free alternative? These methods have little in common with one another and women have many reasons for choosing them. Some have experienced side-effects from hormonal contraception, or fear side-effects, and that decides the matter for them. Protection against sexually transmitted infections is a good reason to prefer condoms. Other women are concerned about hiding their contraceptive use from their partner or family and therefore prefer their menstrual cycle to continue as before.

Condoms

These prevent the sperm cells from entering the uterus. The condom serves as a barrier and hence this is also known as a barrier method. Today, the condom is the only easily available contraceptive method that can be used by men.

The condom is a kind of bag made of latex or similar material that is pulled onto the erect penis and collects the sperm when the man ejaculates. After sexual intercourse, it's important to hold the condom firmly in place when the penis is being withdrawn so that it doesn't end up left inside the vagina, sperm and all. Once that's done, it's just a matter of taking off the condom, tying a knot in it and throwing it straight in the bin. Don't throw condoms down the loo. They have a habit of floating back up again when you least expect it and that's no fun – either in shared accommodation or at your parents' house.

The condom is also the only contraceptive method that protects you against sexually transmitted infections. In other words, condoms protect you against both disease and pregnancy. That makes it sound as if you should be able to drop everything else and just use condoms the whole time, but unfortunately, many people have accidents when they only use condoms. They can split, slip off or be destroyed and so many people opt to combine condoms with other contraception.

Many people use condoms incorrectly, which means there's a greater chance of things going wrong. With this in mind, here's our recipe for perfect condom use.

Condom course

1. Check the date-stamp; an old condom is easier to break.
2. Open the condom package carefully – mind you don't scratch the condom with sharp nails, teeth or jewellery.
3. Once the penis is stiff, place the condom on top of it like a Mexican sombrero.
4. Trapped air may cause the condom to split, so make sure you squeeze the top of the condom as you roll it down the length of the penis.
5. Hold the condom firmly in place when withdrawing the penis from the vagina, otherwise sperm may run out of it.

6. A condom should remain in use throughout the whole of intercourse to protect against pregnancy or sexually transmitted infection, but must be used only once.

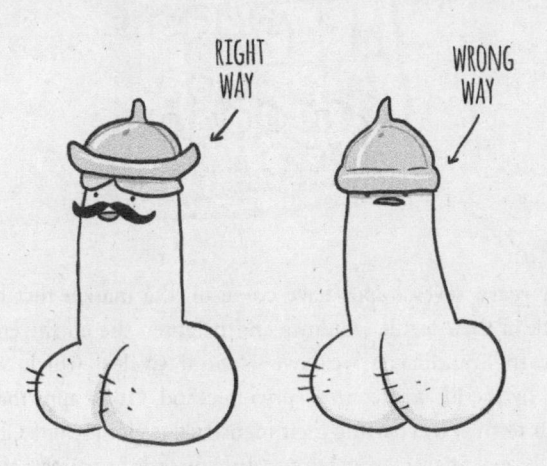

There are other types of barrier methods that can be used by women. We've already spoken about the diaphragm, which for better effect should always be used with a spermicidal cream. There's also a kind of reverse condom, which lies like a bag inside the vagina, instead of around the penis.

Fertility-awareness-based methods – find your fertile window
The phase in which you can become pregnant during a menstrual cycle is called the fertile window (see p. 117). Some methods of contraception involve finding out when your fertile window is in order to avoid having sex when there's a higher chance of becoming pregnant.

There are different ways of doing this. You can use a menstrual calendar, measure your body temperature every morning or examine your own cervical mucus. People often combine these methods for greater reliability.

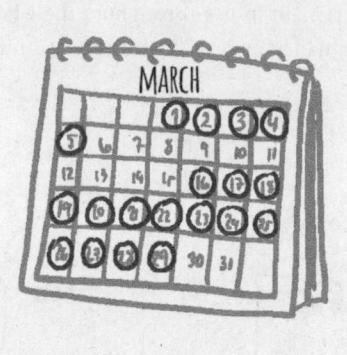

In recent years, several apps have come on the market that help women keep track of their fertile windows and heighten the effectiveness of these methods. In Scandinavia we have Natural Cycles, which was recently approved by the EU as a contraceptive method. Other apps that help users track their fertility by charting their menstrual cycles include Glow, Kindara and Clue. Apps can use earlier temperature records to estimate the likelihood of pregnancy and eliminate some of the possibility of miscalculation. A study financed by Natural Cycles found that their app increased effectiveness in typical use of the basal-body-temperature method from 75 per cent to 92.5 per cent, meaning 7.5 per cent of users became pregnant in the course of a year. There are still only a few studies on these apps with a representative group of participants, so we'll have to see if these numbers hold up in a more diverse group of users.

These methods are too unreliable to be recommended to women who absolutely do not want to become pregnant, because they require a lot from the user. According to the World Health Organization (WHO), 24 per cent of women (that's one in four!) who use methods based on fertility awareness will become pregnant within a year with typical use.

Still, these methods may work well for women who use these methods perfectly, as you can see in our table on the effectiveness of contraception (see p. 136). They are also great at making women more aware of how their bodies work and can be of significant help to women who are trying to become pregnant, as they can use the methods to identify their fertile window, making it easier to conceive.

Women who calculate ovulation with a menstrual calendar should use the information in the section on the menstrual cycle as their starting point (see p. 62). Ovulation generally happens at the same time every cycle, around 14 days before menstruation.

The starting point for those who use the temperature method is that a woman's body temperature alters slightly over the course of the menstrual cycle – by 0.3° Celsius to be precise! As you may recall, the menstrual cycle has two phases. One or two days before phase 2, your body temperature rises 0.3° Celsius and remains elevated for around ten days. At the beginning of phase 2 large amounts of the luteinising hormone are released into the bloodstream, triggering ovulation, which generally occurs one or two days later. In other words, ovulation occurs between two and four days after the body temperature rises. By measuring your temperature every day over a prolonged period you can find out when in your cycle you usually ovulate and use that as your basis for working out which days you are most fertile.

In fact, you can also tell from your cervical mucus when you are ovulating. For this to work you need to examine your discharge every day and look for changes. Just before ovulation your discharge becomes slick and slimy so that you can stretch it between your fingers, generally several centimetres. When ovulation has just occurred, your discharge will become white and creamy. This method requires you to be very familiar with your discharge, and to spend time studying how it alters over the course of your cycle. You should be aware that there are other reasons for the changes in discharge apart from shifts in your cycle. For example, various diseases can affect the consistency (see p. 47), making it difficult to judge where you are in a cycle.[9]

Perhaps this sounds complicated – and indeed that is the problem. That is why these methods aren't a great option for all women. We recommend types of contraception that are secure for everyone and are less prone to human error.

Women who use fertility-based methods need to live an extremely orderly life with plenty of time to examine mucous or record their temperature every morning, must have a will of steel when it comes to resisting sex at the wrong time (or like using condoms) and must be prepared for the possibility of getting pregnant. If this sounds like you – and if you have an aversion to other birth control methods – go ahead and give fertility-based methods a try. But if you wish to avoid pregnancy at all costs, we advise you to choose something else.

If you already struggle with remembering pills, it is unrealistic to make the fertility-based methods part of your daily routine. Even if the available apps make this aspect easier, there are still many opportunities to get it wrong; there's a lot of measuring and recording involved and there's a leeway of several days. The method is also less reliable in women without regular cycles. The menstrual cycle can be altered by external factors such as stress, weight change and illness. Young women often have more irregular cycles than older women, so this method is even less suitable for them, in addition to the fact that young women often live less organised lives.

Copper IUD

The copper IUD is a hormone-free alternative that we can get behind. Fewer than 1 per cent of all women who use the copper IUD become pregnant in the course of a year. Like the hormonal IUD, the copper IUD is a little T-shaped object that is inserted in the uterus by a doctor or health professional. The difference is that this IUD is coated in copper threads. You can keep it in your uterus for up to five years and it gives good protection against pregnancy the whole time. Two threads hang from the base of the copper IUD and stick out through the opening in the cervix so that you can check with your fingers whether it's in place. The doctor uses these threads to remove it. There are several types of copper IUD, and there is little difference between them when it comes to quality.[10]

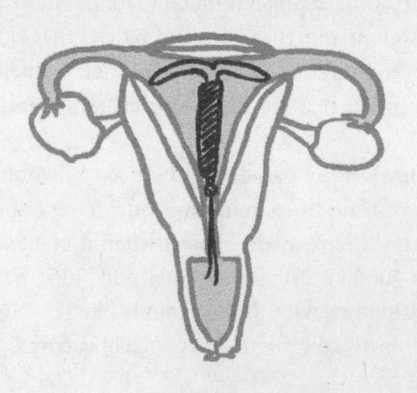

We don't know exactly why and how the copper IUD prevents pregnancy. What we do know is that the copper IUD causes a mild inflammation in the uterus, which alters the environment in there and somehow or other prevents pregnancy.[11] One theory is that the uterus begins to emit spermicidal substances because of the inflammation, or it's possible that the copper itself kills the sperm.[12] Another theory is that the presence of the copper IUD prevents fertilised eggs from being able to attach themselves to the uterine wall.

Women who use copper IUDs ovulate as normal every month, unlike many of those who use hormonal contraception. The copper IUD doesn't have any effect on the pituitary gland or the ovaries, it only affects the uterus. You won't get any hormonal side-effects from a copper IUD, but that does not mean that it is free of side-effects. Many women experience heavier bleeding and more severe menstrual pains than before. Two to ten out of every 100 women choose to remove the copper IUD in the first year as a result of these problems, and the copper IUD is therefore not usually advisable for women who already suffer from such problems anyway.[13]

There are many myths about the copper IUD. The most widespread one is that you can't use it if you haven't previously given birth – not true. It's perfectly fine to use both the hormonal IUD and the copper IUD even if you haven't had children, and you're welcome to try the copper IUD even if you're young. The copper IUD is a long-standing and well-established form of contraception, and they have become smaller and more reliable over the years.

From a purely practical standpoint it can be unpleasant having a copper IUD put in, since it must be inserted through the narrow cervix channel into the uterus. Many experience this as short-term menstruation-like pains. It may be worth taking painkillers in advance. It's also important to try and really relax. Discuss this with the doctor who'll be inserting your copper IUD.

If you can't feel the threads at the bottom of the copper IUD you should contact your doctor as this may mean that it has been pushed out of your uterus and then you're no longer protected against pregnancy. Apparently 5 to 10 per cent of users find that it falls out in this way. In very rare cases you may have become pregnant if you cannot find the threads – as in the event of pregnancy they can, in fact, be drawn up into the uterus.

EMERGENCY CONTRACEPTION – PANIC STATIONS

Sunday morning. You had sex yesterday evening and you didn't use reliable contraception. You have no particular desire to get pregnant and it's so scary it makes your stomach ache. You're not the first person to experience this and you won't be the last either. Sometimes things go wrong and that's why (in many countries including the UK), emergency contraception is readily available. This is something you can use after having had unprotected sex or if you've experienced contraceptive failure.

The definition of contraceptive failure varies depending on the type of contraception. It may be a missed pill, a vaginal ring that has fallen out or a condom that has split. It's important to become familiar with the method you're using so that you know when you've had contraceptive failure. For example, how much time must pass between two contraceptive pills before it's considered to be contraceptive failure? How long must the vaginal ring have been outside your vagina? Ask your doctor, nurse or midwife about the rules for contraceptive failure with your method of contraception.

Contraceptive failure when you're on hormonal contraception – for example a missed pill – may result in ovulation. Many women don't bother with emergency contraception after contraceptive failure because they don't understand that they risk getting pregnant. It may be several days since they had sex when they forgot their pill. But remember that the sperm cell can survive five days inside the uterus while it's waiting for an egg. This means you can get pregnant from sex you had up to five days ago if you experience contraceptive failure that leads to an ovulation today.

In Norway, where we practise medicine, people call emergency contraception the 'regret pill'. We should stop calling it that. 'Regret pill' is a prim term that suggests pursed lips and raised eyebrows. It implies you've done something you should regret – but you really haven't. You've just had sex, and if it was a positive experience there's no reason to regret it. And by the way, that feeling you get when you pick up the blister pack to take today's pill and discover you've missed three pills in the past week isn't regret: it's panic. So we've opted to call it the 'panic pill' in this book.

We're not especially keen on the British term for it either – 'the morning-after pill'. It sounds nice and easy, as if you can take the pill every morning after sex instead of using contraception. It's important not to resort to panic pills too readily either. They're not as effective as regular contraception and there are a few side-effects, although admittedly not dangerous ones. Emergency contraception should only be used when other contraception has failed – it shouldn't replace regular contraception.

There are three kinds of emergency contraception: two different pills and the copper IUD. The first type of pill contains a substance called levonorgestrel, which is a type of progestin (synthetic progesterone). In other words, it contains the same substance as hormonal contraception, although the progestin dose is much higher. The second pill contains a substance called ulipristal acetate, which influences the way natural progesterone functions in the body.

Panic pill type 1: levonorgestrel
The pill containing the levonorgestrel progestin, Levonelle, is the emergency contraception most commonly sold in the UK, and it's available over the counter in any chemist.

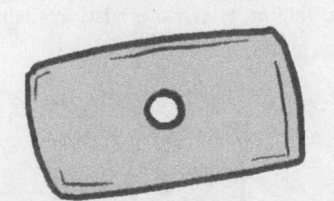

It works by postponing ovulation. The problem is that it is not effective if you've already ovulated, or if you're just about to ovulate. As you may remember from the chapter about the menstrual cycle (see p. 61), women experience a dramatic increase in the levels of luteinising hormone (LH) just before ovulation. Once the rise in LH is already under way, pills containing levonorgestrel won't be able to stop ovulation.

It's difficult to know whether you've ovulated or not. As ovulation may vary from cycle to cycle, only women with totally regular cycles know more or less when they ovulate.

Although this pill isn't entirely reliable, it does reduce the chances of becoming pregnant, so it's definitely sensible to take it, and the sooner you take it the better. It's best to take it within 24 hours of having unprotected sex or experiencing contraceptive failure. That said, it can be effective for up to three days (72 hours) after unprotected sex or contraceptive failure, but the chances of it being effective decrease as more time passes so it's a good idea to keep one in your toiletry bag at all times.

It's perfectly fine to take a pill containing levonorgestrel several times in the course of a single menstrual cycle, but as we said earlier it's best not to use this as your main form of contraception.[14]

Advantages Availability, doesn't affect other contraception, may be taken several times in a cycle.
Disadvantage Less reliable.
Remember Do a pregnancy test after three weeks!

Panic pill type 2: ulipristal acetate
In the UK, pills containing ulipristal acetate are sold under the trade name ellaOne. This pill is effective for up to 5 days (120 hours) after unprotected sex or contraceptive failure. ellaOne is also available over the counter at chemists.

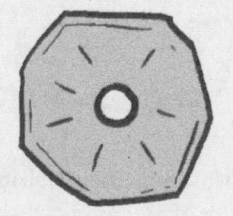

Like panic pills containing levonorgestrel, ulipristal-acetate (ellaOne) pills postpone ovulation. The difference between the two types of panic pill is that this variant can be taken much closer to ovulation and still be effective. You can take it right up until ovulation. ellaOne is effective even if the rise in LH is already under way in your body; however, if you've already ovulated, it will not work. So this pill will prevent more pregnancies. Of course, there is one major disadvantage with this pill too: it reacts badly with hormonal contraception. First and foremost, it affects the way your regular contraception works in your body after you've taken it. This means you must use condoms after taking it because there's a chance that your hormonal contraception won't work. How long you have to do that for will depend on which contraception you use.

At the same time the type of hormonal contraception you use can influence how effective the emergency contraception pill is. So, it goes both ways. This means that you shouldn't use hormonal contraception after taking ellaOne. In fact, new research shows that use of hormonal contraception can disrupt the pill's effect on ovulation, preventing it from being postponed, after all. You should wait until five days after taking ellaOne before starting or continuing to use hormonal contraception.[15]

Emergency contraception using ulipristal-acetate pills should only be used once in any menstrual cycle, because no research has been done into the use of several pills in a single cycle. This doesn't mean the pill is dangerous, but simply that nobody knows whether it works more than once a cycle. Since the pill influences other hormonal contraception, it can also affect the use of panic pill type 1 (levonorgestrel, or Levonelle) if you try to take it right after using ulipristal acetate (ellaOne). If you've already taken ulipristal acetate, it's best to use the copper IUD if you experience another failure.[16]

Advantage Better and longer effect than the levonorgestrel pill.
Disadvantage Reacts badly with hormonal contraception.
Remember Do a pregnancy test after three weeks!

Copper IUD as emergency contraception
Although the copper IUD is the safest form of emergency contraception, it's rarely used. We recommend considering the copper IUD if you need emergency contraception because it is said to be 99 per cent effective for this purpose. It works by preventing fertilised eggs from attaching themselves to the uterus.

The copper IUD must inserted into the uterus by a health professional, so after you've had unprotected sex, request an emergency appointment at your doctor's surgery or family-planning clinic and explain what's happened. You can also go to an out-of-hours surgery or a young people's clinic. The copper IUD is effective for five days (120 hours) after unprotected sex or contraceptive failure. It works because the fertilised egg doesn't attach itself to the wall of the uterus before the sixth day after ovulation, so in some cases it's possible to insert a copper IUD more than five days after intercourse, if you know when ovulation occurred. The copper IUD must be inserted no more than five days after ovulation.

The good thing about the copper IUD, apart from the fact that it's extremely effective as emergency contraception, is that you can then leave it in your uterus and use it as regular contraception. If you don't get on with it, it's also quite possible to have it removed after a short time.[17]

Advantages Highly reliable, can serve as contraception for the next five years.
Disadvantage Availability, as it requires a prescription and must be inserted by a doctor, nurse or midwife.
Remember Many people think they're perfectly safe after taking the panic pill, but that isn't true! Emergency contraception reduces the risk of getting pregnant, but it doesn't work nearly as well as regular contraception. It's very important to take a pregnancy test after using emergency contraception. We recommend that you take the test whether you have menstrual bleeding or not. If your partner or a female friend is the one who's taken the panic pill, remind her to take a test.

For the pregnancy test to be reliable you must wait at least three weeks after using emergency contraception before taking it. There's no point doing one immediately after using emergency contraception, because it's impossible to detect whether you've become pregnant or not so soon afterwards.

Emergency contraception also has side-effects. The most common one is irregular bleeding. Panic pills postpone ovulation and that also delays your period. It isn't dangerous to have irregular bleeding, but it can be a nuisance. Luckily, it's not a long-term problem and will pass. Some women also find that panic pills make them nauseous and if you vomit shortly after taking one, you'll have to take another one. Follow the instructions on the patient information leaflet and from your doctor or pharmacist.

The copper IUD doesn't contain hormones, but even so, it's usual to have changes in your regular bleeding pattern at the outset. If you want to keep the copper IUD as your regular contraception and experience bleeding changes, we recommend that you see how things are going after three months as the bleeding often stabilises over time.

CONTRACEPTION

ARE SOME METHODS OF CONTRACEPTION BETTER THAN OTHERS?

We talk a lot about how different we are and how different methods of contraception are good for different women, but that doesn't mean that all types of contraception are equally good. There's a reason why leaves and honey in the vagina have gone out of fashion, and methods based on fertility awareness are responsible for masses of unwanted pregnancies. That's just the way it is.

Women who use the contraceptive implant have the lowest risk of becoming pregnant, closely followed by the hormonal IUD. In other words, these two types of contraception are the best. A lot of people wonder how this quality is measured. How do we determine how effective the different types of contraception are? And what does it actually mean to say that the implant is better than the Pill? Let us clarify: when we say 'best' we just mean how well the method of contraception works, or how good it is at preventing pregnancy. We're not talking about *side-effects* or how many people like the method of contraception. Whether you like the method or not is personal. But how well it prevents pregnancy can be measured objectively, simply by seeing how many women have become pregnant while they've been using the particular method of contraception in a study. It's far from certain that you'll prefer the contraceptive method that is objectively the best. The aim is to find a method of contraception that is as reliable as possible and that you are also happy with.

Researchers use something called the *Pearl Index* when they're assessing and comparing different methods of contraception. The Pearl Index is a measure of how *effective* a given method is. By effective, we mean how well it works in preventing pregnancy – it's not a question of dangerous and harmless. Contraception isn't dangerous. So, the Pearl Index is a measure of how many women become pregnant while they're using the method of contraception. In strictly concrete terms the Pearl Index is the number of women in a group of 100 users of the contraception who become pregnant in the course of a year.* If, for example, you want to investigate the effectiveness of

---

* There's a common misconception that the highest possible index is 100, as if it was a matter of percentages. But if all the women in a study became pregnant in the course of their first cycle, the Pearl Index would actually be around 1200. It's pretty confusing and actually not especially important unless you're a total nerd. Like us.

133

a new kind of contraceptive pill, you ask a group of women to test the pill and then see how many of them do and don't become pregnant while they're using it. By using results from many such studies statisticians can rank the methods of contraception according to how good they are. But what causes the difference between the methods of contraception?

Two factors contribute to how well a method of contraception works. The first relates to how it is used, because it's possible to use some of the methods of contraception incorrectly, which makes them less effective than those that cannot be used incorrectly.

Take the withdrawal method, for example. The aim is for the man to withdraw from the woman's vagina right before he comes, so that his sperm ends up on the mattress, on her tits or in other fun places. But as many of us have found out, it's only too easy to pull out *after* rather than *before* coming. In the heat of the moment it's so tempting to carry on just a *little* longer and if you mess up one time, that can be enough to get you pregnant. This possibility of using the withdrawal method incorrectly makes it difficult to rely on and it is far from popular among health professionals and users who do not wish to become pregnant. Human capacity for error always comes into play even though perfect use would have been entirely effective. The contraceptive pill, one of the most common methods of contraception, is also an offender when it comes to user error – in fact, user error is its middle name. It's incredibly easy to miss a pill or two. Every woman who's ever woken up in another person's bed far away from her toothbrush and pack of pills knows that. Many of the women who get pregnant when they're using contraceptive pills do so because of the pill-free week. They get out of the routine of taking a pill every day and then they mess up on how long the break should be. Missing a pill can happen to anybody. All of us can have an absent-minded day and some people are absent-minded every day. Prolonging the pill-free week is one of the riskiest things you can do as you are much more likely to ovulate if you don't restart after seven days.

The contraceptive implant, on the other hand, is more effective because it sits in your arm and does its job without you having to do anything at all. It's impossible to forget the implant other than when you need to change it and that's only once every three years. So, there's no user error with the implant. It works perfectly, regardless of your routines and your memory.

One factor that contributes to how good the method of contraception is therefore relates to how it is used and not the method in itself.

Some people may think it's unfair to say that methods of contraception are bad just because the users mess up. After all, that isn't the method's fault is it? You may well think that way, but we take the view that there's no point respecting the non-existent feelings of methods of contraception. Studies show that we humans often end up doing things incorrectly whenever there's any possibility of doing so, and this has an impact on the effectiveness of the method of contraception. In any event the aim is to prevent you from becoming pregnant, not for the method of contraception you like best to win a popularity contest.

The second factor that determines effectiveness is the actual quality of the method of contraception. Many people think that sterilisation is the most effective thing you can do if you don't want to have (more) children. When a woman is sterilised, her Fallopian tubes are cut so that the egg cannot pass from the ovary to the uterus, but even after sterilisation one in 200 women becomes pregnant in the following year. Both the contraceptive implant and the hormonal IUD are more effective than that. This type of error, which is to do with the effectiveness of contraception itself and not the person using it, is called method error.

Pretty much nobody becomes pregnant using the implant, but nothing is black and white in medicine. Someone somewhere will become pregnant regardless of which method she's using. Unfortunately, you can never say never as long as you're a woman who has sex with a man; but you can say 'almost never' and that'll just have to do.

Since there are two different kinds of error connected to methods of contraception, user error and method error, their effectiveness is also measured in two different ways. We distinguish between 'perfect use' and 'actual use' of a method of contraception. Perfect use means that the person using the method of contraception has used it in a completely error-free way. There is no user error, no missed pill, no late withdrawal and no vaginal ring falling in the loo during a boozy night out on the town. On the other hand, actual use describes the result when women do their best to use contraceptive methods correctly, as users of contraception generally do, but still end up making the odd mistake here and there.

The difference between perfect and actual use can be anywhere between major and non-existent, depending on how many mistakes it is possible to make when using the method of contraception concerned. If your life has a good routine, if you're not the least bit scatter-brained or absent-minded and if you have steely control over, for example, your contraceptive pills, it may be that your risk of pregnancy lies closer to the Pearl Index for 'perfect use' than 'typical use'. You're the only one who knows yourself well enough to know that. But if you have a slightly more unpredictable lifestyle, it may be worth considering a method of contraception that works regardless of how many mistakes you might make. Methods of contraception without user error, for example the implant and the copper IUD/hormonal IUD, are equally effective when it comes to perfect and actual use because actual use is perfect without you having to make any effort at all.

So, which methods of contraception are best? Below you'll find a table with a selection of the different methods. The figures are provided by the World Health Organization (WHO). They were updated in 2015, but may change as researchers find new methods of contraception or carry out new research into existing methods.

It may be helpful to know how well the different methods of contraception perform in tests when you're making your choice. However, we advise as many women as possible to try the most effective methods: the ones that have a long-acting effect and no possibility of user error.

Effectiveness of methods of contraception[18]

	PERFECT USE How many become pregnant?	TYPICAL USE How many become pregnant?	Effectiveness of method of contraception
Contraceptive implant	0.05%	0.05%	99.95%
Hormonal IUD	0.2%	0.2%	99.8%
Sterilisation, men	0.1%	0.1%	99.9%
Sterilisation, women	0.5%	0.5%	99.5%

	PERFECT USE How many become pregnant?	TYPICAL USE How many become pregnant?	Effectiveness of method of contraception
Copper IUD	0.6%	0.8%	99.2–99.4%
Contraceptive injection	0.3%	3%	97–99.7%
Contraceptive pill	0.3%	8%	92–99.7%
Condom	2%	15%	85–98%
Withdrawal	4%	27%	73–96%
Fertility-awareness-based methods		24%	76%
Menstruation calendar	5%	12%	88–95%
Basal-body-temperature method	1%	25%	75–99%
Cervical-secretion monitoring method	4%	14%	86–96%
No protection		85–90%	15%

PERIODS ON HORMONAL CONTRACEPTION

Hormonal contraception affects your menstrual cycle. You'll notice it because your monthly bleeding will alter. Most women get lighter or shorter bleeding, but that's not true for everybody. Bleeding may also become irregular or disappear entirely. A lot of women find this bit spooky because there are a lot of myths about losing or skipping periods. Doesn't the bleeding come because it's natural, many people think. Don't our bodies need it? Should we really be messing about with Mother Nature in this way?

As you may remember from the chapter on periods there's nothing to suggest that menstrual bleeding in itself constitutes an advantage for you. That's certainly true if you're using hormonal contraception. Your menstrual cycle on hormonal contraception is no longer a normal cycle and most types of hormonal contraception will actually stop the menstrual cycle entirely. The bleeding that happens is no longer normal menstruation, either, but what we call *withdrawal bleeding*.

Periods and combined pills

Let's start with what happens with your period if you use combined pills. The researchers who designed contraceptive pills over 50 years ago built in one pill-free week every month precisely so that women could have withdrawal bleeding. They thought it would be easier to accept the Pill as a method of contraception if the hormones produced something resembling a normal menstrual cycle, with regular bleeding every fourth week. But even though the contraception imitates a natural cycle, it isn't a 'natural' one. Nor is the bleeding natural and there's nothing unnatural about skipping it. Usually it's oestrogen that causes the endometrium to grow and this mucous membrane is what later becomes your period. The oestrogen in the combined products makes the endometrium grow a little bit each month so most women who use combined contraceptives will have withdrawal bleeding when they take a break of seven days or fewer from hormonal pills, the contraceptive patch or the vaginal ring, even if they don't have a normal cycle. Endometrial growth is less than normal and that's why it isn't necessary to bleed as often as when you're not using contraception. Once a month may be unnecessary for many women. If you're using combined products you can skip menstruation as many times as you like or even use the pills continuously and have the bleeding whenever it suits you. It isn't dangerous and it will work. The progestin in the combined products binds the endometrium so that it doesn't bleed out. If you're using combined products and skip the withdrawal bleeding often enough, you'll probably eventually have what's called *breakthrough bleeding*. The progestin binds the endometrium for as long as it can, but in the end it becomes too much. Breakthrough bleeding means that you bleed while you're on hormones – in other words, outside the short hormone break you can take when you're using the Pill, the vaginal ring or the contraceptive patch. This can involve either spotting, sometimes described as irregular light bleeding – generally just spots on your knickers – or heavier menstruation-like bleeding. This is normal and all it means is that it's time to take a break for a maximum of seven days; then you can go back to skipping the withdrawal bleeding again. Many women think the monthly bleeding you get when using hormonal methods can show whether you're pregnant or not and that if you skip it for too long, this may conceal a potential pregnancy. But that isn't quite right. In fact, it's possible to stop bleeding entirely when using combined products even if you do take a pill-free week in between. This needn't mean you're pregnant. What's more, it's possible to have light bleeding during pregnancy. Bleeding on hormonal contraception is often light and not the same as a regular period. So, you may be pregnant even if you get light bleeding in the pill-free week. The central message must be that you should rely on the method of contraception you're using. Combined contraceptives are effective if used correctly, but if anything changes and you suspect pregnancy the only way to check this is by taking a pregnancy test.

A lot of women suffer from frequent breakthrough bleeding and this can be a nuisance over the long term. Some may find it helps to change their contraceptive method. If you're on the Pill, it may help to change from a variant with a low dose of oestrogen to one with a slightly higher dose. Pills with the highest oestrogen dose are best at controlling the bleeding. For example, many women will experience better bleeding control on Microgynon or Marvelon than on Loestrin 20. You can discuss with a doctor which type you should switch to.

Periods on progestin contraception
These are very different from periods on combined contraceptives. The main difference is that you can't decide what your cycle will be like, and can't change or control it along the way. This is because you take the same dose of hormone every day, without taking a break. If you do take a break, you lose your protection. This means that you'll have bleeding when the progestin can no longer bind the endometrium, and that can happen at any time. All bleeding when you are on progestin contraception is, in

practice, breakthrough bleeding since there's no right time to have with-drawal bleeding. Progestin will bind the uterine lining, or endometrium, making it more difficult for it to bleed out. At the same time the mucous membrane becomes thinner than usual. Since there's no oestrogen in progestin contraception there's nothing to tell the uterine lining that it should grow. As a result, there's no certainty you'll have any bleeding at all, although many women do. After all, oestrogen occurs naturally in the body, too.

When you start using progestin contraceptive it's a bit like playing Russian roulette with your menstrual cycle. You don't know in advance what it will be like but it will be one of three alternatives: regular bleeding, no bleeding or irregular bleeding.

Implants and hormonal IUDs

A lot of women think that if you use the implant or the hormonal IUD you stop menstruating regardless, and many choose this method of contraception for precisely that reason. But that isn't quite true. A lot of women end up without bleeding, but there's also a possibility you may end up with extremely irregular bleeding or a totally regular cycle. Whatever happens, the amount of bleeding will be less than it was without hormonal contraception.

As with the combined products, bleeding while you're on progestin contraceptive doesn't rule out pregnancy. We've had questions from girls who religiously take a pregnancy test every third month because they've stopped having periods as a result of contraception. This is unnecessary and expensive. Bleeding, or the lack of it, is not a good indicator of pregnancy when you're using progestin contraceptives. Take a pregnancy test if you've experienced contraceptive failure or are uncertain whether you're protected against pregnancy.

The copper IUD

Although it isn't a hormonal method of contraception, you may have side-effects related to your period. Unlike with hormonal contraception, which leads to lighter bleeding, many will find they have heavier bleeding and more severe menstrual pains when they use the copper IUD. This is particularly true for women who have previously suffered with heavy, prolonged or painful bleeding. As many as one in ten women opt to have the copper IUD removed in the first year as a result of these problems.[20]

Sometimes it's not convenient to have a period. That may be because you're going on a beach holiday, a cabin-to-cabin skiing trip with your partner or because you can't deal with the blood and pains in the last week before your exam. These are things all women who menstruate will relate to, particularly those who suffer heavier bleeds and a lot of pain. When it's not convenient you can try to postpone the bleeding.

It's always easiest to postpone bleeding if you use combined contraceptives – in other words, combined pills, the contraceptive patch or the vaginal ring.[21] You can also use prescribed medication that's designed to postpone your period.[22]

Here's what to do if you use combined products

Monophasic-type combined pills Normally you'll take your hormone-containing pills for 21 or 24 days before taking a hormone-free break of either seven or four days, depending on which type of monophasic pill you're taking. During these pill-free days you'll have bleeding. If you want to skip the bleeding you can go straight onto a new pack once you've finished up all the hormone-containing pills in your current one. So, if you're using a pack that contains 21 hormone pills (for example Microgynon or Marvelon), you won't have the usual pill-free week. If sugar pills are included, making a total of 28 pills in the pack, you can throw away the sugar pills and start straight onto a new pack. If you use Eloine or Zoely, which operate with 24 hormone pills and a four-day break, you can skip the break and go directly to a new pack of 24 hormone pills. If you're taking multiphasic pills such as Synphase and Qlaira you can also skip your period, but with these you'll need a slightly more thorough explanation. We encourage those of you using these to visit a doctor or nurse if you have questions and to check the patient information leaflet for instructions.

Vaginal ring Normally you keep a vaginal ring in for three weeks before taking a week's break, which we can call a ring-free (or hormone-free) week, when you'll have bleeding. If you want to skip bleeding you can insert a new ring into your vagina after three weeks without having a ring-free week.

Contraceptive patch This is normally changed once a week for three weeks before having a patch-free fourth week, during which you'll have bleeding. To skip the bleeding put a new patch on in the fourth week instead of having a patch-free week.

This is how to proceed if you don't use combined products

The medication Primolut-N contains a hormone that postpones menstruation. This may be a solution for women who don't want to start using contraception that contains oestrogen, but nonetheless wish to skip their period for a short time of up to two weeks.

You start to take Primolut-N at least three days before your period is due: one tablet three times a day. This means you must have a pretty good idea of when your period is due. Without a regular cycle, it will be difficult to use this medication successfully. After that you take three pills a day for as long as you want to postpone your period, up to a maximum of 14 days. Once you stop taking the pills, you'll have bleeding after a couple of days. In other words, you can't postpone your period indefinitely.

Primolut-N can be prescribed by a doctor. Most women can use it, but some should avoid it; this is something your doctor can clarify for you. While you're taking Primolut-N it's important to use condoms to protect against pregnancy because the medication isn't a contraceptive.

WHAT'S THE BEST WAY TO USE CONTRACEPTIVE PILLS?

The Pill can be a lot of trouble, but is still a popular method of contraception. As you've seen in an earlier section, it's possible to become pregnant while you're using contraceptive pills, mainly because it's so easy to use them incorrectly. What's cool is that there's a way of using contraceptive pills that involves less risk of pregnancy, fewer bleeding abnormalities and lighter bleeding. This method works for all combined products. In other words, you can do the same with the contraceptive patch and the contraceptive implant. People using multiphasic pills must follow separate instructions from a doctor, nurse or midwife.

Contraceptive pills and other combined products are effective provided you use them correctly. As you know, combined contraceptives are designed with a break built in. You use the hormones for three weeks (21 days), followed by a week (seven days) without hormones, either without any pills at all or taking sugar pills. During the seven days you'll have *withdrawal bleeding*. If you're using Eloine or Zoely you'll take hormone pills for 24 days and have a four-day break.

The numbers 21 and 7 or 24 and 4 are immensely important when it comes to combined contraception because they mark two important *limits*.

When you use combined contraception, you must take hormones for *at least 21 or 24 days* for the contraceptive to be effective. If you use hormones for fewer than 21 or 24 days in a row – for example if you forget the two last pills in the pack and end up with 19 or 22 days instead of 21 or 24 – there's a danger that you'll lose your protection and ovulate. Then you could become pregnant. So, 21 or 24 days of hormones means *at least* 21 or 24 days. There's no problem with using hormones for longer – as long as you're over the limit you can take the pills for 30, 50 or 100 days in a row. It's entirely up to you.

The number 7 (or 4 if you're using Zoely or Eloine) is a limit that means the break can *be a maximum of 7 or 4 days*; it must not be longer. If you take a longer break from the hormones than this, you will not be protected against pregnancy. There's no problem with taking a break of, say, three days. If, for example, you have short bleeding, for only two days, you can start on hormones again after just a two-day break. But you must never take a break longer than seven or four days (depending on which type you are on). If you do, you may ovulate and then you're in danger of becoming pregnant.

As long as you use hormones for at least 21 or 24 days, and take a maximum break of seven or four days on monophasic pills, contraceptive patches or the vaginal ring, you can actually use combined products as you want. Since so many unplanned pregnancies result from messing up on the pill-free week, it can only be a good thing to keep the number of pill-free weeks to a minimum. This will, in fact, make the contraception more effective.

You'll probably have breakthrough bleeding once you've been skipping your period for long enough. You can solve this by using combined pills continuously and taking breaks when you need to. That way, you can tailor your cycle to suit you, with as few periods of bleeding as possible.

Take hormones continuously until you have bleeding and then take a break to get the bleeding over with. That break may well be shorter than seven or four days. After the break, start taking hormones again and use them right up until you have new breakthrough bleeding. This is absolutely fine as long as you never take fewer than 21 or 24 pills. If you have bleeding after, say, ten days of hormone pills, you must carry on until you've taken 21 or 24 to be protected against pregnancy.

HORMONAL CONTRACEPTION – BUT ISN'T IT DANGEROUS?

You probably noticed ages ago that 'natural' is the new ideal. Strange words like detox, parabens, juicing and superfood have become commonplace. The message of the self-proclaimed health gurus is clear: 'artificial' additives are no good for your body. You shouldn't mess with them.

Overnight, green juice has become the hottest fashion accessory, and at the same time, hormonal contraception has gone out of vogue. Young women have become afraid of using contraceptive pills because they're worried about sinister side-effects. More and more, we hear people saying they have hormonal-contraception intolerance, as if it was an allergy. Others ask whether it's healthy to take a hormone break, a detox, to flush the *unnatural substances* out of their body.

At a time when there's a growing focus on the pure and the natural, many people also feel doctors aren't taking their concerns about side-effects seriously. They feel that the medical profession trivialises their problems or tries to sweep them under the carpet. The result is that many women have a nagging uncertainty about how safe their method of contraception actually is, and end up seeking out information from unreliable sources.

Around one third of all women stop taking the Pill within the first six months of starting it.[23] Of these, around half do so as a result of what they experience as side-effects.[24] It can be frightening to feel that your body is changing if you don't understand why it's happening or what it means. We think you ought to have proper information about both the positive and negative sides of hormonal contraception in order to make good choices for your body. Knowledge breeds confidence.

At the same time, it's important for us to add some nuance to the scary image that has emerged in recent times. Now and then the media can give the impression that we don't know about the side-effects linked to hormonal contraception, as if we were playing Russian roulette with the health of young women. Fortunately this is wrong. You can be confident that the pack of contraceptive pills you pick up at the chemist contains one of the most carefully studied medications in the world. The researchers have fantastic amounts of statistical material to examine since many millions of women have taken the Pill over vast swathes of the planet from as far back as the 1960s. Serious, unknown long-term effects from hormonal contraception would have been discovered if they existed, particularly when you consider that the first pills that came on the market contained up to five times as much hormone as the ones we have today.

What is a side-effect?
Before we can start to talk about individual side-effects you need to understand what a side-effect is. A certain medication is designed to have a particular effect on the body and that's why we take it. In the case of hormonal contraception, the reason we take it is that we wish to prevent pregnancy. Side-effects are all the other effects the medication has on the body, which may be both positive and negative. For example, many women find that they have far fewer spots when they use hormonal contraception. This is a side-effect that is perceived as a positive. Blood clots, on the other hand, are a side-effect nobody would want to have.

In the film *Sliding Doors* (1998) we follow Gwyneth Paltrow's two parallel destinies: in one scenario she catches her train to work one morning, in the other she misses it. This little detail has major consequences for the way her life turns out. This is also the way our body works. Our body is so complicated and complex that it's impossible to affect a single function without creating ripple effects in other parts of the body at the same time.

A side-effect doesn't mean that a medication is harmful. It means that it's working. If anybody ever claims that a medicine or treatment has no side-effects, you should take it with a pinch of salt. It means either they're lying or that the substance has no effect whatsoever.

Doctors and health authorities are very concerned about side-effects. We know they are a necessary evil, but the aim is to keep them at as low a level as possible. This is why it's extremely difficult to get medications approved for sale. The producer must first prove that the positive effects of the medicine will have the greatest possible likelihood of outweighing the negative effects. Years of studies and controlled experiments lie behind any new medication, precisely because we must know for sure what side-effects you can expect when you take it.

After a medication comes on the market it's carefully monitored by the country's regulatory body (in the UK, it is the National Institute for Care and Excellence, or NICE), which is independent of the pharmaceutical industry, so that any unknown side-effects can be detected early on. If you experience a side-effect, both you and your doctor can report it to the medical regulator – and we absolutely encourage you to do so. If there's any suspicion of a serious side-effect having been overlooked – for example that the use of the Pill over many years causes cancer – new studies are launched.

The way this is often done is to compare large groups of people who have taken the medication with equivalent groups who have not done so. Then studies look at whether there are more people with the potential side-effect among those who took the medication. If it turns out, for example, that there are as many people with cancer in both groups, they know that the pills do not cause this form of cancer, because in that case more of it would be seen among the people who had taken pills.

The nocebo effect

Why don't people automatically believe it when a lot of women report the same side-effect from the medication? Don't the health services trust women when they say they've experienced a side-effect? One of the reasons why they can't take it as given that side-effects exist without further investigation is something called a nocebo effect.

Most people have heard of placebos – where people experience real, positive effects from something that doesn't actually work just because they expect and hope that it will. For example, there's a reason why many medicines come in brightly coloured capsules: it has been found people simply become even healthier if the pills they take look sophisticated! This is also one of the reasons why doctors often keep a stethoscope in sight around their neck. The stethoscope creates associations of healing and professional competence in the patient. This alone can contribute to improving patients' health.

The nocebo effect, from the Latin for 'I will harm', works the opposite way. Here, a sugar pill will cause physical problems because you believe it contains active substances. In fact, around a quarter of all patients experience negative side-effects when they receive placebo treatment, in other words, no treatment at all.[25] The same thing can happen if a doctor tells a patient that a medication may have a possible negative effect. More people report this effect than usual without it actually being the medicine's fault. It can often be as simple as people attributing normal symptoms to the medicine. One study by Reidenberg and Lowenthal found that only 19 per cent of healthy people who weren't taking any medicines had been entirely problem free for the previous three days, but 39 per cent had experienced fatigue, 14 per cent complained of a headache and 5 per cent said they felt dizzy.

A study from the University of Yale found that highly educated women over-estimated the dangers of hormonal contraception. At the same time they were unaware of all the positive health benefits it offers – for example, reduced risk of ovarian and endometrial cancer.[26] These negative expectations can become a self-fulfilling prophecy.

With this in mind, it may be easier to understand why doctors are sceptical when a lot of women suddenly report a new side-effect from an old medication such as the Pill. This may simply be the result of too much negative publicity.[27] More research is the way to find out whether it's a real side-effect that has not been discovered before or just a nocebo effect.

Everything has a risk

Begin by taking out the patient information leaflet for your hormonal contraception, if you use it. There you'll find a long list of side-effects, sorted according to how common they are. First come the most common, which apparently affect between one in ten and one in 100 users. These include symptoms like headaches, mood swings and tender breasts. After that come the side-effects that affect between one in 100 and one in 1,000. The further down the list you get, the more disturbing the reading.

The first thing to be aware of when you read this list is who wrote the patient information leaflet: the producer of the medication. The thing people initially think is that perhaps the producer's trying to hide side-effects from us, but the opposite is true. They lay it on thick when it comes to possible side-effects so that they can't be taken to court by dissatisfied customers. Some of the effects that are included in the patient information leaflet are things that have been reported by women using the hormonal contraception, but haven't necessarily been proven to have been caused by the medicine. We'll come back to this later. Others are side-effects that we know to be caused by the hormonal contraception.

The other thing you must be clear about is an understanding of the word risk. When we hear the word risk it's easy to think that it's something dangerous, but it is, in fact, only the chance of something happening.

The time has come for a short course in statistics. When we talk about side-effects, what is known as *the relative risk* often hogs all the attention. Relative risk is how much the chance of having a side-effect increases when you take a medication compared with when you don't take it. So, for example you may read about the danger of blood clots being between two and four times higher for contraceptive pill users than for those who don't use them. This sounds dramatic. Just imagine the tabloid headline: 'Life-threatening Pill! Four times the likelihood of blood clots!' But it's actually not that dramatic at all.

The fact that is most interesting for us as individuals is something called the *absolute risk*. But the tabloids aren't as concerned with this figure because it would often result in boring headlines: 'Minimal chance of blood clots from the Pill! Meet the girl who was incredibly unlucky and got one anyway.' Absolute risk is the actual likelihood that there will be a side-effect when you use, say, the contraceptive pill, without any comparison with people who aren't taking it. This gives a much more understandable and realistic picture of the danger you're exposed to.

What's the likelihood that you'll have a blood clot when you're taking the contraceptive pill? The *relative risk* indicates that users of the Pill are at between two and four times *higher risk* of developing blood clots than those who don't use the Pill. However, the likelihood that you'll develop a blood clot, *the absolute risk*, is somewhere between 0.0005 per cent and 0.001 per cent per year. This means that between 50 and 100 out of every 100,000 women on the contraceptive pill will develop a blood clot every year. So, in other words, even if you take the Pill you'd have to be incredibly unlucky to develop a blood clot.

NORMAL SIDE-EFFECTS OF HORMONAL CONTRACEPTION

Now that we have a little bit of background information about side-effects, we can start to deal with hormonal contraception in particular. Let's begin with the most common things: the side-effects that affect between 1 and 10 per cent, such as headaches, dizziness and tender breasts. These are not dangerous side-effects, but they can still be a nuisance. Nobody gets all of them and many women don't experience any of them. The fact that one to ten people have the side-effects also means that 90 to 99 people don't.

It's also important to be aware that there's no connection between the common and the dangerous side-effects. If you suffer a common side-effect you are not at greater risk of the dangerous ones.

The common side-effects tend to pass after several months' use, so we recommend trying a new method of contraception for three months before giving up. If you still find you're having problems with the side-effects after three months you can try another brand or another form of contraception.

The fact is that people react differently to different brands and methods. A product that gave your friend a pounding headache may be perfect for you. You'll only find out if you try it for yourself. As we explained earlier, there are different subtypes of progestin in the different products and they act on each of us slightly differently. There's also a difference between using a method of contraception that contains only progestin, such as the hormonal IUD and the implant, or a combined product that also contains oestrogen. Even if you had many side-effects with one product, this doesn't mean that you're 'intolerant' of hormonal contraception in general. There's a high likelihood that there are other kinds that won't cause you problems. You simply need to ensure that you choose a method with a different variant of progestin; your doctor can help you with this.

Contraceptives that contain oestrogen have some particular, common side-effects.[28] In fact, these are very reminiscent of the symptoms you can experience when you're pregnant! First on the list are nausea and dizziness. As with pregnant women they pass pretty quickly, but if you're very bothered by this at the start it may be sensible to take the pills at mealtimes or before going to bed.

Oestrogen can also lead to increased discharge. It should not look or smell any different from normal, there's just more of it. A few people also experience leg cramps. We don't know why that happens, but we do know it isn't dangerous. One less common side-effect is that small amounts of milk may seep out of your nipples.

Another side-effect of oestrogen-based contraception is pigmentation. Although this is one women experience on oestrogen contraception, it's probably mostly caused by the progestin in the contraceptive. Pigmentation, technically known as *melasma*, manifests itself in darker brown patches on the skin. These occur when sunbathing, either outdoors or in a solarium. It's normal to have this kind of pigmentation during pregnancy, when it's also caused by the hormones. If you have this problem a high-factor sun lotion helps prevent pigmentation.[29] Another alternative is to try a contraceptive containing a different progestin and see if that helps.

Oestrogen also has positive effects. You may have heard people saying that pregnant women glow. Clearer skin is, in fact, a positive effect of oestrogen. If you have problems with acne, combined products can help. Contraceptives containing only progestin can, however, have the opposite effect, causing greasy skin and hair, and acne. This is a factor that may be important for some people when choosing a method of contraception.

Contraception containing oestrogen is, in fact, often used as part of the treatment for girls with polycystic ovary syndrome, a pretty common condition that we'll come back to in a later chapter.

Another positive side-effect of contraceptives containing oestrogen is that they give you the option to take control of your period. This means you get less period pain, spend less money on tampons and often stop being a hysterical period harpy or a chocolate-guzzling cry baby as a result of PMS.

A further common side-effect early on is *oedema*, which is the medical term for swelling. Simply put, this means that water accumulates in your body. Both oestrogen and progestin may be to blame, so all hormonal products can have this effect, not just the combined products. Fluid retention is one of the reasons why some women feel they're putting on weight when they start using hormonal contraception, but you haven't got fatter, you just have extra water in your body!

There's a myth that hormonal contraception causes you to put on weight. Among the reasons why this arose is that many women start using contraception during a phase of life in which the body is undergoing dramatic change: puberty. Another reason may be that a lot of women put on a bit of weight when they find a partner. And then they think these extra partner pounds are down to contraception, forgetting that suddenly they're spending a lot more time on the sofa cuddling, with a bag of sweeties on their lap and five seasons of *Game of Thrones* on the TV. You don't, in fact, gain weight from hormonal contraception, but it's all too easy to lay the blame there.[30]

Your breasts may also retain fluid, becoming larger and sensitive. Another slightly odd effect is that contact-lens users may find their lenses suddenly don't seem to fit. This is because a little extra water is retained in the eye too, so the cornea on which the contact lens lies changes shape. The increased amount of water in the body may also lead to headaches.

Many women who use the Pill, patch or ring only have headaches during the week of bleeding, in other words, the week when they stop taking hormonal contraception.[31] This is very common and it's a bit like the headache you get when you haven't had your regular morning cup of coffee. The headache is a sign that you're missing something you're used to getting; in this situation it's hormones. To reduce these pains, you can simply skip or shorten the hormone-free interval to a few days. As we mentioned earlier, there's no particular reason why you should have a seven-day break. Providing you don't stop for more than seven days you can decide that for yourself. You don't have this option with progestin-only products.

If you use contraception that only contains progestin, for example an implant, hormonal IUD and oestrogen-free contraceptive pills, you won't get the oestrogen-linked side-effects we spoke about earlier. Nor will you have any of the positive effects of oestrogen (such as clearer skin and control of your period). Progestin can actually cause bad skin and, in some cases, increased hair growth.

Perhaps the most important side-effect is that all women experience a change in bleeding when they use these methods of contraception. This is quite harmless, but some people find it a nuisance. The changes concerned vary according to the person and the type of progestin contraception used and you simply won't know how you'll react until you've tried it. Some women stop having periods entirely, while others may have more frequent light bleeding or irregular bleeding. Most have lighter bleeding than before, but it may last either for more or fewer days. When you've been using the contraceptives for three to six months, things tend to stabilise so that you learn to recognise your unique pattern.

Despite the changes in bleeding that often occur with the implant and the hormonal IUD these are still the two contraceptive methods we most warmly recommend. They have the best Pearl Index scores and are therefore the most effective means of preventing pregnancy. The hormonal IUD also has incredibly low hormone doses compared with all the other forms of contraception. Some people think the hormonal IUD supplies the body with more hormones because it works for several years but that's not true. The hormone concentration in the blood from using the smallest hormonal IUD is, in fact, so low that it's equivalent to taking one single mini pill *every other week*![32] Some people think the low hormonal concentration reduces the chance of side-effects, but that has not been proven. Even so, it might be worth trying if you've had a lot of trouble with the other forms of contraception.

THE RARE SIDE-EFFECTS

Now we're going to go right to the bottom of the list of side-effects on the patient information leaflet. These are the side-effects that make the front pages of the tabloids a couple of times a year because nothing sells newspapers like fear of disease and death. Well, apart from sex perhaps. If you're in any doubt about it, remember that there is no conspiracy between doctors and pharmaceutical companies to threaten the lives of healthy, young girls with hormones. There's even been a study to test it! A bunch of researchers from Harvard followed 120,000 women for 36 years to research the long-term effects of using the Pill. They concluded that Pill users die just as often (or just as rarely if you like) and from the same causes as women who don't use hormonal contraception.[33] In any case we can strike death off our list of concerns.

Blood clots

All the same, the use of contraception containing oestrogen does have serious side-effects that we need to talk about, although they are extremely rare. The one that generally attracts the most attention is blood clots.

Blood clots occur when our blood coagulates, creating one or several lumps in a blood vessel. The lumps stop the flow of blood in this vessel, most commonly in the large veins in the legs and the pelvis – doctors call this *deep vein thrombosis*. Veins, as opposed to arteries, are the blood vessels that carry blood from your organs and extremities back to the heart for reoxygenating.

The reason why we can get blood clots in our legs is that it's hard work for the blood to beat gravity when it's being dispatched back to the heart. The blood relies on assistance from contractions in the muscles to get up speed, a bit like a pump. When we sit still for long stretches, on a plane journey, say, the blood may flow too slowly. If you're very unlucky it may begin to coagulate, or clot. If you get a blood clot in your leg you'll notice it swelling up, and becoming red and painful.

The main reason why people are afraid of blood clots in the leg is that parts of the clot may come loose. Then they'll be swept away with the bloodstream back to the heart and onwards, out into the lungs. Since the blood vessels in the lungs are narrower the clot can get stuck there, causing respiratory problems. This is known as a pulmonary embolism. Although it can be serious, it is rarely fatal. One sign of having a blood clot in the lungs is if you experience sudden stabbing pains in your chest, which worsen when you breathe in. We all get a little stabbing pain in our chest now and again, usually owing to tenderness in the small muscles between the ribs, but the pains caused by pulmonary embolism don't go away. At the same time, you may become short of breath and develop a cough. If you suspect you have a blood clot, it's important to go to your nearest A&E or out-of-hours surgery for treatment ASAP.

As you've already learnt, there's a difference between the types of hormones that the contraceptives contain. Only contraceptives that contain *oestrogen* increase the risk of blood clots. This includes regular pills, the contraceptive patch and the vaginal ring. As we mentioned in the section about risk, the risk of blood clots rises two to four times when you're using combined contraceptives. The reason why we say two to four is because it depends on which type you're using. Of the oestrogen-based contraceptives available today, the ones containing the levonorgestrel type of progestin involve the lowest chance of blood clots. There are four different types of pills containing levonorgestrel on the market in the UK – Microgynon, Rigevidon, Ovranette and Levest. They are all identical, just made by different pharmaceutical companies. If you're going to use contraceptive pills for the first time, we would recommend one of these types.

Some women shouldn't use oestrogen-based contraceptives at all because they have a significantly increased risk of blood clots. The most important group are women with genetic disorders that affect the blood's ability to coagulate, for example a condition known as the Leiden mutation. This is why the doctor will ask you whether your parents or siblings have had a blood clot when you're going to start using combined contraception.

As we mentioned earlier, the risk of healthy young women developing blood clots is incredibly small, regardless of whether they use oestrogen-based contraception or not. If 100,000 women take the Pill, somewhere between 40 and 100 will suffer blood clots over the course of a year's use. If they hadn't used the Pill, between 20 and 50 would still have got blood clots.[34]* It isn't true that the oestrogen in contraceptive pills is more dangerous than the 'natural' oestrogen in the body. Pregnant women who produce masses of oestrogen are at greater risk of blood clots than users of contraceptive pills. For comparison, up to 200 out of 100,000 women have blood clots while they are pregnant or in the period after the birth.[35]

In other words, the likelihood of having a blood clot is greater if you have an unplanned pregnancy than if you are using contraceptive pills. The natural increase in hormones your body undergoes in a pregnancy is much

---

* The numbers vary from study to study and depending on which age group and population type are being studied. The underlying risk of blood clots rises notably with an increase in age and weight, and among smokers.

more substantial than the increase we cause in order to prevent one. This is one of the most important reasons why we should accept this slightly increased risk of blood clots when using contraceptive pills. It is quite simply much more dangerous to become pregnant.

Stroke and heart attack

Two other serious side-effects of oestrogen-based contraceptives are stroke and heart attack. These are diseases that affect the arteries – the blood vessels that carry oxygen-rich blood from the heart to our organs. When one of these blood vessels is blocked because of a blood clot or a burst blood vessel, the tissue to which the blood vessel leads can die of lack of oxygen. If it's an artery supplying the heart muscle part of the heart dies due to lack of oxygen, which can lead to a heart attack. If it's an artery supplying blood to the brain, a stroke can result. Obviously, the consequences of such damage can be considerable.

A study in which all types of Danish women were examined between 1995 and 2009 found that the risk of stroke and heart attack was around twice as high among users of oestrogen-based contraceptive pills.[36] However, remember the difference between relative and absolute risk: although a doubling sounds dramatic, these are diseases that rarely affect young women. Even with a doubling in risk, the likelihood that you'll have a heart attack or stroke is minimal.

To illustrate this, we'll go back to the same study. Of the 100,000 women who used contraceptive pills for a year, around 20 had a stroke and 10 had a heart attack. This study looked at all types of Danish women: fat and thin, smokers and non-smokers, old and young. If it had only examined healthy young women, the risk would have been even lower.

Some women shouldn't use oestrogen-based contraceptives because of their risk of stroke and heart attack. This applies to smokers over 35, women with high blood pressure or heart disease, or those who have had diabetes for more than 20 years. Another group who should not use oestrogen-based contraceptives either is women who suffer migraines with aura. If, however, you have migraines *without* an aura, it's fine for you to use them providing you're under 35.

If you're exposed to too many risk factors that can lead to a stroke and heart attack – for example overweight, high cholesterol and smoking – your doctor may advise you to choose another form of contraception to be on the safe side. To cut a long story short, if you're young and healthy, there's no need to worry about stroke and heart attack risks even if you use oestrogen-based contraception.

Cancer

The last side-effect we need to talk about is cancer. There are still people who believe that contraceptive pills are carcinogenic. Let's start off by stressing the fact that using contraceptive pills and other hormonal contraception does not increase the likelihood that you will suffer from cancer over the course of your life.[37] In fact, several things indicate that, on the whole, contraceptive pills reduce the risk of cancer.[38] They seem to *protect* against cancer in the gut, bladder, endometrium and ovaries. Many of these types of cancer are common among women.

The use of contraceptive pills may protect against ovarian cancer for 30 years after you've stopped taking the pills.[39] If this figure is correct, the researchers think that contraceptive pills will prevent 30,000 cases of ovarian cancer worldwide every year in the coming decades! Population-based studies indicate that contraceptive pills prevent cancer of the endometrium in the uterus for at least 15 years and that the risk of acquiring this form of cancer is almost halved by comparison with women who have not used hormonal contraception.[40] Some researchers have delivered the message clearly: contraceptive pills prevent gynaecological cancer and this positive side-effect outweighs all the negative effects.[41]

However, it seems that contraceptive pills may somewhat increase the risk of cervical cancer. The best study that has been done in this area showed that ten years' use of contraceptive pills would increase the incidence of cervical cancer from 3.8 to 4.5 per thousand women.[42] The risk increased the longer you used the contraceptive pills, but fell again once you stopped. Ten years after you stopped taking the Pill, the risk was at the same level as before you began.

The problem is that it isn't possible to say for certain that the contraceptive pill itself is what increases the risk of cancer, because women who use it are also more prone to infection by HPV – that is, the virus that causes cervical cancer. It is easier to become infected with the virus because many women become a bit more relaxed about using condoms with new partners when they're taking hormonal contraception. It has also been found that women using this kind of contraception have more sex – after all, that's why they're using contraceptives in the first place.

The increasing use of HPV vaccinations should lead to a dramatic decrease in cervical cancer over the next few years, but it's still sensible to continue having regular cervical smears from the age of 25.

Breast cancer is the last form of cancer that people wonder about when it comes to links with use of the contraceptive pill. We know that some types of breast cancer are what is called 'hormone sensitive' – meaning that they like oestrogen, which they need in order to grow. Combined contraceptive pills contain oestrogen of course, and that might lead you to think that oestrogen-based hormonal contraceptives help 'feed' this type of cancer. Luckily, that's not quite how it works. Most of the major studies that have looked at breast cancer and use of the contraceptive pill haven't found any link, with a few exceptions. Individual studies have found a slightly increased risk among women who used the first high-dosage contraceptive pills in the 1960s and 1970s. However, experts think today's contraceptive pills and other combined products contain such low doses of hormones that there's little likelihood they affect the risk of breast cancer.[43]

To sum up: contraceptive pills and other combined products appear to protect women against a number of common or serious types of cancer. This is something to take into account when you're looking at the overall picture for hormonal contraception. Unfortunately, these important, positive side-effects get too little attention in the media in comparison to the rare, dangerous ones.

WHAT WE'RE NOT SURE ABOUT

If you've read the patient information leaflet that comes with your contraception, perhaps you're surprised that we appear to have skipped two important side-effects: mood swings and reduced sexual desire. We haven't done this because we think they're unimportant – quite the opposite. The thing is that these are the side-effects researchers are most uncertain about.

And yet these two possible side-effects are the ones that have been gaining increasing attention among women in recent years, so we think they deserve thorough consideration.

The natural sex hormones influence areas in the brain that are involved in regulating both mood levels and sexual desire. It's a well-known fact that women's moods can swing according to the hormonal swings of the menstrual cycle. For example, some women find they're especially horny around ovulation.[44] It has even been observed that women are more unfaithful around this point in their cycle, too![45]

With this in mind, it isn't so odd to think that contraceptives, which alter the sex hormone balance, might also have an effect on the psyche and sexual desire. Broad agreement has also gradually emerged among women and many doctors that hormonal contraception can cause mood swings, irritability and, in the worst case, depression. Mental and other non-specific side-effects are among the main reasons girls cite for giving up on contraceptive pills.[46]

Despite this agreement among women, the researchers are struggling. Several studies have tried to prove that hormonal contraception has a negative effect on girls' moods, without success. There may be several possible explanations for this.

First possible explanation: the research isn't good enough

An incredible amount of research has been done into contraceptive pills. Over 40,000 articles have been written in the last few decades. The problem is that many of the studies are often of poor quality, especially those dealing with side-effects. Despite the low quality, it's not very likely that this has led to side-effects of hormonal contraception being overlooked or understated. Perhaps that sounds odd, but the *bad* studies are precisely the ones in which you find most side-effects, not the good ones. Most of the few good studies that have been undertaken tend instead to show few or no side-effects. So, the very many bad studies probably give us an exaggerated idea of the scale and severity of these side-effects.[47]

The problem with many of the bad studies is that they've often taken women using hormonal contraception and asked them about side-effects without controlling the findings against women who aren't using it. When you do that you can't actually draw any conclusions, because it's highly possible that all you've done is measure how common these symptoms are in the general population.

Imagine, for example, that 10 per cent of all women have a headache once a month, but don't usually give it any special thought. If somebody were to ask them how often they had a headache, they'd have to guess. Then they take part in a study in which they will take contraceptive pills every day and keep a journal of all possible side-effects. So, in this study, one in ten women will automatically report a headache, even though it has nothing to do with the contraceptive pills. This will not be discovered because there's no comparison with women who don't use contraceptive pills. Instead, it seems as if the contraceptive pills cause the headache. These kinds of studies are rife and are where hormonal contraception has most often been found to have effects on the psyche and sexual desire.

In the field of medicine there's one kind of study that is the best. Naturally it has a fancy name – a randomised controlled study – and it's the absolute gold standard. In these studies, a group of people is randomly divided into those who do and those who do not receive a treatment. Those who do not receive treatment are known as the control group. Ideally, the study should also be blind; in other words, the patients (and preferably the doctor and researcher, too) don't know which treatment they're receiving. Only in such studies is it possible to say anything about causal links or prove whether or not a medication is the cause of a given symptom.

As far as we know only four such randomised controlled studies have so far been carried out into contraceptive pills and non-specific side-effects such as mood changes.* Two of them found no significant difference in mood changes between those who did and didn't receive the contraceptive pills.[48] One study found that use of the Pill led to an improvement in symptoms of depression.[49]

---

* One weakness of these studies is that they were carried out on groups who were using hormonal contraception for reasons other than to avoid getting pregnant, for example because they had problems with acne or severe menstrual pains. Consequently, it's conceivable that these women are different from other women who use hormonal contraception and that this affects the results. For example, might women who have more problems with acne be more depressed?

In the last study, which looked at women from Edinburgh, Scotland, and Manila, in the Philippines, a reduction in depressive symptoms was found among the women who received mini pills, while those who were given both placebo and combined contraceptive pills had a minimal increase in depressive symptoms.[50]

The one exception is a small Swedish study. A group of researchers in Uppsala invited a group of women who had previously experienced psychological side-effects from contraceptive pills to take part in a placebo-controlled study.[51] Half of the patients were given contraceptive pills and half sugar pills, without knowing which group they were in. The study found that, on average, those who received contraceptive pills experienced greater mental deterioration than those who didn't. In addition, images were taken of the women's brains as they looked at photographs intended to evoke feelings. Changes in activity in parts of the brain that we know work with our feelings were seen among some of the women on contraceptive pills. However, there is one big BUT here: this applied to only one third of the Pill users. Two out of three of the women taking contraceptive pills experienced *no* mental deterioration or changes in brain activity while taking them, even though, by their own account, they tended to react adversely to hormonal contraception. These findings may indicate that contraceptive pills have a genuine negative effect on the psyche of a small group of women. But this applies to far fewer women than the number who *feel* this to be the case. That brings us to the next possible explanation: the power of chance.

Second possible explanation: the power of chance

We humans come equipped with a brain that likes to impose order and system on the world around us. We try to sort our sometimes chaotic environment by seeing connections between events even when they don't exist. If two events are linked in time, we draw the conclusion that one caused the other. For example, you start taking contraceptive pills and three months later you suddenly notice you're a bit down. Mustn't it be because of the contraceptive pills? After all, you've never experienced this before, as far as you recall.

But this need not be the reason at all. Depression is a surprisingly common complaint in the population. Roughly one in five women experience proper depression over the course of her life, and many more experience depressive feelings and thoughts.[52] Depression is an illness with many complex causes. Personality type, biological changes in the brain, heredity and life problems can all play a role. Because so many elements are involved it's rarely possible to point to a single concrete cause.

Depression, mood changes and irritability are such common phenomena in the population that this is likely to be a trick of chance. If, in addition, you've heard that contraceptive pills can cause mood changes and depression, it's even more likely you'll draw this conclusion, given the nocebo effect we spoke about earlier (see p. 146). Rumours of mood changes spread like wildfire among female friends on internet forums and suddenly you start to see your own experiences in a new light.

This is shored up by many large population-based studies.[53] In Finland, Australia and the USA, studies of this kind have been carried out, resulting in negative findings. The Australian study followed 10,000 women for three years. There was no difference in the frequency of depressive symptoms among those who did and didn't use contraceptive pills. In addition, the study found that the longer the women had used contraceptive pills, the less likely they were to have depressive thoughts.[54] The American study followed 7,000 women from 1994 to 2008. Here, in fact, the study found that women who used contraceptive pills had fewer depressive symptoms and were less likely to have attempted suicide in the last year than women who did not use hormonal contraception.[55] They found the same thing in the Finnish study – women who used hormonal contraception were simply *less* depressed than the others.[56]

The problem with these studies is, of course, that there may be underlying differences between the women who use contraceptive pills and those who don't. It may be the case that all women who experience a deterioration in their moods stop taking contraceptive pills, while the ones who continue to take them are the ones who don't have negative reactions. In this way, a negative effect may potentially be masked.

Given this criticism, researchers in Copenhagen carried out a very large population-based study of 1 million Danish women aged between 15 and 34, whom they followed from 2000 to 2013.[57] This study found that use of hormonal contraception was linked to an increased risk of needing antidepressants or receiving a diagnosis of depression compared with those who did not use hormonal contraception. The effect appeared to be greatest among the youngest girls, aged between 15 and 19, while the risk fell markedly once they hit 20 and continued to decrease with age. Women over 30 experienced almost no increase in the use of antidepressants or incidence of depression while using hormonal contraception. The researchers think the brain becomes less sensitive to hormone swings as people age.

This same study also observed that the risk of depression and use of antidepressants became steadily lower the longer women spent on hormonal contraception. The risk was seen to be greatest after six months' use, after which it began to fall again. After four years on hormonal contraception there was no difference between users and non-users when it came to the risk of suffering from depression.

The researchers also found differences between the various forms of contraception. Contraceptive pills were the type that appeared to give least increased risk of use of antidepressants, whereas, for example, mini pills, the vaginal ring and long-acting methods of contraception were linked to a greater rise in risk. Although it's impossible to say anything for certain based on just one such study, this underscores why women should have a low threshold for switching their method of contraception if they experience adverse side-effects. There's a difference between the side-effects the different methods of contraception give women, so it's important to try things out.

Having said that, we advise some caution when interpreting this study. There has already been a lot of scare propaganda in Denmark warning women against hormonal contraception *because it leads to depression*. Believe it or not, you can't actually claim that on the basis of this study. What the study shows is that more girls who use hormonal contraception start taking antidepressants than those who don't use it. Nobody has proved that the hormonal contraception is the *cause* of the depression. This may sound like nit-picking, but it's an important distinction. To be able to say anything about causal links you have to use totally different research methods – back to the randomised controlled studies. As we've already discussed, the few such studies that do exist have not shown anything approaching the same results. The Danish study is a solid piece of research that will very probably lead to further serious research in the field, but until we have more studies showing the same results, we cannot conclude that hormonal contraception *causes* depression in certain women.

There's no getting away from 'relative' versus 'absolute' risk, either. Some newspaper articles describing the Danish study reported that teenage girls have an 80 per cent higher risk of depression. This sounds horribly frightening, as if you're almost guaranteed to become depressed if you start taking the Pill while still of school age. The truth is quite different. Every year, one in 100 teenage girls in Denmark who are *not* using hormonal contraception are prescribed antidepressants for the first time. By comparison, 1.8 in 100 of those who do use hormonal contraception are prescribed antidepressants. *So we're talking about an increase of less than one extra person.* Of the girls using hormonal contraception, 98 of them have no depression and one would have become depressed in any event. These are the figures you should keep in mind – not the alarming headlines describing 80 per cent increases. Once there's a proper presentation of the facts on the table, you can choose whether you still think this is reason enough not to start using hormonal contraception. We won't meddle with that choice.

What's the conclusion?

Now, we've been through a lot of studies and presented contradictory results. It may be difficult to digest all of this, and we're very aware of that. Even so, we think it's possible to draw one important conclusion from these studies: hormonal contraception cannot possibly have any major negative effect on the psyche of most women. If such a side-effect does exist, it applies to a minority of women who are, for one reason or another, prone to react adversely to the hormones. We hope to become better informed about who these women are in the future. Perhaps it's worth exercising caution if a lot of people in your family have been struggling with depression or if you have had depressive tendencies yourself in the past.

For the rest of us, it's time to stop worrying – and perhaps to take it with a pinch of salt when we hear stories about ghastly psychological side-effects from hormonal contraception. Feelings aren't the same as facts.

Hormonal contraception and sexual desire

We use hormonal contraception to be able to have just as much carefree sex as we want, but what if it makes sex uninteresting? Is it true that contraceptive pills kill sexual desire? Many women seem to think so. In a Swedish survey, almost 30 per cent of the women using hormonal contraception thought that one of its side-effects was reduced sexual desire.[58]

The largest systematic review of hormonal contraception and sexual desire was carried out in 2013.[59] It combined the findings of 36 studies involving a total of 13,000 women, 8,000 of whom used contraceptive pills. Most of the women found that their sexual desire was unchanged (64 per cent) or indeed increased (22 per cent) after they started using contraceptive pills. Several studies observed an increase in sexual desire while taking contraceptive pills; this is believed to be because the contraception eliminates anxieties about pregnancy – a massive passion-killer for women the world over. As we discussed in the section about desire, sexual desire is, put simply, a function of the balance between brake and accelerator. So, the researchers don't think that the hormones *directly* increase sexual desire. On the other hand, 15 per cent of the women experienced reduced sexual desire while using hormonal contraception. We cannot say for certain whether the hormones are to blame.

What is known, however, is that the levels of active testosterone in the body are reduced when using hormonal contraception. As we know, testosterone is the male hormone par excellence, but we women also produce a small dose of it. Bodybuilders who take testosterone to increase the size of their muscles often feel very horny (often with the tedious combination of micro-penis and poor-quality sperm). Could it be that the opposite happens to women on hormonal contraception – that we lose our desire because of having too *little* testosterone?

The testosterone reduction occurs to varying degrees from one woman to the next and is also dependent on the type of contraception she uses. Hormonal contraception contains different progestins, which have different effects on testosterone. Those containing *drospirenone*, like Yasmin, reduce the testosterone level. That may lead to less acne, but also, perhaps, to reduced sexual desire. The *levonorgestrel* progestin contained in Microgynon and the hormonal IUD, however, has an effect that is more like testosterone and is therefore less likely to cause reduced sexual desire.

The problem with the testosterone theory is that no clear connection has been seen between the testosterone level in the blood and the degree of sexual desire experienced. Some women with relatively high testosterone levels struggle with sexual desire, while others with low testosterone don't notice a thing. It's evidently not simply that sexual desire is proportional to testosterone levels. Even so, people have tried giving women testosterone to increase sexual desire although without achieving any miraculous effects.* On average, they had one extra 'satisfying sexual event' a month (they're great at talking dirty in the research world).[60]

That said, there's a lot we don't know about female sexuality. There's no certainty that we'll ever find a good answer when it comes to the impact of hormonal contraception on sexual desire. Because what actually is sexual desire for *you*? It's horribly difficult to research sexual desire because there's no good measure for what it is. What's more, sexual desire is influenced by so many factors in life that it's complicated separating out what is caused by contraceptive pills and what is just the effect of a fading love affair.

As you've probably already grasped, the world of research is full of uncertainty. What we can say, however, is that there's little to suggest that hormonal contraception has a strongly negative effect on sexual desire in most women.[61]

It's possible that your contraception may have reduced your libido, but it's not common. It's much more common for sexual desire to ebb and flow over the course of a relationship or for stress to rob us of the excess energy we need for sexual fun and games.

Our advice, before you throw your contraception pills in the bin or make an appointment to have your contraceptive implant removed, is to assess

---

* The testosterone supplement was primarily tried out on postmenopausal women or women whose ovaries had been removed after cancer. Little is known about the long-term risk of testosterone use and if a woman becomes pregnant while she's taking testosterone, the foetus may be damaged. In one of the few randomised studies on younger women (aged 35–46) the testosterone supplement was found to have little or no effect on sexual desire. However, the placebo effect was high.

whether there are other aspects of your life that may be contributing to your reduced sexual desire. You can also try to switch to a method of contraception containing a different progestin.

TIME FOR A HORMONE DETOX?

Sex is not a constant benefit for most of us. When you're in a steady relationship, perhaps you have sex several times a week. But then the relationship ends and your single life is less like an episode of *Sex and the City* than you'd hoped. You begin to feel like an elephant on the savannah, searching for water at the height of the dry season. No Cosmopolitans, no eye-candy, not a cock in sight. The contraceptive pills become a bitter daily reminder of your involuntary celibacy and seem to taunt you from the bathroom cabinet: 'Ha! You won't be getting any today either!'

At the same time, perhaps you've heard that hormones aren't good for you, that they're unnatural substances.[62] Why subject your body to sinister hormones when you're not even getting sex as compensation? You think: 'Let this period of being single be a time for detox, cleansing and health! Time for a break from hormones!'

Stop right there. This isn't actually as smart as it sounds. If you've found a hormonal contraceptive that works for you it's plain silly to stop just because you've become single. Most people who start taking hormonal contraception have certain side-effects at the outset, but these most often pass or become milder after several months. The body adjusts to a new hormonal balance and settles down. When you stop, it'll take time for your body to return to a new balancing point, only to experience the same side-effects when you start again.

Blood clots are, in fact, the main reason we don't recommend taking a break from hormonal contraception. Some studies indicate that the risk of blood clots is greatest in the first months after you start taking contraceptive pills, and decreases sharply over time.[63] If you use contraceptive pills on and off every time you meet a new man, your body won't have time to return to balance. The result is that your dream guy won't just give you butterflies in your stomach, but also a higher risk of blood clots.

If blood clots are the dangerous, but rare side-effect of taking a hormone break, there's another one that's much more common. Lovers turn up when you least expect them and your doctor isn't available 24/7. It's no surprise that taking a break from the Pill often ends up giving you more of a detox than you'd bargained for. A nine-month detox, in fact. One in four girls who take a six-month break from contraceptive pills end up having an unplanned pregnancy within half a year.[64] Quite naturally!

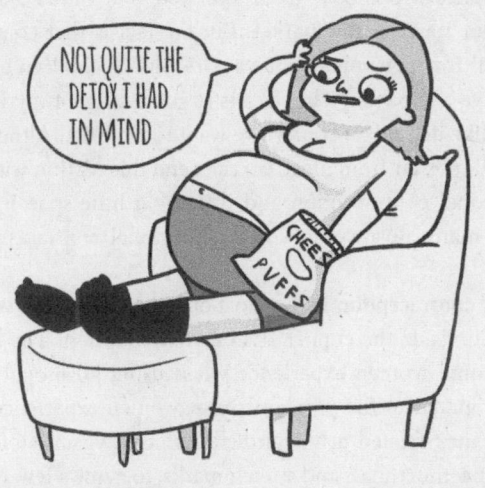

Some women are afraid that long-term use of hormonal contraception may make it difficult to become pregnant later in life. Luckily this is total nonsense, although it can take a few months for you to start ovulating again when you come off certain hormonal contraceptives. In fact, the likelihood of infertility is lower among women who've used hormonal contraception because they appear to have less chance of suffering pelvic inflammations if they're infected with sexually transmitted infections.[65] Unfortunately there are women (and men) out there who can't have children for various reasons. The problem is that you won't know whether you're one of them until you stop using contraception and try to have a baby yourself. If you're 35 and fail to get pregnant it's easy to blame the contraceptive pills you've been using since you were 15. Research shows, however, that contraceptive pills have no impact on women's fertility, whether they've been using them for one or ten years.[66] However, age does have a lot to do with it.

IN DEFENCE OF HORMONAL CONTRACEPTION

Recently, there's been a lot of public discussion about the troublesome aspects of hormonal contraception. We absolutely agree that it's a shame we don't have more options to choose from and we'd very much like to see better alternatives for men on the market. But the fact is that contraception is a necessary evil for us women, since sex results in children and we are the ones who have the babies. This fact isn't going to go away no matter how much we dislike it. And, of course, we want to have sex. Although the world of contraception is far from ideal, we can't end this section without speaking up for hormonal contraception and offering a little speech in its defence because the many positive aspects of hormonal contraception are often overlooked.

Hormonal contraception is the most effective protection we have against pregnancy, alongside the copper IUD and sterilisation. The harmless side-effects that some women experience when using hormonal contraception are small compared to the problems most women experience during pregnancy: pregnancy-related pelvic-girdle pain, massive amounts of discharge, swollen legs, haemorrhoids and stretch marks, to name a few. Not to mention the dangerous if rare side-effects. The danger of blood clots is much higher when you're pregnant than when you're using hormonal contraception.

Far too few people grasp the positive effects of hormonal contraception. We've already mentioned them, but there's no harm in repeating them.

- Hormonal contraception appears to offer protection against some of the most common forms of cancer in women: colorectal, ovarian and endometrial cancer.
- Hormonal contraception reduces menstrual pain, leads to shorter and lighter bleeding and decreases your chances of developing anaemia, which is a major problem for many women.
- With combined contraception products, you can manage the bleeding so that it comes when it suits you.

- Hormonal contraception protects against pelvic infections – an important cause of childlessness in women – by making the mucus plug in the cervix thicker and more impenetrable to bacteria.
- The chance of developing benign breast lumps – a cause of anxiety and surgical procedures for many young women – is reduced.
- Hormonal contraception is also good at treating two common and troublesome female diseases: polycystic ovary syndrome (see p. 194) and endometriosis (see p. 190).

It may be a good idea to remember this list when people portray hormonal contraception as woman's mortal enemy. The contraceptive pill has been and continues to be one of the world's most vital discoveries when it comes to women's equality.

CONTRACEPTION GUIDE

Do you think it's difficult to choose contraception? With 11 types to choose from, it can get a bit much. But don't despair. We've prepared a contraception guide just for you. Since effective contraceptives are prescription-only, you'll have to make your choice in consultation with a health professional (doctor, midwife or nurse) anyway, but it might be good to formulate some thoughts beforehand. Based on what's most important for you, you can now choose the methods of contraception that suit you and find out which ones you'd be best off avoiding. You're probably concerned about a combination of the points below, so it's a question of choosing the best alternative.

The most important thing for me is to avoid pregnancy

If the most important thing for you is not to become pregnant, you should choose the most effective method of contraception there is – the so-called long-acting methods. At the top of the list you'll find the contraceptive implant and the hormonal IUD, closely followed by the copper IUD. Combined products, such as contraceptive pills, are also effective if you use them correctly.

Suitable Long-acting contraception with a low Pearl Index: contraceptive implant, hormonal IUD and copper IUD.

Unsuitable Methods with a high Pearl Index, especially those that are based on fertility awareness.

I'm at high risk for blood clots, stroke or heart attack

If you're at high risk for any of these diseases, you must avoid oestrogen. You can still choose the methods of contraception that are best at preventing pregnancy – progestin-only products such as the contraceptive implant and the hormonal IUD. If you like taking contraceptive pills, there are also oestrogen-free pills on the market such as Cerazette.

Suitable Oestrogen-free methods such as a contraceptive implant, hormonal IUD, oestrogen-free contraceptive pills and copper IUD.

Unsuitable Combined products such as combined pills, contraceptive patch and vaginal ring.

I want lighter bleeding

Periods can be a 'pain', especially for women who have heavy, painful bleeding. In some women it's so severe that they bleed themselves to anaemia and/or have to spend a week in bed each month because of the pain. If that sounds like you, it's handy to know that some methods of contraception can reduce bleeding. A general trait of all hormonal contraception is that the overall amount of blood is smaller. To find which one works best for you, you should experiment, by trial and error, in consultation with your healthcare professional. The copper IUD often increases both bleeding and pain, so it isn't advisable for you.

Suitable Hormonal contraception in general, particularly the hormonal IUD and combined products.

Unsuitable Copper IUD.

I want to control the bleeding

As you may remember from the section called 'Periods on hormonal contraception', contraception containing oestrogen can be used to control your bleeding. Progestin products do not offer any menstrual control. If you're already using oestrogen contraception without positive results, you can switch from a product with a low dose of oestrogen to one with a slightly higher dose. You can, for example, switch from the Loestin 20 to the Microgynon pill and this change doesn't increase your risk of blood clots.

Suitable Combined products such as combined pills, contraceptive patch and vaginal ring.

Unsuitable Progestin products.

I have trouble with acne

If you have trouble with acne, oestrogen can help; in other words, you might consider combined products in consultation with your doctor or health professional. Progestin is often blamed for causing acne. If you're already using a combined product, you can try changing to another one containing a different progestin or a higher dose of oestrogen. Remember that it can often take up to three months for you to see any effect.

Suitable Combined products such as combined pills, contraceptive patch and vaginal ring.

Unsuitable Products containing the same progestin you've already tried out.

171

I want to hide my method of contraception from other people

For some women, it's important to hide the fact that they're using contraception. Some forms of contraception, such as the contraceptive implant, the copper IUD/hormonal IUD or the contraceptive injection aren't visible because they're inside your body. If you're concerned about hiding your contraceptive from your partner or family, you may wish to use a method that won't alter your pattern of bleeding, since changes in menstruation can affect your sex life or mean that you need more or fewer sanitary towels and tampons than normal. One alternative may be to use combined products or the copper IUD. These often give a regular cycle, although the total bleeding may alter. If it isn't a crisis for you to become pregnant, you can also try fertility awareness to reduce the risk of pregnancy. But remember that one in four women who use such methods of contraception end up pregnant over the course of a year.

Suitable Invisible contraception such as implant and hormonal IUD, or contraception that gives you a fixed cycle, such as combined products.

I want to protect myself against sexually transmitted infections

The condom is the only contraceptive method that protects you against STIs. We recommend that you use the condom together with another means of contraception until you and your partner have tested yourselves for STIs.

Suitable Condom together with another contraceptive method.

Unsuitable Not using a condom.

I'm taking other medicines – so can I use hormonal contraception?

Medicines affect each other. If you're taking medicine for, say, epilepsy or mental illness, this can affect your contraception or vice versa. Your doctor will keep track of this. Perhaps she may give you a tailor-made solution.

Suitable Your doctor will help you find the best solution if you're taking other medicines.

I have endometriosis

If you have endometriosis or suspect you may have because of severe pains, hormonal contraception is the first step in your treatment. Since the aim is to stop having periods, you will not take breaks.

Suitable Continuous use of combined products or insertion of a hormonal IUD.

I have polycystic ovary syndrome or extremely irregular periods

If you have fewer than four periods a year WITHOUT using hormonal contraception, you should start using hormonal contraception to expel the uterine lining at regular intervals. If menstruation is extremely rare, you can, in fact, experience excess growth of the uterine lining and that isn't good for you over the long term. Once you've had a couple of breakthrough bleeds on hormonal contraception, the problem is solved and you can start to skip bleeding as you wish.

Suitable Combined products: combined pill, contraceptive patch and vaginal ring.

The contraception I'm using reduces my sexual desire

It isn't certain whether hormonal contraception causes reduced sexual desire and, if so, which mechanisms are to blame. One theory is that this is caused by less active testosterone. Different types of progestin have different effects on testosterone. Those with drospirenone, such as Yasmin, reduce the testosterone level. That can reduce acne, but also sexual desire. However, the levonorgestrel progestin found in Microgynon and the hormonal IUD has an effect that is more similar to testosterone and is therefore less likely to reduce your sexual desire.

Suitable Products with the levonorgestrel progestin, such as Microgynon and the hormonal IUD. Hormone-free contraception such as the copper IUD.

Less suitable Products containing the drospirenone progestin, such as Yasmin.

173

ABORTION

Abortion, the practice of intentionally terminating a pregnancy, provokes strong feelings. On the one hand, it's about a woman's right to choose when it comes to her own body, to choose whether she wants to give birth to a child. On the other, abortion is also about the beginning of a new life and what rights this potential child should have once it has been conceived. There is no easy moral answer to the question of abortion. There will always be a losing party, either the pregnant woman, the father of the potential child, the health professional who carries out the abortion or the foetus.

For us, the woman's rights have the greatest weight – it's the woman who will undergo the physical and mental strain of pregnancy and birth. It is also often the woman who is left with the responsibility for care and provision of support. A child results in greater emotional, economic and social upheaval for the woman, and it's the women who have least to begin with who are often the ones who are hit the hardest. It ought to be the woman's choice whether she wants to take on these burdens, since they fall on her to such a great extent. There are no other areas of policy where we think it's acceptable to impose such considerable personal cost on a citizen to satisfy society's moral norms as when we oblige a woman to give birth to a child she doesn't want to have.

That said, there must be limits. Most people agree that at some point in the pregnancy, an abortion cannot be based solely on the woman's choice, and that the foetus is no longer a foetus, but a child, with rights that outweigh the preferences and rights of the pregnant woman. Where that limit is set varies from country to country, but the upper limit is rarely challenged, whatever it is. In most countries where abortion is legal and accessible, most abortions take place early in the pregnancy, while the rare late-term abortions that are carried out are often done so because of serious or life-threatening abnormalities in the foetus or to save the mother's life.

There are, for example, very different ways of regulating abortion – ranging from total prohibition in Chile and Malta, to Norway, where women have a right to abortion on demand up to and including week 12. In England, Wales and Scotland they can have an abortion up until week 24, whereas

Canada has no abortion law, but it is considered a medical matter between a woman and her doctor. There are also major differences between how available abortion is even where it is allowed: it may be so expensive or offered in so few places that many women do not have real access to it. This is, for example, the case in many states in the USA.

Regardless of your personal feelings about the question of abortion, it is an indisputable fact that it does not help to prohibit or complicate access to it if you want to reduce the number. We often find that the countries with the strictest legislation also have the highest incidence of abortions, while those with good access to legal abortion often have low abortion rates. Throughout all time and in every corner of the world women with unwanted pregnancies have taken matters into their own hands, despite threats of punishment and social ostracism – not to mention the risk of exposure to serious injury or death. The thought of giving birth to an unwanted child can be so unbearable that it outweighs the dangers and threats of legal prosecution.

Knitting needles, wise women, steep staircases and poison are still last resorts for women in some parts of the world where abortion is illegal or inaccessible. Every year, 20 million women feel obliged to undergo unsafe abortions – that's almost one in ten pregnancies worldwide. Of these women, 50,000 die totally unnecessary deaths.[67] Some 6.9 million women require treatment by health services for complications resulting from dangerous abortions.[68] Access to safe abortion would have spared those women. Legal and safe abortion is, in other words, essential for safeguarding women's health. Prohibiting abortion doesn't save any potential children; it just harms desperate women.

That said, abortion is no easy way out. We maintain that few women want to have an abortion or consciously use it as an alternative to contraception. It's often down to bad luck in the form of unprotected sex at the wrong time, contraceptive failure, poor access to modern contraception or – in the worst case – assault and sexual violence. If the goal is to keep abortion figures low, the most effective measure is to ensure easily accessible, effective contraception, and to provide good sex education. Unfortunately, restrictive abortion laws often go hand in hand with poor access to precisely these two aspects of health provision. It's like an ostrich sticking its head in the sand and thinking the problem will go away just because it doesn't have to see it.

How are abortions performed?

Regardless of whether you live in a country where abortion is easily accessible or not, it's good to know a bit about how abortions are performed within the health system. Practice varies from country to country when it comes to how abortions are carried out – whether at a hospital or specialist clinic – and what rules apply. But the methods are the same. If you find yourself in the position of having an unwanted pregnancy, it's good to be able to focus your thoughts on more important things than finding out practical details.

How far along am I?

A common source of confusion when it comes to abortion is how far along you are. Many countries have abortion laws that involve time limits; for example, abortion on demand is allowed up to and including week 12 (in England, Scotland and Wales it's 24 weeks; women from Northern Ireland need to seek abortions in England). But when are you 12 weeks pregnant? You'd think it would be calculated from the date you had unprotected sex, but incredibly enough, that's not the case. Instead, it is calculated from the first day of your last period. This is because that's the last point in time you knew for sure that you weren't pregnant. Seen from this perspective, the law considers you to be 'pregnant' for two weeks before you even had the intercourse that made you pregnant. Not entirely logical, but that's the way the rules work.

Before you have an abortion, most doctors will give you an ultrasound. A little probe, the thickness of a thin carrot, is inserted in your vagina to see how many weeks along you are. If you are 12 weeks the foetus will be up to 6.6 centimetres long, any longer and you are more than 12 weeks pregnant. The examination makes sense because a lot of women have irregular periods or don't remember the date of their last period. The ultrasound examination is the legal answer to how far along you are, if there's any doubt about the matter.

Two methods of abortion

There are two ways of carrying out an abortion: with pills or with minor surgery. Abortion with pills is called a medical abortion, while the other method is called surgical abortion or curettage.

Medical abortion This starts with you taking a pill, normally at a hospital, clinic or at your doctor's surgery. The pill contains a substance called *mifepristone*, which tricks the body into thinking you're no longer pregnant. All the complicated processes that make sure the fertilised egg grows into a foetus and then a baby come to a halt. The abortion has been set in motion, but it is not complete, so the foetus remains in your uterus. Although the process is not complete, this doesn't mean that you can have second thoughts after taking the first pill – as a rule, the foetus will not develop any further in the normal way. When you've taken the pill, you have to wait one to two days. It's perfectly normal to experience mild nausea, light bleeding and menstrual pains during this time, but otherwise, you can carry on with life as normal.

Then, after roughly two days, the abortion must be completed with a second dose of medication. If you're a healthy woman who's been pregnant for less than nine or ten weeks, it's fine to do this at home. If you do, it's important to have an adult with you, such as a friend or your partner. This is to be on the safe side in case of complications – although they are highly uncommon. If you prefer, or you've been pregnant for more than nine to ten weeks, you'll be admitted as an outpatient to a hospital or a clinic and take the last round of abortion pills there. In countries where abortion is illegal, it has gradually become more and more common for women to carry out abortions by obtaining misoprostol online or by other means.

The method is the same regardless of where you do it. You insert four pessaries of *misprostol* in your vagina or place tablets under your tongue. The *misprostol* causes the uterus to contract and squeeze out its contents – a bit like when you have your period, just that this time there's also a tiny little foetus in your uterus that will come out along with the blood.

Once the abortion is under way, you'll have heavier bleeding than with a normal period. The blood that comes out will be clotted and red. If you're afraid of seeing the foetus, all there is to say is that the earlier you have the abortion, the less of a chance there is that you'll see anything. Most abortions in Northern Europe happen before the ninth week of pregnancy, when the foetus will be a 1.5-centimetre-long transparent tadpole surrounded by mucus and blood. Any pictures you've seen on the internet of sweet little mini-babies are thoroughly misleading and designed to make women feel guilty about having an abortion.

For 95–8 per cent of all women, the medical abortion is over in a matter of a few hours.[69] You must remember to take painkillers, as instructed by your doctor, because it may hurt. If you still suffer severe pains, fever or extremely heavy bleeding after an abortion, you must ring the hospital or go to your nearest A&E. People often say that if you bleed through a night sanitary towel in less than two hours, you should contact the doctor.

After the abortion, it is quite normal to bleed less heavily and have a bit of pain for two to three weeks. In that case, it's important to use sanitary towels and not tampons in order to prevent infection. In addition, you should not have sex while you're still bleeding. As long as you're bleeding, it means that the uterus is still getting rid of the remains of the pregnancy, and any bacteria that may find their way up the vagina can easily progress further into your system. It isn't common to develop infections after an abortion, but it's still important to take precautions.

Now and then you read scare stories in the media about women who had a medical abortion and discovered that they were still pregnant several months later. If you follow the instructions you are given by your doctor, this is very unlikely. One in 100 patients has been seen to remain pregnant after a medical abortion. You will be able to tell if this has happened because there will be no proper bleeding after you've inserted the last tablets in your vagina. If that happens, you should contact the hospital again quickly. The pills you've taken will halt the pregnancy, and it isn't good to go round with the remains of it in your uterus. All women who have an abortion should take a pregnancy test a month later to ensure that the pregnancy is completely terminated. In addition, you should contact the doctor if your period has not returned four to six weeks after the bleeding stops.

Surgical abortion A surgical abortion involves a slightly different process and must be carried out at a hospital or abortion clinic. You'll most often be given two pessaries to insert in your vagina on the morning you're scheduled to have the abortion. These cause the cervix to dilate. If you're going to be given a general anaesthestic during the abortion, you'll have to fast from midnight the night before the procedure. This means that you shouldn't eat, drink or smoke. Many places carry out abortions using only local anaesthesia.

The operation itself lasts around ten minutes. The doctor accesses the uterus via the vagina and then the cervix. After that, she will suction out the foetus and the placenta using a little aspirator and then she will gently scrape the uterine lining to ensure that everything has been removed (curettage). Following the abortion, you'll have to remain at the hospital for a few hours so that the doctors can check that everything's going well. After that, you can go home – normally the same day.

Just as with medical abortion, you may bleed and have pains for a while afterwards. The same rules apply for sanitary towels and sex, and here, too, you should contact the doctor if you become unwell, bleed heavily or don't start your period again within six weeks.

As with all surgery, there's a small risk of complications linked to the anaesthesia or the procedure itself. This very rarely includes damage to the uterus, bladder or urinary tract, but it is because of these very rare complications that medical abortion is recommended in many countries. It's always best to avoid surgery, but all in all, surgical abortion carried out by health professionals is very safe. Many women prefer a surgical abortion to avoid the lengthier process involved in a medical abortion.

Some people may have heard that surgical abortion can make it more difficult to become pregnant later on. This impression stems from a rare condition called Asherman's syndrome, which can come about if the surgeon needs to scrape out a great deal of tissue from the uterus and in doing so damages the deepest layer of the uterine lining. Then you may get uterine scarring and adhesions, which may make it difficult to get pregnant later. Gynaecologists these days are very aware that this might happen and do everything they can to be on the safe side. In other words, it's unlikely that an uncomplicated curettage will have any effect on your chances of becoming pregnant later. But the more times you have curettage, the greater the risk.[70] This is one of the reasons why abortion should never be used as a means of contraception.

Unplanned pregnancy can be a pleasant surprise too

Discovering that you have an unplanned pregnancy can be a shocking experience. Of course, for some people it comes as a pleasant surprise, but it isn't unusual to feel a touch of panic as well. Pregnancy can set in motion many emotional processes that you may not have been prepared for. If that happens, it's good to have somebody to talk to. Everybody you meet in the health service has a duty of confidentiality and can offer you guidance through the process, whatever you might choose to do – whether you end up having an abortion, keeping the child or going for adoption. It's also sensible to talk to your partner, friends and family to seek advice and care, whatever you choose to do.

TROUBLE DOWN BELOW

Our genitals are just like the other parts of our body. Provided everything's working as it should, we don't give them much thought. But as soon as something starts to go wrong, it can become an all-consuming business. Any woman who's struggled with menstrual pains, or had a severe yeast infection, knows all about that. That's when we may curse the day we were born women. What wouldn't we give to exchange our monthly cramps for the occasional kick in the balls?

This part of the book will deal with all the things that can cause trouble down below. We're absolutely certain that most women will experience some of these conditions over the course of their lives. Fortunately, most gynaecological ailments are not life threatening, but we can't deny that some may seriously reduce the quality of life for those affected. The world of medicine has fallen short in many aspects of female health and we can only hope that sometime soon this will change, that women's disease will be a prioritised field.

While we were working on this chapter, we did wonder whether we might not end up creating more anxiety than necessary. By talking about rare and dangerous diseases whose symptoms are often vague, might we be exposing women to new and unnecessary concerns? We hope and believe that's not the case. Remember that your body is always giving off small signals indicating wellbeing or ailments. We're supposed to notice the fact that we are alive – we're not machines, after all. But some of us are more alert to these signals than others, and that can lead to health anxiety. We think the best medicine for this kind of anxiety is more knowledge. More knowledge can give you security, but scaring yourself silly by googling vague, common symptoms can only worsen the fear. The trick is to distinguish between normal phenomena that we all experience now and then and those that may be signs of something more serious.

In our work as sexual-health writers, we've discovered that there's a remarkable lack of knowledge out there about quite common female illnesses and complaints. A lot of women are struggling with diseases that those around them have never heard of, and they often feel lonely and don't know where to find help. For example, we'd never heard of endometriosis before we started studying medicine. But even so, one in ten women is walking around with this disease, and many are struggling to adapt their everyday life to the pain. That's not the way it should be. Imagine if one in ten men had to take a week off work each month because of excruciating pain in their balls. It would be a national issue, covered on the curriculum at every school.

In other words, it's also about time we spoke up about *our* problems. That's the only way we can ensure that women get the help they need. Perhaps more resources could also be assigned to research into female diseases so that we can find good treatments in the future – we can always hope.

We'll start with the most common problems of all: bleeding disorders.

BLEEDING ABNORMALITIES – PERIODS UP THE SPOUT

Periods are a significant part of life for most women. From puberty until we are somewhere between the age of 45 and 55 (more or less) our menstrual cycle follows an eternal circle, month after month. We are used to it being one of the more reliable elements in our lives. With that in mind, it's no wonder you get worried and confused when something happens to your period and the cycle is different from what you hear it *ought* to be. *Help, what's wrong*, you think – and you're not the only one. It's odd that changes in blood and mucus from your uterus should feel so alarming, but it's easy to believe something's wrong with the *very core of your womanhood*. Your thoughts become all tangled up in your head. Is there something wrong with me? Won't I be able to have kids ten years from now, as planned? Is it cancer? Is it a disease? Seriously – help!

There are a lot of different types of bleeding abnormalities. They may involve pain, irregularity, problems with the amount of flow or your period may quite simply stop. Let's start with the most common ones.

When your period stops
One of the most common, and perhaps most frightening, things is when your period vanishes without a trace, or *with* just a trace. Sometimes you're

left with trace bleeding, or spotting, even though your usual menstrual bleeding has vanished into thin air.

When your period disappears for more than six months in the instance of women who previously had regular periods or nine months for those who were irregular, we call it *amenorrhoea*.[1] All we mean by regular periods is that your menstrual cycle is equally long every time and that your period arrives at the same moment each time around, so that you can predict when it will come by using a menstrual calendar. Amenorrhoea comes from the Greek, meaning literally 'without the monthly flow' – and that's exactly what it is.

It's common for women's periods to stop. As many as 8 per cent of all women between the ages of 16 and 24 experience this every year, and there can be different causes.[2] The first thing you need to think about is that your period stops when you're pregnant. *But I used a condom, didn't I?* you think, when you're three days late. You're not ready for kids right now, and the panic is close to the surface.

A pregnancy test at the right time can rule out pregnancy. It's incredibly important to check if there's any possibility of it. Was there a contraceptive failure? A missed pill? Did you rely on withdrawal or fertility awareness? Buy a pregnancy test – it's reliable three weeks after unprotected sex or contraceptive failure. If you haven't had sex or if you use safe contraception that can't be used incorrectly – for example, the contraceptive implant or the hormonal IUD – there's another issue. Take a pregnancy test if you're in any doubt. However, there are other possible reasons why your monthly bleeding has vanished.

One rare, but funny cause of missing a period is travel. We don't know why it happens, but long plane journeys, especially if you cross several time zones, can mess with your menstrual cycle, causing the bleeding to come at the wrong time, as if it had jetlag, too. But two much more common reasons for losing your period are weight changes and lots of exercise. It's difficult to define just how sigificant the weight change must be or how much you need to exercise for this to happen. Professional athletes often have amenorrhoea, but you don't have to be a professional to exercise your period away. An anorexia diagnosis based on the strictest criteria requires your periods to have stopped, although that doesn't necessarily mean you have anorexia if you lose your period because of weight changes.

Illness is also a common cause, as is mental stress. Your general state affects your period. Perhaps you've got too much on at school, or you've been exposed to major psychological traumas such as war, accident or a death in the family.

Put simply, your period is a sign that you have energy to spare. For you to become pregnant, your body must be strong enough to bear it. Pregnancy is a strain and if, for one reason or another, you don't have the energy reserves you need to carry a baby, your period often stops to protect you from a pregnancy for which you're not ready. Everything's connected. Body, mind and period are no exception. If your period stops and you're not sure why, then a trip to the doctor is perfectly reasonable.

Illnesses that can lead to loss of menstruation include polycystic ovary syndrome (see p. 194) and metabolic diseases. It may also be good to remember how contraception affects periods (see p. 137). Progestin products such as the hormonal IUD, the contraceptive injection, the oestrogen-free pill and the implant often cause periods to stop over time. This is quite normal and doesn't mean there's anything wrong. As we've explained, the bleeding that comes when you use contraception is not a normal period, but what's known as withdrawal bleeding. Unlike a regular period, it's not a sign of having energy reserves. If you stop bleeding because of hormonal contraception, you don't have amenorrhoea.

Finally, it's good to know that irregular menstruation is completely normal in the first couple of years after you start having periods – and that also includes your period stopping for a while. It takes a bit of time for your hormones to settle into balance and for ovulation to happen on a monthly basis. It'll sort itself out.

It hurts!

More than half of us suffer from severe menstrual pains: unpleasant, cramp-like aches in our lower belly. Some women also have pains in the small of their back, their thighs or their vagina. As long as you've ruled out the possibility that the pains have any special cause – for example, an illness that causes more severe menstrual pains – this is known as primary dysmenorrhoea. If the pains have an underlying cause, they are called secondary dysmenorrhoea. Dysmenorrhoea comes from the Greek, meaning 'painful monthly flow'. The pains are worst in the first few days of menstruation and are often accompanied by other ailments, such as nausea, vomiting and diarrhoea. Up to one in six women suffer such severe pains that they need to take a couple of days off work or school every month.[3]

Menstrual pains are caused by contractions of the uterus. That little hollow bundle of muscles clenches itself tight towards the end of each cycle to push out the endometrium, the inner uterine lining that emerges as menstruation. The uterus is strong – a bit too strong for its own good, perhaps. It squeezes so tight that it can't catch its breath and that hurts! Now, of course your uterus doesn't actually breathe – only your lungs do that – but all the cells in your body need oxygen. Without that, they'd suffocate and die. The oxygen is carried in the bloodstream and what happens during menstrual cramps is that the uterus clenches its muscles too tightly and simply shuts off its own blood supply in the process. It is that eager to get rid of the old endometrium. It's the lack of oxygen to the tissue that's the cause of the pain.

But hold on a minute – haven't you heard about something like this before? If you work in the health service or if, for example, you have a grandparent with a condition called angina, this might sound unmistakably familiar. Indeed, pain caused by lack of oxygen is exactly what people get when the blood vessels in their heart are blocked. They can experience chest pains during physical activity. If Grandad goes up the stairs, his heart needs more oxygen, but his narrow vessels can't manage to transport the blood quickly enough, so the heart suffers 'hypoxic pain'. The same thing happens in your uterus when it's grinding away.

You can also get chest pains from a heart attack. In that case, there's so little oxygen that part of your heart suffocates and dies. If you're starting to get a bit worried now, let us reassure you: menstrual pains aren't the same as a heart attack – they're not dangerous! You won't lose parts of your uterus as a result of the cramps, although it is a bit odd to think that lack of oxygen is the cause of the pain in both cases. So, it isn't the same, but it's similar.

So why is it so painful for some people, while others think periods are a breeze?

The answer is thought to lie in how active your enzymes are. Enzymes are small proteins that ensure that all the chemical processes in your body follow their proper course. One group, called COX enzymes, is involved in producing substances called *prostaglandins*. Among other purposes, prostaglandins are sometimes given to pregnant women to trigger childbirth. What they do is cause the uterus to contract, which in turn causes the lack of oxygen we've just been talking about.

Some experts think that women who have particularly painful periods have especially active COX enzymes.[4] As a result, they produce more prostaglandins than other people. This, in turn, results in stronger contractions of the uterus just when it's struggling to relax between contractions. The prostaglandins also make the nerves in the genital area hypersensitive to pain.

In case you've been wondering whether you have a low pain threshold or find people don't believe you when you describe your pains, here's a little comparison with childbirth that should shut most people up. It has been observed that the uterine contractions of women with dysmenorrhoea can reach a pressure equivalent to 150–180 mmHg.[5] Now perhaps that doesn't mean anything to you, but for comparison, the pressure during the pushing stage of childbirth is around 120 mmHg. During childbirth, women have three to four rounds of uterine contractions every ten minutes. During her period, a woman with dysmenorrhoea may have between four and five such rounds. In other words, the pressure during awful period pains is at least as high as during birth and the pains come at slightly shorter intervals. So now you can understand how it can be so painful. Fortunately, these horrible pains usually ease off over the years.

You may use painkillers for menstrual cramps, but it is important to use them properly. Ibuprofen directly inhibits the COX enzymes, ensuring that fewer prostaglandins are produced. This is why ibuprofen and similar meds, known as NSAIDs (Non-specific Anti-inflammatory Drugs), are the most effective medication for menstrual pains. If you tend to have severe period pains, you should start taking ibuprofen a day before your period, or at least immediately you notice the slightest sign of discomfort. After that you should take painkillers every six to eight hours in the first few days of your period. Far too many people wait until it's really hurting before they take painkillers and then, unfortunately, they'll have much less effect because the prostaglandins have already been produced.[6] Other than that, most forms of hormonal contraception also have a good effect on period pains. Contraceptives are also a more long-term solution, since you use them continuously.

Finally, we must point out that some people may have different, underlying causes for the pain. This is particularly true for women who find that the pain changes or increases suddenly or sneaks up on them over time. *It wasn't like this before.* This may indicate that you have knots of muscle in the uterus, known as *fibroids* (see p. 198), or endometriosis (see p. 190), in which cells like the uterine lining are growing outside the uterus. It is also possible to have increased period pains as a result of a copper IUD (see p. 140). If this applies to you, it's time to switch to another method of contraception.

If you experience sudden, severe pain, you might think about more serious, acute conditions. For example, it's possible for a pregnancy to develop outside the uterus. This can happen if the fertilised egg doesn't make its way down to the uterus the way it should. Then the foetus begins to develop, say, in the Fallopian tubes, where there isn't room for it – this is called an ectopic pregnancy. Pregnancy outside the uterus can manifest itself as severe menstrual pains, sometimes concentrated on one side. In that case, a trip to your out-of-hours surgery or nearest A&E is essential as this is a potentially life-threatening problem.

Irregular periods
In your first years of having periods, your last years of having periods and when you're using hormonal contraception, it's normal for your periods to be a bit irregular. It takes time for your cycle to stabilise after you start menstruating and when you're on hormonal contraception, you no longer have a normal period, because your cycle isn't the way it was before. With the exception of these situations, your cycle should stabilise, settling into a regular length of between 25 and 35 days – more or less.

But if you've been having periods for several years and the bleeding is still (or suddenly becomes) as unpredictable as the plot of the 2014 film *Gone Girl*, you should pay attention. Irregular bleeding can involve many things. It may be spotting – small drops between each period – bleeding at unexpected times or bleeding that happens after or in connection with sex.

As well as vanishing, your period may also be delayed or arrive unexpectedly as a result of stress, weight changes or excessive exercise. Things like that influence our hormones. Other causes may be underlying illnesses such as polycystic ovary syndrome or metabolic diseases.

Cervical cancer or STIs (sexually transmitted infections) may cause the cervix to become tender and bleed slightly. If that happens, intercourse can trigger light bleeding during or after sex. So, bleeding associated with intercourse should be checked out by a doctor.

If you're using combined contraceptives (combined pills, contraceptive patch or vaginal ring) and suffer from irregular bleeding, it may be a good idea to talk to your doctor or nurse. It could help to switch to a product with a bit more oestrogen. There are two different doses of oestrogen in contraceptive pills. For example, Loestrin 20 is a low-oestrogen dose pill, whereas Microgynon or Marvelon contain a bit more oestrogen. Otherwise, the pills are the same. Many women find irregular bleeding stops when they switch to a product that contains a bit more oestrogen.

Too much blood!
As you can see from the different sizes available on the tampon shelf at the supermarket, your female friends won't necessarily bleed as much or as little as you. For some women, even the thought of the tiny mini-tampons is too much. Women who bleed the least need only stick a paper tissue in their knickers, and that solves the problem. Others must change the more absorbent super-plus tampons every few hours and the fear of bleeding through makes them yearn for even higher absorbency levels – super plus, plus, plus, plus, plus. You get the picture.

Blood loss over the course of a cycle tends to vary a lot from one woman to the next, but the average is between 25 and 30 millilitres – or around the size of a single espresso at your local café. It's also within the norm to bleed a double espresso.[7] Are you one of those women who's hooting with laughter now? *A single espresso? Over the course of the whole period? Ha ha – pathetic! A double a day at least!*

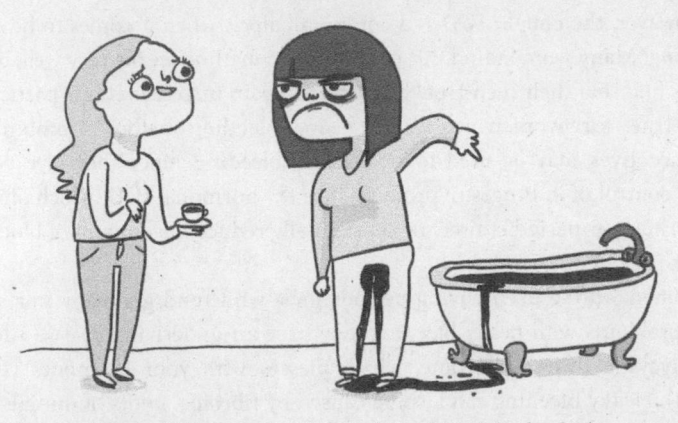

Some people's periods are more like Lady Báthory's bathtub than something from your local coffee shop. Lady Báthory was a serial killer from Transylvania who was said to bathe in the blood of virgins to keep herself young. But no. Nobody bleeds a whole bathtub's worth of blood over a single cycle, although it may almost feel that way when the bleeding just won't stop and the blood charges through tampons, knickers, trousers and straight onto your mother-in-law's white sofa. In fact, it would take approximately seven women's life-long production of period blood to fill up a bathtub with a volume of around 200 litres. Still, a lot of women have such heavy periods that they end up suffering from anaemia and need to take iron supplements. Then they get sluggish and pale, often have headaches and just can't be bothered to do any of the stuff they like. Periods like this can really make you lose your sparkle!

Menstrual bleeding is considered to be unusually heavy if either you bleed for longer than eight days per cycle or the volume is more than 80 millilitres – so more than two and a half single espressos.[8] Not exactly a bathtub, but a lot of blood all the same.

It's common for young girls to bleed more in the early days after they start their periods. Things can improve over time and it's rarely a cause for concern. However, some girls have such heavy bleeding that it may be sensible to check it isn't caused by an underlying disease. Certain blood disorders can, in fact, cause you to bleed more, or more easily, than other people – but this is very rare.

However, the copper IUD is a common culprit when it comes to heavy bleeding. Many women find this contraceptive method works very well, but others find that their menstrual bleeding and pain increase. This is particularly true for women who had heavy bleeding before. Combined contraceptives may be used to treat heavy bleeding, since they give you better control of it. Progestin products, like the hormonal IUD, which often eliminate your period entirely or substantially reduce the amount of blood, are also winners.

Women who've been having periods for a while and gradually start to have problems with heavy bleeding may have an underlying disease such as polycystic ovary syndrome, which messes with your hormones (see p. 194). Heavy bleeding can also be caused by fibroids, knots of muscle in the wall of your uterus (see p. 198). You can read more about these diseases later on in the chapter.

ENDOMETRIOSIS – A BLOODY CHARTER HOLIDAY

The pain of periods is something we take for granted, but some women have such severe period pains that they have to put their whole life on hold. Several days a month they lie there, curled up on the sofa with hot-water bottles, snacking on painkillers as if they were sweets. That's not the way it should be. If that's how it is for you, it's possible you may be suffering from something called endometriosis, a condition that affects around one in ten women. A third of those who struggle with this severe pain in the lower belly and genitals have endometriosis.[9*] Of course, this does not apply to pains in the vulva itself, which we'll come back to later.

As you may have gathered from the name, endometriosis involves the endometrium, the mucous membrane that lines the inside of the uterus. This is the membrane that builds up every cycle as your uterus prepares to receive a fertilised egg. It is expelled from the uterus in the form of menstruation if you don't become pregnant. But you knew that already. What's different when it comes to endometriosis is that those who suffer with it

---

* It is difficult to know just how many people are affected, because many women don't have symptoms and the diagnosis can only be established through an operation.

also have cells from the uterine lining *outside* their uterine cavity. In some cases, the cells of the uterine lining have gone astray into the muscle wall of the uterus, and then it's known as *adenomyosis*.

It's not quite clear how these cells end up outside the uterus. One leading theory is that the period has run the wrong way, in other words, up the Fallopian tubes instead of out of the cervix, and so ended up in the inside of the abdomen. This happens to all women to a certain degree when they have their period, but it seems there are some susceptible women whose bodies can't manage to get it all cleaned up. When that happens, small groups of mucous-membrane cells misunderstand where they belong, and settle down in, say, the ovaries, the pelvis, the gut or other places in the abdomen. Most often, these endometrial cells are found close to the internal pelvic organs, but in some very rare cases they can be found as far up as the sacs that surround the lungs. This has prompted some to wonder whether there may be other mechanisms causing endometriosis apart from periods gone astray. Perhaps there's a kind of stem cell (the cells that can become whatever cell they want to) that has developed wrongly in the wrong place? Or perhaps cells from the uterine lining are transported in the bloodstream to other parts of the body? Perhaps we'll find the conclusive answer in a few years.

The colonies of endometrial cells haven't forgotten where they come from, or their purpose, even though they've found a new home, just like British pensioners on the Costa del Sol. They behave as if they were living in the uterus. This means that they react to the hormones in the menstrual cycle just like ordinary endometrial cells. Incredibly enough, this means that every month, you also have a mini-menstruation outside your uterus.

A misplaced period is not popular. The immune defences put up a particularly stubborn fight when endometrial cells settle down in an otherwise quiet and orderly neighbourhood. Because the body has strict rules about what should happen where, when these colonies of endometrial cells begin to bleed in a place where they don't belong, rebellions quickly follow. The new neighbours don't have a clue what's going on when they suddenly get hit by an unexpected shower of blood and naturally enough they call the police – our immune cells – which arrive at top speed to clean things up. The result is that you get an inflammation in the tissue that surrounds the endometrial colony. And inflammations hurt.

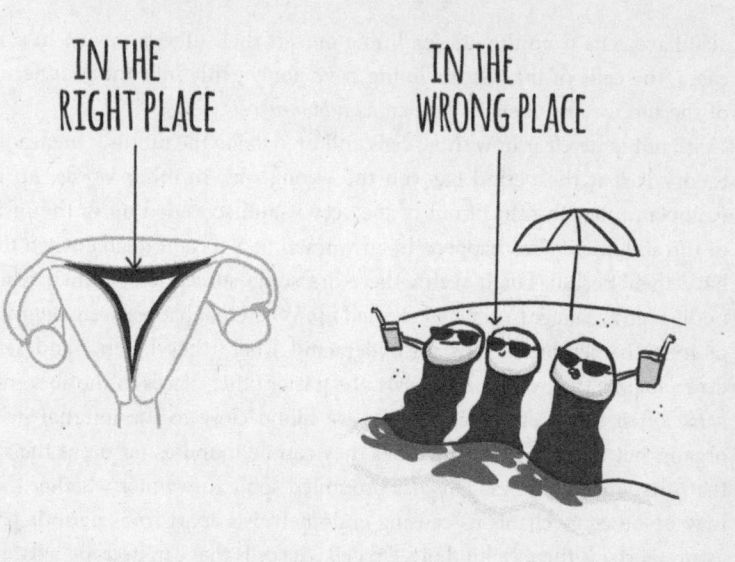

IN THE
RIGHT PLACE

IN THE
WRONG PLACE

Most people will find it difficult to distinguish these pains from severe, but normal period pains, since the endometrial colonies are most often located close to the uterus, although some women will also find they have pain in odd places. For example, if the colonists have settled near the urinary tract, it may hurt to pee, or if they're happiest in the rectum, pooing will be painful.

The one thing all these types of pain have in common is that they're cyclical – meaning that they follow a fixed pattern. They often begin one or two days *before* menstruation and may continue for several days after it has ended. One way you can differentiate endometrial pains from ordinary menstrual cramps is that they usually develop gradually several years after you first start your periods, as if your menstrual cramps are steadily getting worse as you get older. Some people do experience the pains from early in their teens, but this is less common. As a result, people tend to be diagnosed with endometriosis when they're in their 20s or older.

Over time, the monthly inflammations around the colony can cause scarring and adhesions inside the body. For example, the ovaries may adhere to their neighbour, the uterus. These internal scars can cause different types of problems, such as chronic, or long-term, pain. Constant, dull pain in the pelvic area is a common problem for women with endometriosis. Many women also experience deep, stabbing pains during intercourse. The pain is in the lowest part of your belly, not in your vagina or vulva.

Another problem is that many women with endometriosis have difficulty conceiving. Endometriosis is responsible for around a quarter of all cases of involuntary childlessness.[10] We don't know quite why people have problems with fertility. Scarring and adhesion can damage the Fallopian tubes and the ovaries, but it looks as though other mechanisms are to blame too. It seems as if both the immune defences and hormones are involved. If you're struggling to get pregnant and have endometriosis, artificial insemination may help.[11] Surgery is available in addition to or instead of artificial insemination. Surgical removal of the colonies of endometrial cells outside the uterus has helped some women become pregnant, both naturally and through artificial insemination. The recommendation is that the operation should be carried out only once, and that women should save it until they're ready for children.

We don't know why some women have endometriosis. To a certain extent it's hereditary, but many other factors seem to come into play. As far as we know, there's nothing you can do to avoid it. It's simply a matter of bad luck. Some grandparents like Costa del Sol, while others are happiest in the countryside, summer and winter. Likewise, some of us have endometrial cells that seem to want to emigrate outside the uterus.

The problem with endometriosis is that there's no sure way of finding out if you have it through simple tests. Blood tests, gynaecological examinations and medical imaging such as MRI scans tell us little or nothing about these charter-hungry endometrial cells. The only way we can confirm or rule out whether women have endometriosis is simply to take a look inside. This is done through keyhole surgery – peering into the abdomen with cameras through a small hole. As with all surgery, complications can arise, so this isn't done unless the problems are major and other causes for the pain have been ruled out.

What doctors will often do instead of surgery is try out endometriosis treatment and see if it works. For most women the treatment is simple and harmless: contraceptive pills without a break or a hormonal IUD and painkillers, like Ibuprofen. By taking contraceptive pills continuously, the endometrium colonies are prevented from bleeding and this can also cause them to shrink over time.[12] Ibuprofen acts on the pains and may reduce the inflammation at the same time. This won't eliminate the colonies, but it can diminish the problem.

If this kind of treatment doesn't work, there are other more sophisticated ways of treating endometriosis, such as surgery or stronger hormonal treatment. This is specialised work. Endometriosis is a chronic (long-term) disease that doesn't pass until menopause. Unfortunately, the treatment doesn't cure the disease. Even after surgical removal, the endometrial colonies may return over time. Nonetheless, you should be aware that there is help out there and ways to reduce your pain. The first important step is realising that it is actually endometriosis you're dealing with and finding a doctor who cares. Awareness of endometriosis is slowly growing and we sincerely hope we are the last generation of women to grow up without having heard of this potentially disabling disease.

POLYCYSTIC OVARY SYNDROME – WHEN YOUR HORMONES GO HAYWIRE

'The only thing worse than periods is not getting periods', as a female friend of ours likes to say. A lot of women worry if their period vanishes or appears more rarely than once a month. One common cause of irregular menstruation or infrequent menstrual bleeding is a condition called polycystic ovary syndrome, or PCOS. You haven't heard of it before? Well, you're not the only one, but there are good reasons why we should all be more concerned about this condition. It is, in fact, the most common hormonal disorder among women of fertile age, affecting somewhere between 4 and 12 per cent of them, many of whom don't know it themselves.[13]

The name of the condition stems from the fact that in PCOS, cysts are often found on the ovaries. These are like small water blisters filled with a transparent fluid, which can make the ovaries look a bit like bunches of grapes. Unlike other types of cysts on the ovaries, these ones are so small that they don't burst, so you won't notice they're there.

Although this is the best-known aspect of PCOS, it's just a small part of the condition. PCOS is a syndrome, meaning that it consists of a bunch of different problems that often, though not always, occur together. The problems are caused by a number of hormonal-system disorders. They don't just mess with the ovaries, but also the pancreas, the digestive system and the pituitary gland, that little scrotum-shaped gland under the brain.

The ovaries store all your eggs and ensure that ovulation occurs each month. If you have PCOS, these tasks may become problematic because both the pituitary gland and the ovaries produce the wrong levels of the hormones that control the menstrual cycle. The result is that you may have fewer ovulations or none at all. You may notice this in your everyday life because your period may arrive more rarely or may disappear entirely.

Since ovulation is necessary in order to become pregnant, many women with PCOS will take longer than normal to conceive, or will need help to do so.[14] PCOS is one of the most common reasons why women have difficulty becoming pregnant.[15] It is also linked to a higher risk of complications in pregnancy, such as miscarriage and gestational diabetes.

It is suspected that women with untreated PCOS face a higher risk of endometrial cancer later in life; this is the most common form of genital cancer among women in the Western world.[16] One review study found that while healthy women have a lifetime risk of around 3 per cent of acquiring endometrial cancer, women with untreated PCOS appear to have a risk of 9 per cent.[17] One of the reasons why untreated PCOS is believed to lead to higher risk of endometrial cancer is that the uterine lining of women with PCOS is being built up all the time, and is not shed through menstruation. As a result, the cells of the uterine lining thicken and can begin to behave abnormally. This is easily preventable by ensuring that the woman has three or four menstrual bleeds over a year, with the help of contraceptive pills or another course of hormones.

Just to be clear, what's happening with this thickened uterine lining is not the same thing that happens when people skip their periods using hormonal contraception. With PCOS, the uterine lining is continuously receiving signals telling it to grow, whereas hormonal contraception prevents the lining from growing. Although the result in both cases is fewer periods, the mechanisms are quite different.

Other symptoms of PCOS

In addition to all the fuss with ovulation, the ovaries – as well as the fatty tissues and the adrenal glands – can produce too much of the male hormones known as androgens. All women produce some male sex hormones, but the balance is normally tipped in favour of the female variants. If the androgens get the upper hand, you may find that hair growth increases in places you're not used to having it, for example beard growth on your face, or a thick 'happy trail' – the broad strip of pubic hair on your belly. The excess hair is called hirsutism and over half of all women with PCOS are troubled by it.[18] A lot of women with PCOS also have problems with persistent acne, lasting well beyond puberty. The way they put on weight will also be affected. Women often tend to put on weight in a pear-like pattern – most of the fat settles around their bottom and thighs – but with PCOS, the male sex hormones mean that women tend to put on weight following the apple pattern – around the belly. You can even end up with a beer gut, one of the most unhealthy types of fat possible. However, androgens also have unnoticeable effects. For example, you may get high levels of cholesterol and fatty acids in the blood, and that's no good for the walls of your blood vessels.

The third place that often behaves abnormally when you have PCOS is the pancreas. This is an organ in the digestive system that produces substances that break down food and a hormone called insulin. Insulin is released after meals and sends the body's cells signals that trigger uptake and consumption of blood sugar. In 50–70 per cent of all women with PCOS, the cells do not react the way they should to insulin signals from the pancreas.[19] The women are insulin resistant and so the pancreas compensates by producing even more insulin, in the hope that the message will finally get through. Aren't people laughing at your joke? Talk louder!

This high insulin level is no good for the body. If you don't get the insulin resistance under control, you may develop type II diabetes over time. Women with PCOS have a much higher chance of developing it than other women with the same weight and lifestyle.[20] US studies have shown that 20 to 40 per cent of PCOS patients are in the preliminary stages of diabetes or have full-blown type II diabetes by the time they reach their 40s.[21] The combination of insulin resistance, abnormal levels of fat in the blood and the increased fat around the belly are key ingredients in the recipe for cardiovascular diseases. These changes can contribute to increasing the risk of cardiovascular diseases when you are older.

PCOS should be taken seriously

So, if you have irregular menstruation, PCOS may be the reason. To check whether you have it, your doctor will do blood tests to measure your hormone levels and examine your ovaries with ultrasound to check for cysts. If you turn out to be one of the women out there with PCOS, there are certain things it's important to think about to ensure your future health.

The most vital advice for women with PCOS relates to weight control and lifestyle changes. If you are overweight, you may have fewer problems if you lose weight. If your weight is normal, you don't need to think about this of course. Losing weight can be easier said than done, but any exercise and healthy eating will improve your wellbeing. Because for up to four out of five overweight women, losing just 5 per cent of their body weight – for example, going down from 80 to 76 kilograms – is enough to return their normal ovulation.[22] In addition, this can reduce insulin resistance as well as the likelihood of diabetes and cardiovascular disease. The problems with increased hair growth and acne also diminish, because the fact of being overweight in itself increases the production of male sex hormones.

We would also advise you to discuss starting a combined product, such as combined contraceptive pills, contraceptive patch or vaginal ring, with a doctor who is knowledgeable about PCOS. This is one of the most important parts of PCOS treatment. The oestrogen in the contraceptive pills will reduce the production and activity of male sex hormones in the ovaries, which will, in turn, help with both hair growth and acne. In addition, it is possible to reduce the development of more cysts and the risk of endometrial cancer. Women who cannot take oestrogen because of a risk of blood clots can use oestrogen-free methods of contraception such as the hormonal IUD or the contraceptive implant, but unfortunately these have no effect on the male hormones.

Think about whether you want children or not. If you do, it may be sensible not to put it off for too long. Many women with PCOS may need help to get pregnant and this process takes time. It may be a good idea to be prepared for that.

FIBROIDS – A UTERUS WITH BALLS

Did you get a bit of an unpleasant surprise last time you were at the gynae-cologist? A lot of us have benign growths, or tumours, known as *fibroids*, in our uterus. It's hardly surprising that your blood runs cold when you hear the word *tumour* applied to your own body, but in this situation you can relax. Just lie back in the gynaecologist's chair and breathe deeply. Fibroids are benign tumours that grow from cells in the muscle walls of the uterus. They have nothing to do with cancer. They are not cancer now and they will never become cancer. Doctors may refer to fibroids as myomas or 'muscle knots', which should make it easier to grasp the difference between benign and slightly less benign tumours.

Fibroids are made of what we call smooth, involuntary muscle; in other words, muscle we cannot control consciously, like the ones we have in our gut and stomach, for example. Fibroids are often spherical and rubbery. If you had one on the table in front of you, you could cut it in two with a knife and see that it's pearl-white inside, and not red as you might have expected. Fibroids look a little like pearls – the real ones that grow in oysters at the bottom of the sea.

Fibroids can grow in various places in the uterus, inside the wall and outside the wall protruding into the uterine cavity. Some women have just one, but it's common to have as many as six or seven.[23] They may be tiny or in worse cases they may grow to the size of a grapefruit. Fibroids don't necessarily grow steadily over time. Some may grow an awful lot in a short time, others will stop when they are one centimetre in diameter – and there are fibroids that shrink and vanish of their own accord.

Fibroids are very common in women up to the age of menopause. Like so much else when it comes to the genitals, they respond to oestrogen, so they only appear after puberty and tend to vanish after menopause. Up to one in two women discover that they have myomas, or fibroids.[24] There are probably even more who have them, but they're often so small that people don't notice them. Since fibroids are benign, there's no need to look for them just to check whether they are there or not. It's fine to have them as long as they're not giving you any trouble.

Most myomas do not have any symptoms, although you may get severe or prolonged menstrual bleeding, particularly if they are growing into the uterine cavity. Bleeding between periods is not common with fibroids. Nor is pain a classic sign, although some women do suffer pressure pain in their pelvis if they grow very big. One exception is if a fibroid begins to break up and die, for example owing to poor blood supply. This can be extremely painful, which can be frightening – especially if it happens during pregnancy – but it isn't dangerous.

If you picture a uterus filled with six or seven pearls the size of tennis balls, it's easy to see why fibroids might also cause other problems. They can, for example, press on the bladder, which lies in front of the uterus, giving you an urge to pee. They can also give you a heavy, bloated feeling, slightly reminiscent of pregnancy, and your stomach can, in fact, grow so that it looks as if you're several months gone.

In a kind of gruesome irony, the myomas can, in the worst case, make it difficult to become pregnant.[25] Fortunately this applies to a minority of women with them, but they're still the cause of infertility in 1 to 2 per cent of women who struggle to have children.[26] It isn't certain exactly what prevents pregnancy in these women, but the position rather than the size seems to be the main cause.[27] Fibroids that protrude into the uterus may make it difficult for the fertilised egg to fasten itself onto the endometrium, because, of course, the inside of the uterus is precisely where it needs to be. They can also block the opening into the Fallopian tubes, so that the sperm are unable to reach the egg, which is impatiently waiting for a nice date to fuse with. If fibroids are suspected to be the cause of the infertility, they may be removed, but it isn't certain how positive the effect is.[28]

One thing we are more uncertain about is how the fibroids affect pregnancy once a woman manages to conceive. Again, it seems to be the ones that grow into the uterine cavity that cause the most problems. Some studies have shown an increased risk of miscarriage, between 22 and 47 per cent, where the fibroids are inward growing.[29] Other than this, the fibroids do not seem to have any major adverse effect on the pregnancy, except that a Caesarean section may be needed if the fibroids are blocking the child's way into the birth canal. So, there's no reason to surgically remove them before having a baby.[30]

It is possible to limit the growth of the fibroids, but how? One simple solution is to try long-acting progestin products such as contraceptives – for example the contraceptive implant or hormonal IUD.[31] If you suffer from heavy bleeding because of the fibroids, hormonal contraception can also help combat this. The use of contraceptive methods with a low dosage of oestrogen doesn't cause the fibroids to grow, so there's nothing to stop you using these products if you prefer.

Generally speaking, fibroids in the uterus are a bit like freckles: you may have a few or a lot, they may be big or small, but they may well not cause any trouble. There's no need to remove them just because they're there. You only need to remove them if they cause problems. And remember: fibroids can almost never become cancer.

VULVODYNIA – UNEXPLAINED PAINS IN THE GENITALS

Are you suffering from pains in your genital area for which neither your doctor nor other health professionals can find an explanation? You are not alone, but the lack of available facts about these pains is frustrating. The pains are there, that's for certain. They take a toll on your everyday life and make it difficult to have sex – but where do they come from? For now, we have little knowledge about this.

All in all, there are many causes of pain in the genital area. Yeast infections and other genital ailments cause persistent burning and itching, and sexually transmitted infections, or STIs, can cause pain during sex. There are painful skin diseases, such as lichen sclerosus, that can affect the vulva and, more rarely, genital cancer can cause pain. Bartholin's glands (see p. 12) may become inflamed and extremely painful – the list goes on. The one thing all these conditions have in common is that they are usually demonstrable. If you see your doctor about the pain, she will examine you and find out the cause of the pain through testing. There's nothing odd about genital pain if you have recurring herpes outbreaks, but what happens if the doctors look and look and can't find anything?

If you have pain in your genital area and cannot find any definite reason for it, this is often called *vulvodynia*. Dynia comes from the Greek word for pain. Vulvodynia therefore means vulval pains.

One thing we should emphasise right from the start is that the pain of vulvodynia is absolutely real, even if the doctors can't find any cause. Many women with this condition are left feeling as though they're not being taken seriously when they can't get any clear answers about what's wrong with them. Perhaps they've gone through lots of examinations and visited one doctor after another without anybody finding anything wrong at all. Does this mean that the pain is all in their mind? Absolutely not – the pain is real. We do take you seriously.

There are several different ways of having vulvodynia, and this can mean two things. Firstly, that there are several unknown conditions that cause vulval pain, but since we still know so little about it, we place them under the same umbrella term. Secondly, the different kinds of unexplained vulval pain may be manifestations of a single condition that produces different symptoms from person to person.

It will be interesting to see what emerges once more research has been done in the field because fortunately medicine is advancing steadily. In the Middle Ages people believed all disease was caused by an imbalance in bodily fluids, and that bloodletting – perhaps with leeches – was the miracle cure for everything from depression to cancer. To give you a slightly more recent example, it's not so long since doctors believed stomach ulcers were caused by lifestyle factors such as stress and coffee drinking. However, a special bacterium called *helicobacter pylori* turned out to be the culprit.

This may prove to be the case with vulvodynia as well. Is it a neurological disease? Does a type of bacteria or virus cause an infection? Is it a reaction to another treatment? We shall see.

Women with vulvodynia may experience different kinds of pain. They may have spontaneous, burning sensations on their genitalia – the general medical terms for these types of pain are *allodynia* and *hyperalgesia*. With allodynia, stimuli that don't usually hurt – for example light pressure or touch – suddenly become painful. The touch of a finger can, for example, trigger burning pain on the vulva. Allodynia often occurs in areas that have been injured in some way. We don't know for sure whether this applies to allodynia of the genital area. Hyperalgesia means that stimuli that are usually painful become even more so. For example, a pinprick that you'd normally shrug off can result in intense pain. Both hyperalgesia and allodynia are *neuropathic pains*. This means that they arise because of an injury to or disease of the peripheral nerves – in other words, the nerves outside the brain and spinal cord.

Neuropathic pains are the most common forms of pain associated with vulvodynia, but we can't say for sure that other forms of pain cannot occur. It is possible that the pains vary from person to person and, as mentioned, we don't know whether all instances of vulvodynia are the same disease. Another important factor is that we all interpret pain in different ways. This applies to all pain, not just vulval pain. Some, for example, may experience the discomfort as an itching, and think that it is caused by something they're familiar with from before, such as a yeast infection. This can result in repeated antifungal treatments even though yeast is not the cause.[32]

There are also variations in where the pain is located, and this is one of the factors that divides vulvodynia into groups. Some people experience pain in the whole of their vulva, that is by the vaginal opening, on the clitoris and on and around the labia. This is referred to as *generalised vulvodynia* and is more common among slightly older women. Others have localised pain in a specific place on their vulva. This is called *localised vulvodynia* and is most common among younger women. Pain is most frequently experienced on the clitoris or right beside the vaginal opening, in the area known as the *vestibulum*, so these two *localised vulvodynias* each have their own name: *clitorodynia* and *vestibulodynia*.

Vulvodynia, and vestibulodynia in particular, was previously known as *vestibulitis*, a term you may have heard or read about in the media. When a medical term ends in –itis, it means we're talking about an *inflammation*. Vaginitis, for example, is the same as vaginal inflammation. Since nobody has managed to prove that any inflammation is present in the genitals when women have vulvodynia, doctors have opted to stop using the term vestibulitis. It is more accurate to call it vulvodynia or just vulvar pain.[33]

There is a difference in the way the pain behaves. Some women have what is called *provoked pain*, while others experience *spontaneous pain*. Provoked pain typically involves neuropathic pain – or hyperalgesia or allodynia. Provoked pain means that it hurts when something comes in direct contact with the genitals. This can occur in slightly different ways. Touch or pressure that would not normally hurt can cause great pain. Examples could include the pressure of a bicycle saddle, intercourse, tampon use and direct contact with the clitoris. You can become so sensitive that even the touch of loose-fitting clothes or underwear can hurt. One test doctors often use to find out whether you're suffering from provoked pain is to press on the painful area, for example on the entrance to the vagina, with a cotton bud.

Spontaneous pain means that the pain happens suddenly without there being any contact with anything at all. This pain is often of the burning kind. You may also experience a mixture of provoked and spontaneous pain. Some women experience a burning sensation constantly, while others have pain now and then.[34] Typically, localised vulvodynia, such as vestibulodynia, most often involves provoked pain, while generalised vulvodynia most often involves spontaneous pain, as well as pain triggered by contact with clothing.[35]

No definite connection has been found between vulvodynia and other genital problems, such as STIs. One popular theory, however, is that there is a connection between vulvodynia and treatment for yeast infections. This doesn't necessarily mean that you'll get vulvodynia from using antifungal treatment. As we explained earlier, many women believe that the vulvar discomfort is caused by yeast infections, and naturally enough, they use antifungal treatment to get rid of the problems. This can make it difficult to decide whether the treatment is causing the problems or the problems result in the treatment.

One study found a relationship between repeated yeast infections and vulvodynia, but the experiment was carried out on mice, so it's difficult to draw any conclusions when it comes to us bipeds.[36] The mice in the study experienced allodynia. The same study also found there was a tendency for the affected area to become extra sensitive. The number of nerve endings capable of perceiving the pain had risen. Based on this study, it may seem as if repeated yeast infections affected the mice's capacity to feel pain from a purely neurological perspective.

Other studies have shown that women with vulvodynia have developed alterations in their genital nerve supply. It may be that some women with vulvar pains have grown more pain-sensitive nerve fibres.[37] But it is unclear what causes these changes.

Good-girl syndrome?

If you've read about vulvodynia in the media, you've probably picked up on the fact that a lot of people focus on the potential psychological aspect of the illness. Many of those treating it, perhaps especially sexologists who deal with the interplay between psyche and sexuality, also highlight this in their work with patients. Might it be that vulvar pain affects women who have sex when they don't actually want to? Could it be that 'good girls' are the ones who are affected, or women who've had bad or painful sexual experiences in the past? What about the women who've been exposed to assault or abuse? All these possibilities have been applied to unexplained vulval pain. But do they hold water?

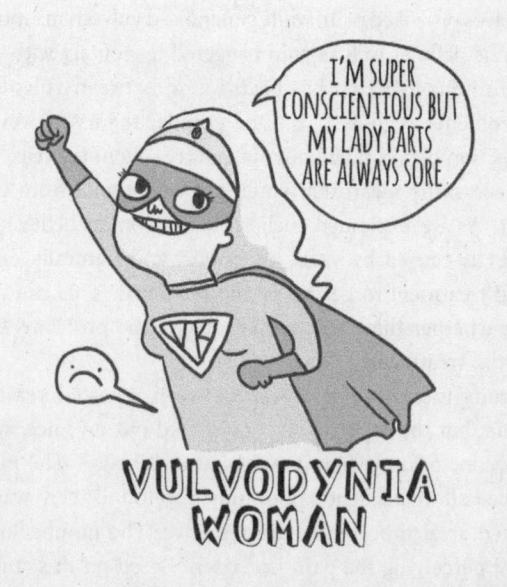

VULVODYNIA
WOMAN

It's easy to slap a 'psychological causes' label on conditions whose physical causes aren't immediately identifiable, but we should be very careful about doing this. If women don't recognise themselves in these descriptions, it can lead to confusion and anger. In particular, the term 'good girl' can create a misleading impression that the woman herself, or her personality, is responsible for the pain. So being capable and conscientious is supposed to lead to physical ailments that hamper your existence – this isn't constructive. That said, genital pains may well turn out to have psychological causes for some women, but that needn't be a source of shame.

A lot of women with vulvodynia use talk therapy as part of their treatment. This can help not only because they get to work on potential psychological aspects of the pain, but also because vulvodynia itself can be a major psychological burden that people may need help dealing with.

We know that all kinds of pain are closely linked to the psyche. Many people who experience pain will gradually develop avoidance behaviour and tensions that can worsen the underlying problem, leaving a person trapped in a vicious circle. The expectation that intercourse will be painful can, for example, cause you to unconsciously tense up your vagina to protect yourself, and then the attempts at intercourse will hurt even more.

It is also well known from pain research that the brain becomes more sensitive to new pain impulses when people live with pain over time – pain simply breeds pain. Relaxation techniques and psychotherapy can help people break out of this cycle of pain. However, this is not the same as claiming that vulvodynia must have a psychological cause from the outset.

As far as we know, there's no research that shows a clear link between vulvodynia and earlier assaults or sexual abuse. Even so, such an experience may be an underlying factor for some women with this condition. Studies that compare the psychological profiles of women with and without vulvodynia yield variable results. One study that compared 240 women with vulvodynia and as many without the condition, showed that it's much more common for vulvodynia to develop among women who have previously suffered anxiety-related conditions.[38] Another study, which compared two smaller groups of women, found no difference in the psychological profiles of women with and without vulvodynia.[39] How far vulvodynia is a disease with a psychological explanation is a matter of debate. It is perfectly possible to suffer from vulvodynia without having a history of psychological challenges or violent sexual experiences.

Since we know so little about what causes vulvodynia the treatment is still experimental and complex. Different methods that help deal with other pain syndromes are attempted in the hope that they will also help here. Nonetheless, the first step is to find a gynaecologist and/or GP with a specialist interest in vulval pain.

As we mentioned earlier, neuropathic pains are involved in some forms of vulvodynia and in this case there are some pretty good medicines, for example special antidepressants and some epilepsy medicines. These medicines, which help combat nerve pain, have proven to be effective for some women with vulvodynia.[40] Other women find that oestrogen helps, for example in the form of contraceptive methods such as the vaginal ring. The oestrogen affects the mucous membrane in the vagina, making it thicker. Analgesic gel may also reduce the pain, and women struggling with provoked pain who still want to have sex may benefit from using the gel during intercourse. In addition to talk therapies, many will find physiotherapy helpful. You can learn special exercises that'll make it easier to relax your pelvic-floor muscles. Many women with provoked vulvodynia also struggle with other conditions involving muscle tensions, for example neck and shoulder pain or tension headaches.

A general piece of advice often given to women with vulvodynia is not to do anything that causes pain. For example, it's important not to force yourself to have intercourse if it hurts. If you want to have sex nonetheless, you can try out other things that don't cause pain, alone or with your partner. Sexologists are good at offering advice and guidance in this respect, and it may be an idea to take along your partner, if you have one, to these appointments. People are also advised to be careful about using perfume, soap and creams on their genitals, as there is some speculation that this may exacerbate the pain.

Vaginismus

Many people discuss vulvodynia in the same breath as a condition called *vaginismus* – yet another difficult and somewhat controversial diagnosis. Vaginismus is where a woman involuntarily contracts or has tensions in the pelvic-floor muscles that surround the entrance of her vagina. These women often refuse vaginal penetration – whether sexual or for gynaecological examinations – because they suffer or expect to suffer pain and discomfort. In other words, vaginismus can be a demanding diagnosis, which complicates sex, tampon use and medical examinations.

Some think of vaginismus as an involuntary muscle spasm that makes the vagina physically narrower. The Norwegian term sometimes used for vaginismus translates as vaginal cramps. Research using equipment that measures muscle activity has found no clear proof that women with vaginismus have 'muscle spasms', nor is there any professional agreement about which muscles might be involved in vaginismus.[41]

The diagnoses of vestibulodynia and vaginismus overlap. The pains of vaginismus are often described as being the same as or similar to the pains women get with vestibulodynia. The pains are mostly located in the entrance to the vagina and are therefore distinct from the deep pain women get when they have endometriosis or an inflamed cervix from STIs. Whether these two diagnoses are two sides of the same coin, or two separate conditions that often occur together is difficult to say.

The treatment for vaginismus is much the same as for vulvodynia. With vaginismus, additional work is often done on training women to be able to tolerate having something in their vagina; this generally starts with the woman herself inserting a very thin object, known as a dilator, whose size is later gradually increased. Analgesic gel is always used during the insertion so that it won't be painful. This element of the treatment can be done in collaboration with a gynaecologist, sexologist or physiotherapist.

Both conditions can be limiting

Vaginismus and vulvodynia take a great toll on a woman's joie de vivre and sex life. For many, a normal sex life becomes impossible while the condition persists and their relationship can deteriorate or fail. Many worry whether they'll ever have a partner or children, whether they'll have to live alone for the rest of their lives. They feel inadequate. The fact that we still know so little about the conditions can lead to feelings of bitterness, and many women may feel stigmatised by their dealings with the health system. One small consolation pending further information is that most women do get better, and many become entirely healthy.

CHLAM, THE CLAP AND THEIR DISTANT RELATIVES

We're major fans of the *Paradise Hotel* reality TV show and hooted with laughter the time one of the male participants claimed he could tell just by looking at girls whether or not they had venereal disease, and so he never used condoms.[42] We don't know what power he is blessed with. Perhaps he got a certificate from Hogwarts School of Witchcraft and Wizardry or is related to one of those TV psychics? One thing's for sure, though, nobody can tell just by looking at women (or men) whether or not they have venereal disease. A lot of people don't even know they've been infected themselves – and that's the core of the problem. People keep on having sex without condoms even though they've got venereal diseases. So, the thing you don't know about then spreads.

We generally call venereal diseases sexually transmitted infections, or STIs for short. STIs can infect you when you have sex or sexual contact with another person who's already got one. The diseases are caused by different types of microorganisms, such as bacteria, viruses and parasites. Some of the STIs can only be transmitted through bodily fluids such as blood and sperm. Others can be passed on through contact between skin and mucous membranes. Some STIs are very common, while others are rarer in our part of the world. It's not unlikely that you'll catch one or several STIs over your lifetime – it's one of the few disadvantages of having sex.

Since sexuality has long been associated with shame and guilt – especially for women – the same has also been true of STIs. Even now, few people are open about their own problems with genital warts and chlamydia. Although these conditions are common and sometimes difficult to protect against, many people are left with the feeling that they ought to have had less casual sex and perhaps avoided exposing their partner to infection. We hope that both knowledge about and normalisation of STIs can eliminate some of these awful feelings of shame. Infection is first and foremost a question of poor condom use and after that, of good and bad luck. It's not a question of your 'personal sexual morality'. Some people sleep with hundreds of people without using condoms and miraculously get away without an infection, while others can have a single one-night stand and end up with genital warts. Shit happens in your sexual life too.

Before we had modern medicine and antibiotics, some of the STIs were linked to more than just shame. They were also the cause of serious suffering and, in the worst case, death. For a long time, gonorrhoea was a common cause of blindness in children, who were infected by their mothers during birth. It was so common that all new born babies in Norway were treated for gonorrhoea with eye-drops as soon as they saw the light of day. In Henrik Ibsen's famous 1881 play *Ghosts*, Osvald, the suffering artistic soul, has syphilis, which ultimately attacks his brain and central nervous system. Today, we can treat syphilis with penicillin, enabling people infected with it to return to perfect health. That wasn't possible in the 19th century and many people suffered like Osvald and died of the disease.

Despite the medical advances, STIs are still a major obstacle to public health worldwide. Since the 1980s, when AIDS took the lives of thousands of young gay men, the disease has rarely been out of the news and with good reason. AIDS, or Acquired Immune Deficiency Syndrome, is a disease that causes the collapse of the immune defences – the body's protection against bacteria, viruses and other junk. The microorganism responsible for this is HIV, the human immunodeficiency virus. In 2015, 1.1 million people died of HIV-related causes, and more than 36.7 million people are living with the virus today. Since the start of the epidemic, 35 million people have lost their lives.[43] Once you've been infected with HIV, there's no way to get rid of it. In the UK, HIV-positive people receive such good treatment that they can live a long and (almost) normal life. With thorough treatment, they will no longer be contagious. So, there are medicines that can hold the virus in check, but unfortunately, only half of the people in the world who are infected have access to these medicines.

In Norway today, neither syphilis nor HIV are widespread, but they do happen. In 2015, 221 people were newly diagnosed with HIV, while 189 were diagnosed with syphilis in 2014.[44] That's an incredibly small number by comparison with other STIs, which can almost be viewed as endemic.

You can check for HIV and syphilis with a blood test, but since they're so rare, there's no need to take tests regularly unless you're particularly exposed to risk of infection.

Chlamydia

The most common bacterial disease is called chlamydia. In Norway in 2014, 292,772 chlamydia tests were carried out, of which 24,811 were positive – in other words, as many as 8 per cent![45] A positive test means that chlamydia was found. In the 15–19 and 20–24 age groups, the number of positive tests is higher than for all the other age groups put together. In the 15–19 age group, 13.6 per cent of the girls tested positive, against 16.1 per cent of the boys. Among the 20–24-year-olds, 10.6 per cent of the women tested positive against 16.3 per cent of the men. We must assume hidden figures are high, since many people don't get tested.

The majority of those who test positive are women – 60 per cent of them, no less. This doesn't mean that women get more chlamydia, but that they're better at getting themselves tested. As you can see from the numbers in the 15–19 and 20–24 age groups, the proportion of boys who have chlamydia when they actually do get tested is higher. This means that more boys than girls are walking around with chlamydia but don't know it.

It seems as if some boys take a chance on the girls taking care of the testing, and assume they'll get a phone call if a past partner tests positive. It's not very classy, not to mention being far from watertight as strategies go. You may well have chlamydia even if your sex partner has tested negative. The risk of infection isn't 100 per cent for every sexual encounter and that's why both partners ought to be tested. In other words, the anti-condom participant in *Paradise Hotel* and a whole bunch of others along with him really need to change their habits. Using a condom is always a smart move when you have sex with a new person, even if you've had a test. There's no guarantee that your partner will have been as smart as you. What's more, now and then we forget condoms – and what's done is done. If you forget to use a condom, it's important to get tested.

Mycoplasma and gonorrhoea

Two illnesses that are a bit like chlamydia are the bacterial diseases mycoplasma and gonorrhoea. Condoms protect you effectively against all three. Gonorrhoea is much rarer than chlamydia. In Norway in 2014, 682 people were diagnosed with it. Just 119 of these were heterosexual women, but an ever-increasing number are being infected.[46]

Mycoplasma is a disease that is often overlooked by GPs. It is a bit like chlamydia's little brother. They're very similar, have the same symptoms and probably the same after-effects – but we'll come back to that later. Even so, there's no routine test done for mycoplasma. It will only be checked if the patient has symptoms. And even then, it doesn't occur to many doctors to run tests. The treatment isn't the same as for chlamydia, so it's important for the disease to be picked up. If you have symptoms, but test negative for chlamydia it may be sensible to ask for a mycoplasma test.

What are the symptoms?

The most common symptoms of chlamydia, mycoplasma and gonorrhoea are a change or increase in discharge, a stinging sensation when you pee and general discomfort or itching of the genitals, urethra or anus, depending on where the infection is located. All three bacterial diseases often attack the cervix, which becomes inflamed and this can make intercourse unpleasant or painful. Some may find they bleed a bit after or during sex owing to pressure on the sore cervix. Generally, we should always be alert to any bleeding from the vagina when we don't know what's causing it – particularly if it's connected with sex. One explanation may be menstruation or the use of hormonal contraception, for example, but it may be caused by STIs or other diseases and so it should always be checked by a doctor.

However, not everybody has symptoms. In fact, only half of all men and as few as a third of women get chlamydia symptoms.[47] Nor is it common to experience symptoms with mycoplasma, and some people don't have any symptoms with gonorrhoea either. So, why should we bother about something if we don't even notice it? Well, firstly, bacterial diseases are extremely contagious. The risk of infection with chlamydia during unprotected sex is 20 per cent.[48] Secondly, there is a danger of long-term damage.

If the bacteria get the chance, they can find their way up through the cervix and end up in the uterus and the Fallopian tubes. There, they can cause inflammation. This is known as pelvic inflammatory disease (or PID), and you can get it from chlamydia, mycoplasma and gonorrhoea.[49*] It is estimated that untreated chlamydia will cause 10 to 15 per cent of people to develop acute PID.[50] The danger is that the inflammation may cause scarring in the Fallopian tubes, which can block them (a common reason why women have trouble conceiving) and it can cause chronic pain.

If you get PID, it is common to feel sick and unwell, and you often get severe pains in your lower belly, vaginal bleeding, fever and increased discharge. Typically, the pains do not diminish or get better, but increase. These symptoms should all be taken seriously and checked by a doctor as quickly as possible, at the out-of-hours surgery if need be.

It is also possible, though not common, to have symptom-free pelvic inflammatory disease, which may only be discovered years later during investigation for infertility.[51] This is yet another reason to get checked regularly after changing sexual partners.

Chlamydia, mycoplasma and gonorrhoea can all be treated with antibiotics.

---

* There is disagreement in professional circles as to how far mycoplasma can cause pelvic inflammatory disease. Research in this field is still sparse, but a few small individual studies suggest this to be the case. Better safe than sorry.

For now, most people who are infected return to full health without long-term damage, but a worrying trend of antibiotic resistance is developing, particularly in cases of mycoplasma and gonorrhoea. Antibiotic resistance means that the bacteria become immune to some types of antibiotics, so that more powerful medicines are needed to get rid of them. In other words, the best option is to avoid getting infected from the outset by using condoms.

Herpes and HPV

There are two more STIs that are even more common than chlamydia – herpes and HPV, both of which are viral diseases. HPV stands for *human papilloma virus* and there are many different forms of the virus. Some types cause genital warts, while others can cause cervical cancer. Herpes is the same as cold sores and is a disease that causes small blisters on the skin.

Herpes and HPV are passed on through contact between skin and mucous membranes. We don't know exactly how many people are infected with the different types, but both are very widespread and it's common for people not to notice that they've been infected.

Because there aren't necessarily any symptoms, many people are infected by a partner who doesn't know that he or she is contagious. This makes it difficult to protect against infection. Nor is it certain that condoms provide good enough protection. If, for example, a man has genital warts or herpes on the root of his penis, he will be able to infect his partner even if he uses a condom as it doesn't cover the infectious area.

You can be vaccinated against HPV and some of the vaccines give protection against both the viruses that cause genital warts and those that can cause cervical cancer (see p. 241). If you have genital warts, they can be treated with cryotherapy (frozen with liquid nitrogen) or swabbed with different medications that make them disappear. In other words, it's very much like the treatment you have when you get a verruca from the showers at the swimming pool. Genital warts are not dangerous and they have nothing to do with the risk of cancer. Warts and cancer are linked to different types of the HPV virus.

HPV infections will often pass of their own accord and so will the warts, but some people are bothered by warts that constantly come back.

Herpes, on the other hand, is a virus you cannot get rid of. Once you've been infected, the virus will remain in your nerve cells in a kind of hibernation for the rest of your life. You may have several outbreaks, which can be shortened with a course of antivirals prescribed by your doctor. However, herpes isn't dangerous and the problems tend to diminish over time.

How can I protect myself against STIs?
Condoms provide good protection against HIV, chlamydia, mycoplasma and gonorrhoea. However, HPV and herpes can be passed on through skin contact, so you can be infected from places that are not covered by the condom.

When giving a woman oral sex, the other partner can use a dam – a thin, transparent sheet of latex that can be placed over the vulva. This will, for example, be able to prevent herpes infection from mouth to genitals or from genitals to mouth. Dams aren't especially practical (and are almost impossible to get hold of – they're called dental dams in the UK as dentists use them for root-canal surgery) so they aren't widely used. You can make your own by snipping the top off a condom, cutting the length of the cylinder and spreading it out so that you get a large, transparent square.

When should I get tested?
It's sensible to get tested for chlamydia every time you have unprotected sex with a new partner, even if you don't have any symptoms. It's also a good idea for both you and your partner to get checked as early in your relationship as possible. Since you can have STIs for a long time without noticing anything is wrong, you may, in fact, both have chlamydia without knowing it. If you're symptom-free, it's normally enough to do a self-test from your doctor's surgery, a young people's clinic or a genito-urinary medicine (GUM) clinic that will involve a urine test or using a little cotton bud to take samples from your vagina or anus. (If you've had unprotected anal sex, it isn't certain that the infection will be picked up unless you also take an anal test, so you should ask for one.)

If you have symptoms, you may also need to have a genital examination. It's up to your doctor. It's important to contact your doctor if it stings when you pee, you have itching, your discharge changes, you have a rash, blisters or unusual bleeding and/or if there are any other things you notice. No tests are run for herpes or the HPV virus unless the patient has specific problems.

It is important to be aware that a chlamydia test is only deemed effective if it is taken two weeks after you were potentially exposed to infection. This means that you can only rely on a negative result if the test was done two or more weeks after the sex in question. You can, of course, test yourself earlier as many people test positive before the two weeks are up, and therefore can start the treatment earlier. If you get a positive result before two weeks have passed, you can be sure that you have chlamydia. However, if an early test comes back negative, you can't be entirely certain of the result until you take a new test, at least two weeks after you were potentially exposed to infection. This two-week rule also applies to testing for mycoplasma and gonorrhoea.[52]

Risk and dangerous holiday sex

Now, we've discussed a long list of venereal diseases, or STIs, but focused on the chlamydia test. What about the other diseases? Some women go to the doctor and ask to be tested for 'everything', but there's no need to be tested for everything every time. Which tests you should have is something you should decide together with your doctor, and this will depend on what risk you've had of becoming infected with a venereal disease.

If you're a heterosexual woman living in the UK and only have sex with heterosexual men living in the UK, you have a lower risk of the serious diseases such as HIV, syphilis and gonorrhoea than if you'd had unprotected sex with sex workers on holiday in Thailand. It goes without saying. Among heterosexuals in the UK, chlamydia is absolutely the most common venereal disease and it's often enough to test for that, as well as gonorrhoea.

However, if you've had unprotected sex while you've been on holiday abroad it's important to tell your doctor. Doctors often forget to ask, so don't expect them to take the initiative. Get yourself tested, even if you only had sex with sweet British boys at the Full Moon Party in Thailand as you haven't a clue who else they've had sex with apart from you on their backpacking holiday. The same applies if you've had sex with somebody who's just back from travelling in a country with a lot of venereal diseases. And just to set the record straight, it's worth being aware that this doesn't just apply to trips to Thailand; many Brits pick up infections in, say, Germany, Spain and Poland, which have quite different incidences of venereal diseases than the UK. If you've sold or bought sex, you should definitely take a broader range of tests. The same applies if you've injected drugs or have had sex with a person who does so.

In the UK, the group consisting of men who have sex with men (MSM) has the highest risk of contracting more serious venereal diseases.* Gonorrhoea and syphilis are much more common among the MSM group than in the heterosexual population. This makes it extra important for these men to get tested. It may be good to remember that this also applies to women who have sex with MSM. If your last male one-night stand also has sex with men, the risk of disease is higher than if he just has sex with other women. The focus on MSM isn't about shaming people – it's a question of pure statistics.

You may have good or bad luck whether you have sex with women, men or men who have sex with men. It won't do any harm to test yourself for the less common diseases, but the risk isn't especially high, so you don't need to do it every time. Remember though, test often, test according to the risk and use condoms as often as possible.

HERPES – IS YOUR SEX LIFE OVER?

Small, painful blisters on your lips or your genitals don't sound much like fun. Herpes is more common than you think and it's infectious, a nuisance and almost impossible to protect against, but fortunately it's harmless. Even so, it seems as if herpes is the venereal disease a lot of people are most frightened of.

Many are scared by the knowledge that you can't get rid of herpes. Once you've been infected, the virus will be in your body for the rest of your life. This raises a lot of questions. Does it mean, for example, that you're always infectious and that you can never have sex with anybody without a condom again?

The sudden appearance of herpes in a relationship also creates a lot of distrust and uncertainty. Who infected whom? Has your partner of three years been unfaithful to you?

There are a lot of myths and misunderstandings about herpes. Anxiety about it is common, both among those who are infected and those who are afraid of becoming infected.

---

* We use the term 'men who have sex with men' in preference to 'homosexual'. It is quite possible to be a man who has sex with men without identifying as homosexual. Sexual orientation is not necessarily the same as who you have sex with.

Herpes is a viral disease that affects the skin and mucous membranes and there's more than one type. Two slightly different viruses may be the culprits: herpes simplex virus 1 (HSV-1) and herpes simplex virus 2 (HSV-2). The herpes virus is transmitted through contact with the skin or mucous membrane, such as kissing or sex. It can also be transmitted indirectly. The classic example is the kindergarten kid who's infected after sucking the same plastic dinosaur as the other children. Over half of the population is probably infected with HSV-1 on their mouth during childhood.[53]

We don't know exactly how many people are infected with herpes in total because there isn't any register. But for once it's almost correct to say that *everybody* has it, unlike that time you tried to convince your parents that *everybody else* had a Game Boy and that you had to have one too. It is believed that as many as 70 per cent are infected with HSV-1 and 40 per cent with HSV-2. You may be infected with both types or just one of them. On top of that, it's possible that an even larger share of the population has herpes. A lot of those who are infected don't know a thing about it, because not everybody gets the associated problems.

Just stop and think about these figures a bit. After all, this means that it's more common to be infected than not. Even so, a lot of people think of herpes as being the end of the world. But more than 70 per cent of the Norwegian population haven't had their lives destroyed or found themselves unable to have sex again!

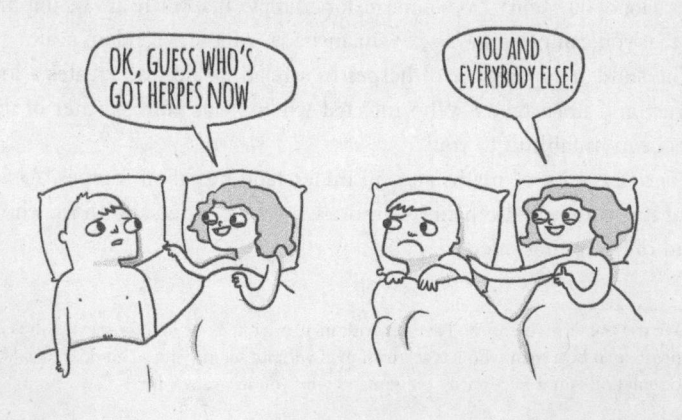

216

But hang on a second. Oral herpes and genital herpes are two different diseases, aren't they? So why are we talking about them as if they were the same thing. A sexually transmitted infection is pretty different from a cold sore, isn't it…?

Herpes is, in fact, the same wherever you have it on your body. Before, it was thought that HSV-1 was mostly linked to oral herpes, and HSV-2 to genital herpes. But HSV-1 can just as easily cause outbreaks on the genitals and HSV-2 can just as easily cause an outbreak on the lips, assuming that this is where you've been infected. You can also get herpes around the anus, on your fingers or (if you're really unlucky) in your eye. That said, HSV-1 on the genitals involves fewer and milder symptoms than HSV-2.[54]

So, genital herpes is also a cold sore, while oral herpes can be a sexually transmitted infection. It's possible to transmit the infection from genitals to lips and even more common the other way. As many as 80 per cent of the young women who contract genital herpes these days are, in fact, infected by HSV-1 from the lips of a partner during oral sex.[55]

Since so many people have herpes without knowing about it, this means in practice that many young women are infected by a partner who doesn't know that he or she has herpes to start off with either. So how are you supposed to protect yourself against it?

Once you've been infected, the virus can cause an outbreak within a couple of days, but it is also possible to be infected without noticing anything. After you've been infected, a gang of herpes viruses will move up the nerves from the area of skin where the infection occurred. They'll settle down to sleep inside a nerve cell a bit deeper in your body, like a bear going into hibernation. And there they will remain for the rest of your life. Now and again, the virus will move down through the nerves and out onto your skin. Then a new outbreak may occur, causing blisters to form in the same place as last time. It is also possible to have a *hidden outbreak* – in other words, the virus may be on the skin without you noticing anything at all. This is like the invisible bear waking up from hibernation.

A visible herpes outbreak starts with discomfort in the form of a prickling, burning sensation on the skin of your genitals or your lips. Then small blisters appear, growing in clusters, several crowded together. After a few days, the blisters dry out and become scabs, which eventually fall off.

The first outbreak is usually the worst. It is known as a primary herpes outbreak and can make some people very ill. They may have fever or problems urinating because the stinging in their genitals is so bad. As with everything else, you should visit your doctor if you get severe symptoms without knowing for sure what the problem is. A primary herpes outbreak will last longer than subsequent ones. You may get new blisters for one to two weeks. The scabs will disappear entirely three or four weeks after that.[56] If you have a dramatic primary outbreak, it may help to know that the next outbreak won't be as bad – if, indeed, you have another outbreak at all.[57] Many people never have any more after the first one.

If you do have a new outbreak, it will always occur in the same place as the first one. The number of outbreaks will usually diminish over the years. There is no medicine that can get rid of the herpes, but there is a course of tablets that your doctor can prescribe to calm and shorten the episode if you notice that it's imminent. In especially troublesome cases involving many outbreaks each year, you can use medication over longer periods to suppress them.

New outbreaks often come at times when your immune defences are low. That's why the common name for oral herpes is cold sore. You often get it when you're ill, for example with a cold. Stress, menstruation or sun can also trigger an outbreak, as can irritation of the skin – for example chafing underwear and waxing or shaving.

There is no vaccine against herpes, as there is with HPV, but there's no need for one either. Herpes acts a bit like a vaccine against itself: if you've been infected with it once, for example as a child, you can't be infected with the same virus on another place on your body later in life. The virus activates your immune defences so that they'll always recognise the same virus and prevent it from settling in new nerve cells. That means you'll only be infected in one place by each virus. If you're infected by one virus on your mouth, you're protected against infection by the same one on the genitals and vice versa.

But as you now know, there are two herpes viruses. If you've previously been infected with HSV-1, you won't be protected against infection by HSV-2. *In theory*, you can get herpes in two places if the two different herpes viruses are involved. However, it must be said that you have a certain degree of cross-protection. If you're infected with virus number two, you often have milder symptoms or no symptoms at all.

Since herpes works a bit like a vaccine, you can't infect yourself. If you have genital herpes, the virus can't move to other places on your body. Watch out, though! That only applies once the immune system has been activated. Your immune defences take a bit of time to build up to recognising herpes, so you can, in fact, infect yourself the first time you have an outbreak with one of the herpes types. So, you should be extra careful about hand washing and hygiene the first time you have an outbreak. Don't rub your eyes when you've got virus on your fingers – just don't!

Even though you can't infect yourself once the first outbreak is over, you can infect other people. The most common question we're asked about herpes is: 'when am I contagious?' Naturally enough, people with genital herpes are scared of infecting others – and how are you supposed to know you're safe? People also wonder if treatment with tablets prevents infection or whether there are special times when they shouldn't have sex.

The answer is that for transmission to occur through skin and mucous-membrane contact, there must be virus on the skin or the mucous membranes. Since herpes tends to lie hibernating in the nerve cells deep in the body, you're not usually contagious. The virus must have moved out from the nerves and onto your skin for you to be able to infect other people. This is something that happens when you have an outbreak. You are most contagious a week before an outbreak, because that's when the virus is gathering on the skin, and during the outbreak itself. The blisters are full of the virus. It may be sensible to avoid sex when you can feel that an outbreak is on the way – which often happens several days before the blisters appear. But of course, it can be difficult to know for certain that an outbreak is imminent a week before it arrives.

Then there are the hidden outbreaks too. The virus can wander out onto the skin without you noticing anything and without you having any blisters – but even so, you are contagious. In practice that means that you aren't normally contagious, but you *can* be contagious at any time. You can never be certain that you're not contagious. There are no safe periods. By now you may be thinking: but that's a total crisis! It is quite simply impossible to be certain that you won't infect other people and that's probably the most difficult aspect of being infected. But think again.

Let's say that you have HSV-1 of the genitals and want to have sex with

219

a new person. There's a 70 per cent chance that your potential partner has already been infected with the virus and is therefore protected against new infection without knowing it. That alone reduces the risk dramatically. If, in addition, your partner has a cold sore on his or her mouth, you can be almost certain that you won't pass the infection on, since oral herpes is usually caused by HSV-1. If your partner is already infected with HSV-1, he or she is protected against fresh infection by you.

Another way of looking at it is that most people will be infected sooner or later regardless. If you don't infect them, somebody else will do so at a later date. Herpes is harmless and most of the people who have the virus will hardly notice.

Herpes in a relationship

Finally, we need to talk a bit about a difficult problem connected with herpes: herpes in a relationship. Let's say that neither you nor your partner has had herpes blisters before. Not on your mouth, not on your genitals. You've been together for three years and have a fantastic relationship. And then it happens. You get a severe outbreak of blisters on your genitals and think the worst. You haven't been with anybody, so your partner must have been, mustn't he or she?

As you now know, you won't necessarily be aware that you have herpes. It's not a given that you had an outbreak of blisters when you were infected. You may have had herpes for a long time without having any visible signs. It's also quite possible you could have been infected by one of your partner's invisible outbreaks. In other words, infidelity need not have come into the picture at all! As we have already said, herpes is common and you don't necessarily know you have it. We have seen relationships ruined by unfounded accusations of infidelity after one partner has a herpes outbreak. Of course, it's possible infidelity may have been involved, but herpes is no proof of that. If you don't have any other reason to doubt your partner, herpes shouldn't be the factor that sows the seeds of distrust.

It's great for people to take responsibility for not infecting their partners with venereal diseases. If we were talking about chlamydia, we'd applaud loudly, but when it comes to herpes, it often just makes us sad. It's so unnecessary for people to be afraid of having sex because of herpes. Herpes isn't HIV, even though both are viruses you can't get rid of. It's quite harmless and it isn't the end of the world to be infected with genital herpes. You're one of many. Yes, in fact, you're one of the majority. It's highly likely it will give you very few problems over the course of your life. And if you do have problems, the chances are that they'll diminish. If you are one of the few unlucky people who have lots of outbreaks, treatment is available.

INTENSE ITCHING AND ROTTEN FISH –
GENITAL PROBLEMS YOU'LL CERTAINLY ENCOUNTER

Something's brewing between your legs. It's red, it smells peculiar or it's itching so much you can't sleep at night. Yeast infections and bacterial vaginosis are common genital problems that aren't caused by sexually transmitted infections. Most women are hit by one or the other, or both, over the course of their lives. Both conditions are harmless, but they can be an incredible nuisance. Since you'll probably encounter these genital problems, it's worth finding out a bit more about them.

Microorganisms such as bacteria and fungi usually trigger negative associations and a yearning for soap and kitchen spray. Who hasn't heard how quickly bacteria can multiply on a dishcloth, or seen how fungus spreads across a wall in a damp cellar? It's enough to give you the shudders – but not all microorganisms are harmful.

Some bacteria are totally necessary for us to function, for example, the gut bacteria that assist our digestion. In fact, we have around ten times as many bacteria as we have cells in our bodies, and that doesn't mean that we are unwell.

The mucous membrane on the vulva and in the vagina is covered with microorganisms that constitute what is known as the *normal flora* of the genitals. They help keep your vagina healthy by supporting the immune system in its battle against alien microorganisms and by keeping the vaginal environment in balance. As you may remember, the vagina is self-cleaning, and, in fact, using soap and especially douches eliminates its natural protection.

The vagina's normal flora varies according what stage of life you are at. Before you enter puberty and after menopause, the normal flora consists mostly of skin and gut bacteria, but when you are fertile your body is influenced by oestrogen. This hormone makes the mucous membrane thick and active, and the normal flora becomes unique to your genitals, and differs from the flora in other parts of your body.

The normal flora of fertile women consists for the most part of different types of lactic-acid bacteria, lactobacilli, which rely on oestrogen for their nourishment and survival. The lactobacilli produce acid like the type you find in natural yoghurt. This ensures that the vagina has a low pH of around 4.5, creating an environment that is inhospitable to bad bacteria types, which aren't comfortable in acidic surroundings. In addition, normal flora contains a couple of other bacteria types as well as a bit of yeast fungus and a bit of virus.[58] All the microorganisms are battling for the same food and a place to live, and since there are so many different types, none of them gain the upper hand. Together with the body's immune defences, the different microorganisms keep one another in check. However, the genitals are vulnerable to problems when the normally protective flora becomes imbalanced.

Yeast infections in the vagina

Let's start off with yeast infections. Around 20 per cent of all women have a kind of yeast known as *Candida albicans* as part of their vagina's normal flora.[59] Many have this kind of yeast in their anus and it may move from there to the vagina, especially if the opportunities for growth there are good. As many as 50 per cent of all pregnant women have yeast in their vaginas.[60] This may be because *Candida albicans* loves oestrogen and the body is extra full of oestrogen when you're pregnant. *Candida albicans* is responsible for the vast majority of yeast infections.

Hang on, though. *Yeast* – you mean like the stuff we put in rolls and bread? Almost! It isn't exactly what you'd find at the supermarket, but it is similar. In fact, one woman with a vaginal yeast infection used the yeast to make sourdough bread in November 2015 and became a genuine internet sensation.[61] The trick was to collect a bit of her discharge using a dildo and to use it to make sourdough. The sourdough worked and she baked a loaf, which she then ate. She said it tasted 'pretty damn nice'.

If you're among the 20 per cent whose vagina always contains yeast, this doesn't mean you have a *yeast infection* – that only happens when the yeast causes inflammation of the mucous membrane. In other words, when you've got it, you'll know all about it.

Also known as thrush, this yeast infection can affect both the interior of the vagina and the inner labia. The itching may be intense and some women find that it stings or burns down below, too. This can make intercourse painful or cause a stinging sensation in your vulva when you pee. The infected mucous membrane becomes red and swollen. Some women also get a whitish, lumpy discharge that can be described as looking like cottage cheese, while others get a runny discharge.

Some women find that when they have a vaginal yeast infection, their male partners develop symptoms on their penis, such as a rash or an itching sensation. Nonetheless, we must stress that a yeast infection is not a sexually transmitted infection. You can still have sex even if you have one or are taking treatment for one. The man's problems don't usually need separate treatment. It's enough for you to get rid of the infection and then his symptoms will pass, too.

Since yeast infection or thrush is so common, you can buy treatment at any chemist without a prescription. There are many types and all of them work equally well. The treatment consists of a cream and vaginal tablets, known as a pessaries, or antifungal tablets you take orally. If you use the vaginal pessary, you should insert it before you go to bed so that it can do its work overnight. If you do it in the daytime, the pessary has a tendency to dissolve and rapidly run out into your knickers. If you use the cream, you need to smear a thin layer of it on your inner labia, all the way from your clitoris to your anus. It may be a good idea to avoid vaginal pessaries when you're having your period, not because it's harmful but because the blood can carry the medication out of the vagina – flush it out, so to speak.

The availability of these over-the-counter treatments lowers the threshold for women to diagnose and treat themselves when they have thrush-like symptoms. The problem with this is that *all that itches is not thrush*! If it itches down below, there's only a 50 per cent likelihood that it's thrush.[62] Different genital conditions can have similar symptoms. So, we recommend in the strongest possible terms that women who suffer new symptoms should visit their doctor. Itching and changes in discharge are vague symptoms that can be caused by anything at all, for example, sexually transmitted infections such as chlamydia and gonorrhoea, and it's worth identifying these as early as possible. Different types of eczema and irritating conditions of the genitals are also common, sometimes owing to residual detergent in your underwear, or the use of perfumed soaps or intimate wipes.

It turns out that women are not good at distinguishing between thrush and other genital conditions, even if they've had thrush before. Women only diagnose thrush correctly in one out of three cases.[63] If, in all these situations, they opt for over-the-counter treatment instead of a trip to the doctor, this leads to a lot of pointless, incorrect treatment that doesn't help eliminate the problems. Unnecessary use of antifungal treatments can also delay diagnosis of the actual problem, which can result in new, additional symptoms. In fact, extensive use of antifungal medications can itself cause an irritation of the mucous membrane that is reminiscent of a yeast infection. In other words, there's nothing stupid about taking a trip to the doctor to make sure it really is thrush – at least the first time you have problems or if you find that the symptoms are constantly recurring.

When you've been diagnosed as having thrush and use antifungal medication, it's important to use the treatment the way your doctor or the pharmacist recommends. Even if the problems go away, you must always complete the course. Continue to use the cream for at least two days after the symptoms disappear. If you finish the treatment too early, there's a risk that small amounts of thrush will remain, and then the infection may flare up again when you stop.

Yeast infections are common. We know that three out of four women get them over the course of their lives. But what causes them? It's actually not that easy to put a finger on it. We know of several things that predispose us to yeast infections. We know that many women develop thrush after taking a course of antibiotics, or because they wash their genitals too often. After all, soap and antibiotics will help eliminate the normal flora that keeps our genitals healthy. We also know that oestrogen has something to do with it. Pre-pubescent and post-menopausal women rarely have problems with thrush since their genitals are not as influenced by sex hormones, whereas pregnant women can be troubled by it frequently. We know thrush often appears at certain points in the menstrual cycle. Women suffer from it most often before menstruation, unlike bacterial vaginosis, which we'll come back to shortly.

People with diabetes are especially prone to it, particularly if their blood sugar is not well controlled. We also see that girls have thrush more often once they've become sexually active, and those who have sex several times a month are somewhat more predisposed to it.

Some women have long-term problems with yeast infections that never entirely go away. It can be a great hindrance for these women. Around 3 to 5 per cent of all women suffer from more than four yeast infections a year.[64] If you're very prone to it, it's important to talk to your doctor, as she may need to do a proper examination and can prescribe an antifungal treatment that is stronger than the ones available over the counter.

Unfortunately, no effective method of protecting against thrush has been found. However, folk remedies are rife, both on the internet and in doctors' surgeries. One common piece of advice is to supplement the lactic-acid bacteria in your vagina with yoghurt, either in pill form or by drinking lots of yoghurt pro-biotic drinks. However, this kind of treatment hasn't been proved to be effective, so perhaps it's a waste of money, unless you're very fond of them.[65]

Other than that, people are generally advised to keep their genital area dry, as thrush likes wet, warm conditions. This means that you should avoid synthetic underwear and tight trousers, and only use panty liners when strictly necessary. Wear cotton underwear because it breathes best and sleep naked so that your genitals get a good airing. None of this has any documented scientific effect, but may be worth trying if you're really bothered by thrush. After all, it's free and has no side-effects.

Bacterial vaginosis

Now we're going to move onto another genital condition that's also incredibly common: bacterial vaginosis, or BV for short. Have you ever heard female genitals described in fish-related terms – as a shrimp-fest or a fish taco? The truth is that healthy genitals shouldn't smell fishy, but BV is to blame for the fact that many do.

BV is caused by an imbalance of the normal genital flora. There is a reduction in the protective lactic-acid bacteria, while the other types of bacteria that cause trouble in the environment flourish. The lactic-acid bacteria keep your vagina acidic, and acidic is good. When you have BV, your vagina becomes a little less acidic, in other words, more alkaline. That's why pH is one of the things your doctor may measure when you have genital problems to check whether you have BV.

There is no single bacteria that's solely responsible for BV: it's a cocktail of different kinds. Some of them usually live in the vagina or in other areas of the body as part of your normal flora. Problems follow if they have moved, or there are too many of them.

Most experts think that only women who have had sex get BV, and that the risk of acquiring it increases with the number of sexual partners but diminishes with condom use. This applies to both women who have sex with women and those who have sex with men. The more partners you have, the greater the risk of BV.[66] So, you might think some of the bacteria come from your sexual partner, but that doesn't mean BV is a sexually transmitted infection. Remember that many different bacteria cause BV. It's not a question of one contagious and harmful bacterium, as with chlamydia. As we've said, everyone's normal flora has its own unique bacteria combination, or balance. So, think of it in terms of mixing up your normal flora with those of several people who have a slightly different combination of bacteria than you. Too many cooks spoil the broth, or in this instance, spoil the balance.

Women who haven't had several sexual partners can also get BV, but they must still have had sex. BV is harmless and so there's no reason to protect a regular partner against infection by using a condom or abstaining from sex while you're being treated. Although it is always worth using a condom if you have several partners, but that's because of the risk of sexually transmitted infections, not of BV.

In addition to the characteristic smell, which is described as *rotten fish*, women with BV have heavier-than-normal discharge. Many describe a greyish, very runny discharge, and need to change their underwear several times a day. The smell can be so strong that it can be detected through clothes. Many women experience a sporadic fishy smell or a worsening of the fishy smell after vaginal intercourse or during and after menstruation. Does that mean that menstruation and sex give you BV? No, but menstruation and sperm can worsen the symptoms if you have BV.

In fact, the smell becomes stronger the more alkaline your genitals become. So it becomes worse if you have fewer lactic-acid bacteria or if an alkaline substance is added to your vagina. Both blood and sperm are more alkaline than the environment in the vagina and will therefore increase the fishy smell. If you get the fishy smell after your period or after sex, it may mean that you have BV without severe symptoms, but which flares up when the environment becomes less acidic.

Perhaps this sounds pretty easy to recognise, but as with thrush, you won't necessarily identify BV by its symptoms. BV can also cause itching as well as other symptoms that make you think it's thrush. Discharge is a common symptom of different sexually transmitted infections, and remember that it's certainly possible to have several things at once! It's always difficult to distinguish genital conditions from one other. The moral is that you must visit your doctor for a check-up if your genitals are different from normal. Notice a change in discharge, itching or a stinging sensation? Then go to your doctor.

Bacterial vaginosis doesn't mean that your genitals are dirty, although that's what a lot of people think when they detect the bad smell. If you try to get rid of the problem by washing you'll only make matters worse by rinsing away the good bacteria that keep your vagina acidic. BV can pass of its own accord, but it's best to get medical treatment. Since BV is caused by bacteria, a course of antibiotics or antibacterial treatments are called for. You can also buy vaginal pessaries containing lactic-acid bacteria, which supposedly help the environment in the vagina. Unfortunately, there is no research proving that this kind of treatment has any effect whatsoever.

WHEN PEEING HURTS

It's no coincidence that urinary-tract infections are described as *peeing barbed wire*. Urinary-tract infections are crappy and as a woman you're particularly prone to them. Our short urethra is to blame. As is the fact that our anus is in close quarters to the urethral opening. Bacteria from our anus work best if they stay where they belong, but it's difficult to fence bacteria in. They can easily climb into the urethral opening and move up through it until they have settled on the mucous membranes inside the urethra and bladder. Once there, they cause inflammation.

You'll notice when you have a urinary-tract infection, or UTI, because it hurts when you pee. It stings, burns and can feel as if what's coming out is barbed wire. It becomes particularly painful towards the end of the flow, when the bladder is emptying itself out entirely and its walls press against each other. In addition, you'll notice that you have a frequent urge to pee, but only produce a little at a time. Plus, you may notice that your urine smells odd, or that there's a bit of blood in it.

The vast majority of urinary-tract infections in young women – as many as 95 per cent – are what we call uncomplicated.[67] This simply means that the infection is considered to be less dangerous and requires simple treatment or none at all. Previously, all urinary-tract infections were treated with antibiotics because people believed the infection would climb up through the system to the kidneys, causing pyelonephritis, but antibiotics are now used more sparingly in many countries. Most urinary-tract infections pass of their own accord, without antibiotics, if you give it a few days, drink a lot of fluid and take a few painkillers if necessary.

Of course, you should always be alert to any deterioration. If you develop a fever or the pain worsens, especially if it moves up towards your back, you must visit your doctor as soon as possible, at the out-of-hours surgery if need be. This may be a sign that the bacteria have caused pyelonephritis and there's a risk that you may end up with a messed-up kidney.

A urinary-tract infection must always be taken seriously if you're pregnant. In that situation, it is automatically considered to be complicated and you need a special antibiotic treatment. They are also considered to be complicated if you have them frequently. Then it's often necessary to investigate more closely what kind of bacteria are involved, and sometimes checks will be carried out to see if you have an underlying condition that makes it easier for you to become infected. Having said that, some women get urinary-tract infections again and again without our knowing why. It is suspected that these women may have slightly different immune defences in the mucous membranes of their urinary tract, which makes it easier for the bacteria to gain a foothold.

Many women desperately seek ways to avoid urinary-tract infections.

Cranberry juice or pills are common folk remedies that have been used for centuries. Cranberry contains a substance that is supposed to prevent bacteria from attaching themselves to the mucous membrane in the bladder. However, a major review of the research by the prestigious Cochrane Library indicates that cranberry has no protective effect.[68] But again: if you like cranberry juice there's nothing to stop you trying it, and there are no side-effects. Other tips are to drink large quantities of water to flush out your plumbing, empty your bladder as soon as you need to pee and, of course, always wipe from front to back after having a poo.

What we do know is that sex increases the chances of getting a urinary-tract infection. During sex a lot of moisture often builds up in the genitals, making it easier for the bacteria to move from place to place, and, at the same time, all that genital-to-genital rubbing and thrusting can push bacteria into the wrong hole. We know the risk of acquiring a urinary-tract infection is 60 times higher than normal in the first two days after intercourse for women under the age of 30.[69]

You've probably heard the popular advice that if you pee after sex you'll have less chance of ending up with bothersome stinging. It's great advice. By peeing after sex, you'll flush out any gut bacteria that have found their way up into the urethra, before they manage to invade your mucous membrane and cause trouble.

An ordinary urinary-tract infection is not a sexually transmitted infection even though sex may be involved – it's just a matter of regular bacteria from your anus being in the wrong place. But chlamydia, gonorrhoea and myco-plasma are also common causes of a stinging sensation when peeing. So, you should be on the alert. However, the bacteria behave slightly differently. The sexually transmitted bacteria thrive in the urethra, but not in the bladder, unlike the butt bacteria. When you have a sexually transmitted infection you don't get the characteristic pain at the end of flow. It's also less common to have a frequent urge to pee. Even so, it isn't easy to notice the difference yourself – so go to your doctor. A urinary-tract infection can resemble chlamydia and chlamydia can resemble a urinary-tract infection. If you're really unlucky, you may get both at once.

DRIP DRIP DRIP – ALL ABOUT URINE LEAKS

It's no fun having to buy maxi packs of incontinence pads at the shop when you're 19-and-a-half years old and childless, but old ladies and women who've had loads of children aren't the only ones who suffer from urine leaks. The technical term for urine leaks is urinary incontinence and it's a common problem in women. Age and childbirth, along with high BMI, are the biggest risk factors, which means that an ever-increasing number of women start to suffer from them as the years go by. That's probably also the reason why many people believe it's uncommon to have urine leaks before giving birth, but women of all ages can be affected.

It's difficult to say just how many women actually suffer from urine leaks. The figures from studies vary and it is believed that fewer than half of all women who have incontinence go to the doctor, which may indicate high hidden figures.[70] One study of Norwegian women found that 30 per cent suffered urine leaks,[71] while a study of women three months after birth found that 20 to 30 per cent were affected.[72] Some international studies have reported anything from 10 to 60 per cent, depending on the severity of the leaks involved.[73]

We know less about younger, childless women and the figures that do exist vary dramatically. One study looking at Australian women between 16 and 30 who hadn't had children found that as many as 12.6 per cent experienced urine leaks.[74] A Swedish study resulted in quite different findings: around 3 per cent of all women aged 20 to 29 had urine leaks.[75]

Regardless of which of these studies comes closest to the truth, we can safely say that urine leaks aren't uncommon among young, childless women.

There are several ways of being incontinent. We distinguish between what is called stress incontinence, urge incontinence and a mixed form, which combines the two.

Stress incontinence is the most common, affecting around 50 per cent of those who suffer urine leaks.[76] This occurs when you leak urine if something causes the pressure on your abdomen to increase, for example when you cough, sneeze or laugh or you jump or run. By comparison with urge incontinence, the amounts involved are small, but the degree of severity varies enormously. There may be a difference between how often you leak and how much you leak once it happens.

Urge incontinence is about *need*. Women who suffer from this form of incontinence have a sudden, strong need to pee right NOW, sometimes followed by a large urine leakage. Around 10 to 15 per cent of all women who have incontinence have only this form.[77] Women with urge incontinence often have an overactive bladder and that means they have a strong urge to pee without necessarily leaking. Women with overactive bladders usually pee more often than other women and need to get up to pee in the middle of the night.[78]

Between 35 and 50 per cent of women with incontinence have a mixed form – both stress and urge incontinence – so the form of the leakage can vary. Sometimes they leak when they jump or sneeze for example, at other times they have a powerful urge to pee and leak a large amount.

Urine leakage can be caused by many things. If you drink more water than you need to it may be a good idea to cut down. Many people think drinking a lot of water is healthy, but, in fact, you don't need more than around 2 litres every 24 hours unless you exercise a lot or live in an extremely hot climate. You get some of this water through food. It's usually unnecessary to drink more than 1.5–2 litres every 24 hours. It may also be a good idea to cut down on diuretic drinks such as coffee and tea.

Sometimes urine leaks are symptomatic of other illnesses. Some women have leakages when they have a urinary-tract infection and some neurological diseases can cause leaks. So, it may be sensible to talk to your doctor if you can't see any clear reason why the leaks have started, for example that you began to leak after giving birth or after you suddenly started drinking 5 litres of water a day. Your doctor can give you guidance and help find a solution.

The fact that you leak urine doesn't necessarily mean you're condemned to use black clothes on your bottom half to hide the leaks as best you can, or to give up running and laughing for the rest of your life. Fortunately, you can do something about it. The first thing people try in order to put a stop to the leaks requires a bit of initiative. A lot of people who suffer from stress incontinence do so because their pelvic-floor musculature is too weak – they may, for example, have been affected after childbirth. The pelvic-floor muscles are the ones you use to stop the flow of urine when you're peeing or to clench your vagina. If your pelvic-floor muscles are stronger it can be easier to prevent involuntary leaks when the pressure on your abdomen increases. There are several ways to train these muscles, but mainly this involves contracting the muscles in your genitals at intervals, the same way as you train any other muscles in your body at the gym. Many women get help from their GP or a physiotherapist, too. There are special exercise programmes you can follow, including dedicated apps specially designed for pelvic-floor training. You can also try vaginal balls or similar tools. The point of vaginal balls is to use your pelvic-floor muscles to keep the balls in place for as long as you can manage. Regardless of how you exercise these muscles you will hopefully notice that you get stronger and have fewer leakages over time.

Pelvic-floor exercises may also have some effect for women who suffer primarily from urge incontinence, but a process called bladder training is even more important. For those with urge incontinence, the problem is not located in the muscles. The bladder muscle contracts at the wrong time, without you having any control over it. That's why women with urge incontinence often pee such large amounts. Bladder training is about teaching yourself to pee less frequently. The point is to pee according to a time schedule and not according to need. You can start by saying that you're allowed to pee, say, every hour. If a sudden urge arises between these permitted peeing times, you mustn't go to the loo, but must hold it in. After a while you gradually increase the interval between each time you're allowed to pee, to two hours, three hours, four hours and so on. Over time this will often help with urge incontinence.

In some situations, medical treatment or surgery may be used to treat incontinence. For some women, quite simple outpatient procedures make the world of difference, but for others exercise alone will do the trick. What helps you best will be a matter of what you want and how serious the leakage problem is, and how much it affects you day-to-day.

HAEMORRHOIDS AND ANAL SKIN TAGS

If you take a look at your anus, you'll quickly see how wrinkled it is. There's a reason why some people call it the balloon knot. The wrinkles are caused by the valves, called sphincters, that clamp the hole together. It must be able to expand a great deal and its extra diameter is hidden by a structure, kind of like a pleated skirt. Normally, these pleats are evenly distributed around the hole to form a relatively flat surface. So, it can strike horror in your heart when you suddenly discover something new and alien hanging out of this hole. You feel as if the new protrusion is screaming out for attention, drawing the gaze towards a hole that a lot of women try to forget about entirely. The likelihood is that it'll be an *anal skin tag* or a *haemorrhoid*, both of which are harmless conditions.

Haemorrhoids are a surprisingly common problem for both women and men. In fact, around a third of adults have them, although that's not reason enough for it to be a regular dinner-table topic.[79] It's possible to have them both inside the rectum and outside, around the anus; but let's stick to the external ones. A haemorrhoid is a haemorrhoid, wherever it is.

A haemorrhoid is a varicose vein in the anus and it looks like a balloon-like, purplish-blue protrusion. You'll almost always be able to push it back into place again (unlike an anal skin tag, see below), but it'll pop out again the next time you poo or do a particularly effortful squat. It'll often itch and may be tender. Sometimes the only problem may be that you'll find fresh blood on the toilet paper when you wipe your backside. This is caused by the simple fact that a haemorrhoid is a blood vessel that's gone astray. Usually the blood vessels around the rectal opening are supported by connective tissue and mucous membranes, so that we don't see them. With age, these supportive structures become flabbier and so increased pressure in the pelvis – for example straining on the toilet, heavy lifting, pregnancy and birth – can cause a small section of a blood vessel to be pushed out of place, like a kink in a garden hose. This kink can easily come under pressure around its root, causing blood to accumulate within it and form a little balloon. This balloon is what we call haemorrhoid.

Haemorrhoids around the anus are not serious, but they can be a real nuisance. Blood vessels don't like being messed about with in this way, so small inflammations can easily arise around the bulge, or haemorrhoid. Then you may find you get a bit of mucus or that it's painful or itchy, so that the mere act of sitting – let alone having a poo – becomes a tiresome business. Some people also find they bleed, either a little or rather a lot.

Fortunately, help is at hand. The most important thing to do, banal as it may sound, is ensure that you have good loo habits. Drink enough water to keep your faeces soft and go to the loo only when you feel an urgent need, to avoid straining. We also recommend leaving your newspaper on the kitchen table. If you sit on the loo for a long time the pressure around the haemorrhoid increases, which can worsen the problems. Good loo habits are often all it takes for a haemorrhoid to slip back into place of its own accord. It's also sensible to push it back into place with your finger when it pops out, so that it has a chance to find its way back to the right spot. It may feel a bit odd poking your finger up the hole like that, but if it's any consolation, doctors do this to total strangers every day of the week.

You can also buy various haemorrhoid creams at the chemist and these tend to work well. If that doesn't do the trick, there are plenty of good treatment options your doctor can help you with, including surgery. And as you may have grasped by now, your doctor is used to doing this!

If the thing sticking out of your butt isn't a haemorrhoid it's probably an anal skin tag. This is simply a slightly larger fold of skin in the anus, which is usually produced by the collapse of a haemorrhoid. When a haemorrhoid forces its way out, this can cause some of the folds of skin in the anal ring to come away from their proper place. Later, when the haemorrhoid retreats, they will combine to form a slightly larger fold which may protrude slightly from the surface. An anal skin tag or two rarely causes major problems, although you may have temporary itching and secretions if the skin fold becomes irritated by chafing by thongs, frequent excretion or similar. Some people may also find it more difficult to keep their anus clean.

However, some people feel that anal skin tags are unsightly. It *is* possible to have tags removed surgically, but you should always give it a lot of thought before opting for surgery because there's always a risk of complications. It's also worth being aware that removal hurts. You'll not only be left with a scar in the middle of your anus, but also, unfortunately, excrement isn't going to hold off just because you're newly out of surgery. Our advice is to relax and leave the anal skin tags in peace unless they cause loads of problems.

CERVICAL CANCER AND HOW TO AVOID IT

The neck of the womb, or the *cervix uteri*, is the gateway between the uterus and the vagina. You can feel it in the uppermost part of your vagina; it's like a bung with the consistency of the tip of a nose that has a tiny little hole in the middle. This is the narrow channel the sperm cells travel through to reach the uterus. Your period comes out of here and when you give birth your cervix can expand enough to let a whole baby pass through. It is also here that you can get cervical cancer.

Cervical cancer is unique in the context of cancer. As early as the 1800s it was discovered that this type of cancer behaved differently from others. It was much more common among prostitutes than in married women and nuns were more or less spared the disease. Could it be a divine punishment for promiscuity?

Nowadays we know that God and punishment have little to do with the matter. Cervical cancer is simply caused by a viral disease that is transmitted through sex! We've mentioned this virus earlier in connection with sexually transmitted infections, namely human papilloma virus (HPV).

HPV is a large family of viruses, several of which give humans warts. Most of them are quite harmless – ordinary skin warts are caused by one type, for example. Some HPV types thrive best in the genitals. They are transmitted through sexual contact and most of us who are sexually active will be infected with one type or another over the course of our lives; more than 80 per cent have had the virus before they turn 50. HPV is therefore considered to be the most common venereal disease and, at any given time, almost half of all people between 20 and 24 are walking around with an infection.[80]

As a rule, there's no cause for concern. Unlike with the herpes infection, your body will most often get rid of the virus on its own, the way it does with a cold. We know this because women who are checked for HPV over time often switch virus type. This indicates that the infections are short lived and that women are re-infected with new virus types when they change partner.

However, some of the HPV types differ from the others in that they can give some people a prolonged infection of the cervix. These types are called high-risk viruses, and the most common are HPV 16 and 18. Over time, if you're unlucky, an infection like this can develop into cancer. Number 16 alone accounts for over half of the cases of cervical cancer and may also cause mouth and throat cancer as well as vaginal, vulval and anal cancer. However, this will take more than an infection. It's very common to be infected with HPV 16, but only very few people get cancer. This means that other factors are needed for the development of cancer – for example, special vulnerabilities in the person concerned or other environmental factors such as smoking, for example. What these other factors are, we do not yet know.

Put slightly differently, almost all the women who develop cervical cancer have an infection caused by the HPV virus, but very few of those with an infection develop cancer.

A long road from sex to cancer

Fortunately, cancer doesn't develop overnight. First the virus will cause you to have cell changes, or *dysplasia* to use the technical term, in the cervix. This involves cells with small defects and abnormalities that prevent them from behaving normally. In the beginning these 'sick' cells are just slightly different, but if the immune defences leave them in peace they can really start to stand out from the crowd. Over time the cells can become more and more altered, until they are completely unrecognisable and start to grow in places they shouldn't. Only then have they become cancer cells.

In most cases, it takes at least 10 to 15 years from the first innocent cell changes to full-blown cervical cancer. In the meantime, it is assumed that they go through various stages of cell changes. During each of these stages, the cells may change their minds or be destroyed by the immune defences.

These cell changes, which *may* be precancerous stages, are the ones it's preferable to discover as early as possible. Through regular screening and cell tests at least every three years (see below), changes can be captured in good time and removed before they pose any threat. This is how to defend effectively against cervical cancer.

Cell changes and cervical cancer rarely involve symptoms or signs that indicate that you are unwell until late in the course of the disease. And that's why regular examination of the cervix is so important. Symptoms of cervical cancer can include bleeding abnormalities, such as bleeding between periods or bleeding associated with sex. Some women experience pain in their genitals or in their lower abdomen either during sex or in their day-to-day life. Others may find that their discharge starts to smell bad and contains traces of blood.

In other words, the signs that can accompany cervical cancer are very non-specific: they are present in a lot of common and less harmful conditions of the genitals. If you have any of these symptoms you should always go to your doctor for a check-up, but you needn't be worried about cancer. It's most probably a matter of an STI, a side-effect of contraception or a condition involving pain during sex; but it is important to check.

Get checked

Will you be turning 25 soon? Then you'll have had an invitation from the NHS to take a cervical smear test. In the UK this is sent to all women aged 25 who are registered with a GP. If there's one offer you really should take up, this is it. Women who have regular smear tests reduce the risk of developing cervical cancer by 70 per cent over their lifetime. That's what we call incredibly cheap life insurance! And it's another reason why it's important to be registered with a doctor. In Norway, this comes from the cancer register.*

Despite this almost half of all Norwegian women between 25 and 34 opt to chuck their letter in the bin. Uptake of screening has fallen from 71 to 57 per cent in this age group. Young people are the ones who aren't getting checked, even though they are more exposed than previously. This has negative consequences. More young women than ever before are getting cervical cancer in Norway. According to the Norwegian Cancer Register there has been a 30 per cent rise in cervical cancer in women under 40 in recent years. In the UK, there has been a 5 per cent rise in the cases of cervical cancer in the last decade.[81]

The reason is that fewer women are turning up for their cervical check-ups at a time when more young women are being infected by the HPV virus that causes cancer.

---

* For some time a pilot project has been under way in certain Norwegian counties, which involves taking an HPV test instead of a smear test. The women who turn out to have HPV 16 or 18 are then recalled for a smear test. It's very possible that this will be the future of screening in Norway, maybe as soon as the next few years. This means that many Norwegian women will be spared unnecessary gynaecological examinations and smear tests, and only those who are at increased risk of having abnormal cells will be checked.

So, the smear test is a simple solution for preventing cervical cancer. After the first invitation, you should have a smear test every three years until you are 49, then from 50 to 65 it's every five years. The NHS will send you a reminder to book a new smear test when three years have elapsed since you last took one. Having the smear test itself involves making an appointment with your GP or the practice nurse. It's also possible to have the test done by a gynaecologist if you'd prefer, but you'll normally need a referral from your doctor, even if you have it done privately.

You shouldn't have a smear test done during your period and you should preferably not have had vaginal sex in the two days before the test. The gynaecological examination only takes a few minutes. The doctor or nurse dilates your vagina with a kind of funnel called a speculum. She will then have a look at your cervix and take a sample with a little brush. The brush is rubbed gently against the cervix, loosening some cells that can then be examined under a microscope at the laboratory. If everything is normal, you will get a standard letter reassuring you of that. If the cervical cells show changes you'll hear from your doctor.

Cell changes don't mean you have cancer
So, you have had a smear test and received a nasty, barely understandable letter from your doctor. You have abnormal cells – but what the heck does that mean?

A repeated theme among women we meet is that they are frustrated and anxious about inadequate information from the screening programme when it comes to the process surrounding cell changes in the cervix. Most young women who are found to have abnormal cells feel quite healthy and have never thought they might get cancer. So, the letter can come as much more of a shock than health professionals realise.

Many women who are told that cell changes have been found jump to the conclusion that they already have cancer and will die. What we would emphasise to such women is that it is very common for young and sexually active women to have slight cell changes in their cervix. Any HPV infection, even the low-risk viruses, may cause changes. This is also why women under 25 aren't checked – incredible numbers would become unnecessarily anxious and might end up being over-treated without improving our ability to pick up new cases of cancer.

In the vast majority of cases, cell changes in the cervix will disappear on their own without any kind of treatment. Like other viruses, they tend to pass. The body's own immune defences are fantastic at tidying things up themselves! Your doctor knows this and that explains why she might not seem especially worried when all you can think about is CANCER.

Just to reassure you a bit more: 25,000 Norwegian women are found to have abnormal cells during their smear test every single year and of these, only 3,000 end up needing treatment for serious precancerous stages. Even fewer, around 300, later develop cervical cancer. In the UK, around 175,000 women have an abnormal smear, but only 15,000 will need any form of treatment.[82]

But let's take a look at that letter from your doctor. What has happened since you took your smear test? The cells that were brushed off your cervix were sent to a laboratory. There, a doctor stained the cells and placed them under a microscope. The doctor looks for cells that appear abnormal. Depending on how unusual the cells look and how many of them there are, the cell changes are classified from mild to moderate and severe. Even serious cell changes can disappear of their own accord but it's still important for all cell changes to be followed up.

As well as looking at the cells, the laboratory may examine the sample by applying an HPV test. Where on the scale the cell changes lie, and the result of the HPV test are decisive elements when it comes to what happens next:

The cell sample shows uncertain or low-grade cell changes

You'll need to go back to your doctor. In the UK, all borderline and low-grade cell-change smears (known as dyskaryosis) are tested for high-risk (HR) HPV – this is called HPV triage. If you are negative for the high-risk HPV, then you have a routine smear in three years. If you test positive for high-risk HPV you need to see a gynaecologist in a colposcopy clinic (see below).

The cell sample shows high-grade or serious cell changes

Your GP will refer you to a gynaecologist who will do two things. First, she will take a look at your cervix with a special magnifying instrument. This examination is called a *colposcopy* and is done to look for changes in the mucous membrane. After that the gynaecologist will take a tissue sample (*biopsy*) from your cervix, which will be sent to an expert – a pathologist – for examination under a microscope. During a smear test only a few cells are brushed off the surface of the mucous membrane, but in a biopsy a tiny fragment of the surface of the cervix is removed to investigate whether there are abnormal cells deep in the mucous membrane. The whole architecture of the mucous membrane is examined.

The biopsy is not as uncomfortable as you think. The surface of the cervix is not as sensitive as your skin, so you'll feel a pinch when the biopsy is taken rather than a sharp sensation. You could be given some local anaesthetic if you need it. After the biopsy, there may be some mild discomfort, but generally you can get on with your day. It could be a good idea to take some ibuprofen ahead of the examination. It is also normal to bleed a bit during the examination so most women need to use a sanitary towel (not a tampon!) for the rest of the day.

When the pathologist examines the biopsy under the microscope, the changes will again be classified according to stages, from light to moderate and severe changes. None of these terms means cancer. Only when the abnormal cells have made their way right through the mucous membrane is it a question of cervical cancer.

If the colposcopy and the biopsy are totally normal or show only slight changes, you can relax. However, you'll have to visit your GP for a new smear test and HPV test within 6 to 12 months to check that everything is fine. In nine out of ten cases, the changes will have vanished or remained stable without any kind of deterioration.[83]*

If any of the examinations confirm that there are moderate to severe precancerous stages, you will, as a rule, be seen in the hospital to remove the small area of abnormality at the surface of the cervix. The procedure is called large-loop excision of the transformation zone (LLETZ) to the cervix and is performed in the outpatient setting for around 85 per cent of women. Some women are advised to have the procedure done under

---

* 60 per cent of slight changes disappear spontaneously, while 30 per cent remain stable. Only 10 per cent will develop further into severe changes and 1 per cent will develop into cancer over the person's lifetime.

general anaesthetic if their gynaecologist feels it may be more appropriate. This is something that can be discussed with her. It's a simple procedure, but it isn't done unless it is necessary.

In the past doctors performed a cone biopsy, which was a larger procedure in which the outer part of the cervix is removed, normally with an electrical loop or sling. But some women who underwent a cone biopsy have been seen to have a slightly higher risk of premature birth or miscarriage in subsequent pregnancies. Although this is only around one to three women in 100.

Most women who have had a loop excision – around 90 per cent – will be totally cured. Following the treatment, you will normally have a smear test either at your GP's surgery or in the colposcopy clinic. At the same time, you are again tested for high-risk HPV. If this is negative for high-risk HPV, then you are cured! You can then have your next smear at the normal recall time, so after three years if you are under 50 years old. If the cell changes have gone of their own accord, or have been removed through loop excision, there's no need to worry about cervical cancer. It's like snakes and ladders: you go straight back to the start.

Nonetheless it's important to remember that you can be infected with HPV again, so it may be sensible to have the HPV vaccine. We'll come back to that. You must also continue to go to your regular screening involving smear tests for the rest of your life. But overall you should focus on relaxing. One positive lifestyle change you can make to avoid recurrence of abnormal cells if you smoke, is to stop now. Smoking is proven to slow down the regression of mild abnormalities. Even for those women who have been treated it is common for smoking to promote abnormalities in the presence of high-risk HPV.

A vaccine against cancer
Now, we talked a lot about how you should relate to HPV infections and cell changes, but imagine if you could prevent infection with the carcinogenic virus in the first place! It is, in fact, quite possible. A few years ago it would have seemed like science fiction, but today there actually is a vaccine that can protect against cancer. It's a medical miracle.

As we explained earlier, there are over 100 different types of human papilloma virus (HPV), and only a few of them cause cancer. There are two

HPV vaccines, Gardasil and Cervarix, which protect against the most dangerous types of HPV – numbers 16 and 18. Between them, these two high-risk viruses cause 70 per cent of all cervical cancers. Vaccination against these viruses gives you almost 100 per cent protection against infection and therefore against the cell changes and cervical cancer caused by these virus types. A new HPV vaccine has recently been approved that protects against nine different virus types. It can prevent 90 per cent of all cervical cancer, but is not yet covered by the Norwegian health authorities.

The Gardasil vaccine also protects against HPV 6 and HPV 11, which cause genital warts. Some studies show that Cervarix also offers partial protection against genital warts. It's important to grasp that there's no connection whatsoever between genital warts and genital cancer, but all the same it's great to avoid having them. Without the vaccine, 10 per cent of the Norwegian population would get genital warts, around 10 per cent of all Norwegian women would have to be treated for serious cell changes and 1 per cent of all women would get cervical cancer over the course of their lives.

In the UK, immunisation against HPV started in September 2008 for girls aged 12 to 13 with a catch-up for girls up to 18 in the following three years. The vaccine is given in three doses over half a year. A vaccine is not a medicine, but it prevents the virus from settling in your body and making you ill in the event of future infection. The vaccine stimulates your immune system to recognise the virus and prepare a battle plan for the quickest and most efficient means of crushing it if it should make an appearance. If you already have an ongoing HPV infection involving type 16 or 18, the vaccine will not eliminate the virus from your body. This is why the vaccine is given to young girls. We want to protect them before they start having sex and potentially become infected with viruses.

The vaccine is approved for girls and boys aged 9 to 26 years, and has proven effective up to the age of 45. There are two reasons for this. First of all, very few of us are infected with *both* HPV 16 and 18. If you haven't yet been infected by these types, the vaccine will have a protective effect. Secondly, most HPV infections pass of their own accord, as we said. Unfortunately, it has been observed that natural immunisation against HPV is poor. This means that even if you've had an earlier HPV infection, you're not necessarily protected against subsequent re-infection by a different sexual partner. An HPV vaccine can help protect you against this kind of re-infection.

For now, boys are not included in the general vaccination programme in the UK, but it's hoped this will change over time. Norway's Public Health Institute recommends the HPV vaccines for both girls and boys. It should be just as effective for men – on genital warts and HPV-associated cancer of the penis, anus and throat/mouth – as it is for women. Some of you may have noticed that there's been an increase in throat and mouth cancer among men. There is speculation that this is because oral sex has become more common, causing men to be infected with oral HPV. A vaccine can prevent infection and the development of cancer here, too. Homosexual boys in particular will benefit from the vaccine since they are not indirectly protected by the vaccination of girls, often known as herd immunity.

Unfortunately, boys and girls born before 1991 who wish to take the vaccine must pay for it themselves, but should you consider paying for the vaccine out of your own pocket?

For every sexual partner you have, the risk of HPV infection is around 10 per cent. Even if you've already been infected with one or more types it's very possible that you won't have been infected by HPV 16 or 18. If you take the vaccine, you'll be protected against future infection by new sexual partners. As we mentioned, studies have shown that the vaccine is effective for men and women up to the age of 45. Since you must pay for this out of your own pocket and it's expensive, you should weigh up the benefit against what you perceive as your own risk of infection. Put simply, this means that the number of sexual partners you've had is significant. The fewer previous partners, the greater the likelihood the vaccine will be effective for you. The number of sexual partners you end up having in the future will also play a role. The more of them there are, the greater the potential risk of infection and the greater the benefit of the vaccine. In addition, women who have been treated for abnormal cells have a low risk of recurrence because they have received the HPV vaccine.

HPV vaccine is safe and effective
In Norway today one in four girls in year seven opt not to receive the HPV vaccine.[84] We don't know why people choose to drop the vaccine, but fear of

side-effects appears to be widespread. There are also some parents who think their 12-year-old daughter won't have sex for many years and so the HPV vaccine is unnecessary. In Denmark, there's been a great deal of media attention around possible side-effects, and this has led to a drastic reduction in the proportion of vaccinated girls.[85] There have also been some scare stories about the vaccine in the Norwegian media recently. There's little reason for this.

In Norway, nearly 500,000 doses of the vaccine have been given to 160,000 girls. Within this total, 645 cases of possible side-effects have been reported, 92 per cent of which were described as not very serious. It was simply a matter of passing problems such as swelling and tenderness around the site of vaccination, fever, nausea and diarrhoea.

Of the few serious side-effects reported since 2009, 52 in total, there are ten cases of chronic fatigue syndrome/ME and five cases of postural orthostatic tachycardia syndrome (POTS). POTS is a condition that causes an elevated pulse rate when you stand up, as well as unstable blood pressure, fatigue and dizziness. The Norwegian Medicines Agency reports that the number of cases is no higher than one would expect in this age group with or without the vaccine and a recent Norwegian study of 175,000 girls showed no increased rate of chronic fatigue syndrome among vaccinated girls.[86] In other words, the vaccine is not believed to have caused these problems.

Nonetheless reports about possible serious side-effects are always taken extremely seriously. After many cases of conditions such as POTS were reported in Denmark after vaccination, the European Medical Agency decided to carry out a safety review. The result of the investigation came in November 2015. The conclusion was that no data point towards any causal link between the HPV vaccine and either POTS or another syndrome called CRPS (complex regional pain syndrome).[87] These are rare conditions, but their occurrence is no higher among vaccinated girls than in the rest of the population. Nor was any link found between the vaccine and chronic fatigue syndrome/ME. More recently, a large cohort study of 3.1 million adult Danish and Swedish women found no association between the HPV vaccine and 44 serious chronic illnesses, including autoimmune and neurological diseases. The only association found was with coeliac disease, although the researchers only found this in the Danish women.[88]

So far more than 180 million women worldwide have been vaccinated against HPV, and no serious safety problems have been identified with the vaccines. Although there will always be a possibility of side-effects when using medication and vaccines, these tend to be mild, temporary problems. The same cannot be said of cervical cancer.

MISCARRIAGE – FROM FACEBOOK TO REALITY

In summer 2015, Mark Zuckerberg, the founder of Facebook, posted a slightly unusual update to his 33 million Facebook friends.[89] He and his doctor wife announced that they were overjoyed to be expecting their first child, a girl, and were ready to make the world a better place for her sake. Yawn, you may think, automatically clicking 'Like'. These sorts of personal announcements are bread and butter on Facebook, a place that has become synonymous with humble-bragging and image-crafting.

But Zuckerberg didn't stop there. He chose to tell his followers about the rocky road to pregnancy, the happy ending and 1.6 million likes – a story about everything we don't normally mention. The couple suffered three miscarriages over several years of trying to become parents. Four pregnancies resulted in one child.

A miscarriage is a pregnancy that stops before week 24 of the pregnancy, when the fertilised egg stops developing or the foetus dies in the womb. You'll most often notice that you're miscarrying because you get pain and vaginal bleeding. That said, there's nothing unusual about bleeding during pregnancy. Around one in four pregnant women bleed in their first trimester, although miscarriage only occurs in one out of ten cases of bleeding.[90] Even so, you should always contact your doctor for a check-up if you bleed at any time during pregnancy.

Miscarriage is one of the most common complications in early pregnancy. It happens in around one out of five *clinical* pregnancies, defined as pregnancies that women themselves are aware of.[91] There are also miscarriages that happen before a pregnancy test can detect that you're pregnant. These types of pregnancy are generally called *chemical* pregnancies. Taking chemical pregnancies into account, it is assumed that only half of all fertilised eggs will result in viable pregnancies.[92] In other words, miscarriage is as common as a successful pregnancy.

Pregnancy tests today are so sensitive they can detect that you are preg-nant incredibly early on, but it's not necessarily very sensible to use this option if you're longing for a positive result. Because most miscarriages happen in the first few weeks after fertilisation, up to the point before your next period is due. Since it's so common for these early pregnancies to end in miscarriage, you can save yourself a great deal of disappointment by waiting to take the test until after the point you'd expected to have your period. If you wait two extra weeks, until week six of the pregnancy, the risk of miscarriage has fallen to 10–15 per cent. A positive result at that point therefore implies that you'll probably be a parent in eight months' time. After eight weeks, the risk is down to just 3 per cent. Once the three-month mark is past, the risk stabilises at a low level of around 0.6 per cent.[93] With every passing week, the chances that everything will be fine become higher and higher.

Fear of miscarriage is the reason why pregnant women often choose to wait until three months have passed and the first trimester is out of the way before telling people about their pregnancy. The idea behind this secrecy is primarily to spare the pregnant woman in case anything goes wrong. It's bad enough to lose a longed-for baby without also having to ring around friends and family to call off the happy news. It's debatable whether three months is a sensible limit. You could just as well set the limit a month earlier, around week eight, if you have to have a limit at all.

Unfortunately, the result of this secrecy is that many couples feel there's something shameful about miscarriage. It's not unusual to hear people commenting after a miscarriage: 'Well, it was a bit odd to tell people so soon,' as if you could kill the foetus in your belly just by talking about it. It's quite absurd. Zuckerberg describes miscarriage as a lonely experience: 'Most people don't discuss miscarriages because you worry your problems will distance you or reflect upon you – as if you're defective or did some-thing to cause this. So, you struggle on your own.'

Zuckerberg isn't alone in the feelings he describes. In a study published in the American journal *Obstetrics & Gynecology*, nearly half of those who had been through a miscarriage reported feeling that they were somehow to blame, or having a sense that they had done something wrong. They felt alone and ashamed.[94] It makes for sad reading, not least because self-blame is caused by a relatively widespread misunderstanding of the causes of miscarriage. In the same US study, it emerged that almost a quarter thought that lifestyle choices, such as smoking, alcohol and drugs, were the most *common* cause of miscarriage. Many people also thought that heavy lifting and stress could lead to miscarriage. On mother and baby forums on the net, coffee drinking and bubble bath are named as other possible causes.

In reality, miscarriage is rarely a result of misdeeds by the mother (or father). The most common cause of miscarriage is serious chromosomal abnormality in the foetus; that is, there's an error in the genetic code that is already determined at conception. Forget the boozing, unhealthy eating or social smoking you indulged in before you knew you were pregnant.

The merging of the mother's and father's genetic material into a joint recipe for a unique person, which must be followed to the letter, is incredibly complicated. It's hardly surprising that errors are constantly happening for no apparent reason. Miscarriage is the body's control mechanism and its way of ensuring that we have healthy children who can live good lives. It can be horribly painful to suffer a miscarriage like this, but it's actually your body doing right by you.

Only when you've had two or three in a row should you consider investigating whether there's something in the mother (or father) that is causing the miscarriages. Before that it is considered quite normal. Where women experience repeated miscarriages, the cause can be anything from anatomical aberrations and hormonal disorders to autoimmune diseases and hereditary blood conditions. These are conditions nobody can be blamed for, but which can hopefully be treated.

Simple bad luck is the most frequent cause of miscarriage, but we do know that a few things increase the risk. The most important factor is the mother's age. A Danish study found that 25 per cent of all pregnancies in 35- to 39-year-olds ended in miscarriage, compared with 12 per cent among 25- to 29-year-olds.[95] By the age of 40 only half of the pregnancies ended in birth, among other reasons because the quality of the eggs starts to become so poor that errors in chromosomes and genes that make the foetus non-viable are more frequent.

We all know there's no place for smoking in a pregnancy. You should stop smoking as soon as you know you're pregnant. But what about the time before you find out? What about that time you smoked at a party when you still don't know? The biggest review of research that has been undertaken found a clear link between smoking and miscarriage.[96] If 100 non-smokers and 100 smokers became pregnant, 20 of those in the first group would miscarry versus around 26 among the smokers.* It is estimated that around one in ten miscarriages are caused by smoking, but it seems as if you have to smoke a great deal – more than ten cigarettes a day – in order to increase the risk to any appreciable extent.[97] So a spot of social smoking in the first few weeks shouldn't be grounds for massive guilt or anxiety.

The same is only true of alcohol to a certain extent. Alcohol is extremely harmful for the foetus, but we don't know how much it takes to cause damage. It's not very easy to check how much pregnant women can drink before the foetus suffers damage or death. It would of course be horribly unethical to ask a group of pregnant women to drink during pregnancy to check how much alcohol was needed to cause miscarriage or foetal injury. Since we don't know where the limit lies, many national health authorities, including the NHS, recommend avoiding alcohol entirely. That way you'll be on the safe side.

However, not everybody agrees that total abstinence from alcohol is the only right way, and this can be confusing when you're pregnant. Nina discovered this herself when she was pregnant and many doctors told her a glass of red wine now and then was perfectly fine. The world-famous economist Emily Oster got sick of the mixed messages and decided to investigate the research behind the advice more closely. In her book, *Expecting better – why the conventional pregnancy wisdom is wrong and what you really need to know* (2013), she claims there is little to support official advice about the *absolute* avoidance of alcohol in pregnancy.[98] Her analysis indicates that it's probably safe to drink one to two units of alcohol a week – a unit is a small glass of wine or one glass of beer – but on two different

---

* The relative risk of miscarriage during pregnancy was 1.32 for smokers compared with non-smokers. In this example we have assumed that the risk of miscarriage for non-smokers is 20 per cent. This may well be too high, but has been chosen to illustrate relative risk in an understandable way.

days of the week. This doesn't have long-term effects on the child's behaviour or intelligence. In her view, the official advice to totally abstain from alcohol is driven by the assumption that women won't be able to limit themselves: if you accept a glass of wine on your birthday, it'll quickly become a whole bottle. We agree with Oster that this underestimates women's self-discipline and most of us manage to stop drinking for the full nine months, after all. If you're curious or sceptical, you can read her book for yourself and see whether you're convinced.

But perhaps it isn't that one glass of red wine with dinner you're worrying about when your pregnancy test comes out positive. Many women are nervous when they find out they're pregnant because of a slightly too alcoholic party or two in the weeks before they knew they were pregnant, where a lot more than one or two glasses of alcohol were consumed. A Danish population-based study from 2012 found that the risk of miscarriage doubled if women had four or more drinks a week in the first three months of their pregnancy.[99] So in theory, a real bender in the weeks before you discover your pregnancy can lead to miscarriage, but this by no means implies that it will necessarily happen. And if it does, it's impossible to put a finger on whether your boozing session was the specific cause. The miscarriage might have happened anyway. Just think how incredibly common it is!

And now on to the rumours that abound on the internet: heavy lifting, stress and normal amounts of coffee drinking do not lead to miscarriage. It seems that you'd have to drink up to ten cups of coffee a day before it *might* constitute a risk.[100] Cross-country skiing champion Marit Bjørgen trained for six hours a day during pregnancy and delivered a very healthy baby. Nor does it seem that vitamin supplements or the like can protect against miscarriage, although you should start taking folic acid, which is a B vitamin, from the moment you find out you're pregnant until at least 12 weeks – and preferably from the time you start trying to get pregnant.[101] It can prevent damage to your child's nervous system.

Mark Zuckerberg has been among those encouraging people to share on social media. A lot of people think it's too intimate and compromising to talk about these kinds of experiences in public spaces, but the man still had an important message. Openness about miscarriage is important in order to make it clear just how common it actually is, as well as the fact that it's an event that affects all kinds of people. There's nothing shameful about a miscarriage and it's usually nobody's fault. One positive side of it is that the vast majority of women who have miscarriages go on to have completely healthy children later.

The three-month rule we mentioned earlier was intended to protect women against the pain of telling others about the miscarriage, but perhaps this rule does more harm than good. It perpetuates misunderstandings and stigma instead of normalising and creating acceptance. The result is that many women are left feeling isolated, with an unjustified sense of shame and guilt, at a time when they're most in need of warmth and consideration from the people around them. So, let's start talking to each other!

THE TICKING CLOCK – HOW LONG CAN YOU PUT OFF HAVING CHILDREN?

When you're approaching 30, it's weird how often even complete strangers feel they have right to get involved in your private life. 'The clock's ticking, dear! Isn't it about time you started thinking about having children?' It's irrelevant to them whether you're single, in a new relationship or married to your job. They'd rather see you drop everything you're doing and force the first man you can lay your hands on to engage in immediate reproduction.

Think about having children, yes. A lot of women think and think without any children coming of it. Even if you want to have children – which is absolutely not a given – there are plenty of potential obstacles. The most obvious one is finding a person you can actually imagine having children with and who is also ready to have children with you. Oddly enough a lot of men head for the hills the minute that sweet girl in the bar starts talking about prams and settling down with stars in her eyes after the second drink.

Unfortunately we can't help you find the perfect dad, but what we can do is give you a little ammunition to use on those busybodies who won't stop going on about babies. Or a dose of reassurance if you're starting to feel stressed. Because although 30 is often presented as a magic limit, that's far from the whole truth.

Let's start with a few facts. Around 75 per cent of all couples who try to get pregnant manage it after six months. Before the year is over, somewhere between 85 and 90 per cent will have become pregnant.[102] *Infertility* is defined as an absence of pregnancy after a year of regular unprotected sex. So, this applies to around 10–15 per cent of all couples, but that's not the end of it. Of the couples who have been labelled infertile, half will become pregnant quite naturally during the second year of trying. They should, in fact, be called *sub-fertile*. They struggle to have children, but achieve it if they try for long enough. So, in all up to 95 per cent of all heterosexual people manage to have children through regular intercourse given plenty of time.

And then there's the matter of age. The average age for first births has steadily risen as women have entered the labour market. In 2014 women had their first child at 30.8, on average.[103] Women want to wait longer before having children than they used to both because they study for longer and want to build a career. At the same time the medical community issues us with warnings, highlighting figures that show a dramatic drop in fertility as we age and urging us to think carefully before we put off trying for pregnancy. There are several good reasons for this – among others, the risk of complications in pregnancy and abnormalities in the children increases as the mother becomes older. We'll come back to that. The question is whether we exaggerate the difficulties of having children once you've hit 30.

Several more recent studies have studied healthy women and their likelihood of becoming pregnant. Although far fewer women become spontaneously pregnant as they get older, the figures are less dramatic than you might often think. One study followed 782 couples who were trying to have a child.[104] The women in the 19 to 26 age group were clearly most fertile – 92 per cent were pregnant within a year – and after that the trend declined. But no major differences were found between the fertility of women in their late 20s and those at the beginning of their 30s – 86 per cent of the women between 27 and 34 were pregnant within a year. By comparison, 82 per cent of those between 35 and 39 became pregnant in the same period. Other studies have found similar figures. In a Danish study of 3,000 women, 72 per cent of all the 35- to 40-year-olds became pregnant in the course of the year, while 78 per cent of those who tried to time intercourse in relation to ovulation became pregnant. The figure for 30- to 34-year-olds was 87 per cent.[105]

What can we take away from this? If all girls tried to become pregnant as soon as they finished school, one in ten would fail. However, 20 years later, this figure rises to somewhere between two and three out of ten. The upside is that the majority manage to become pregnant well into their 30s! If we must talk about an age limit, 35 is closer to the truth.

For most people who are struggling for pregnancy, age is not a direct cause. First, we should point out that the problem lies with the man in a third of cases, because the man's age also plays a role. The woman has the problem, or is part of the problem, in the rest of the cases. And what's wrong then? The biggest source of infertility is disorders in the hormones that control ovulation. It's often down to polycystic ovary syndrome, where the hormone balance is not as it should be (see p. 194). The next most common cause is damage to the Fallopian tubes. This may be caused by past sexually transmitted infections, such as chlamydia, where the bacteria have caused inflammation and scarring of the Fallopian tubes. The problems may also be caused by endometriosis, which is the condition where cells from the uterine lining grow in the wrong place (see p. 190). Finally, fibroids – those myomas in the uterus – can prevent pregnancy. These are the most common causes of problems with pregnancy, not age.

However, the problem with increasing age is a higher risk of miscarriage. As we mentioned earlier, the risk of miscarriage is twice as high for women over 35.[106] Naturally this means that those of them who are expecting children experience miscarriage more often than the women who get pregnant young.

Age has a clearly negative effect on your chances of getting pregnant, and the risk of miscarriage, pregnancy complications and chromosomal errors such as Down's syndrome increases. But most women will not have any problem having healthy children 'the old-fashioned way' well into their 30s. The likelihood that you're one of the women who will struggle is, of course, impossible to determine based on the statistics, but it may be that you would have struggled to have children even if you'd tried as a 28-year-old. If you suspect that you have endometriosis or polycystic ovary syndrome, or if you've had chlamydia several times, it may be sensible not to postpone trying to get pregnant for too long. You may also need a bit of extra help and time to succeed.

GENITAL MUTILATION

Every year many millions of girls are mutilated for life. Their genitals are cut, sewn up or pricked with needles. Genital mutilation is a cultural practice that exists in several corners of the world, but which is fortunately becoming less and less common. Today it occurs most frequently in parts of Africa, the Middle East and certain Asian countries, but there was a time when people also practised genital mutilation in the West. From the mid-1800s, many gynaecologists in the USA and the UK cut away women's clitorises to cure them of masturbation, because masturbation could, of course, lead to hysteria, epilepsy and low IQ.[107] Cutting women's genitals has always been and continues to be a brutal effort to control female sexuality.

In Norway and the UK, a lot of effort has gone into preventing girls from an immigrant background from being mutilated and it seems that the work has been paying off. But for many women the damage is already done and that's why we've included this section. We also think it serves as a reminder of how female genitals are still considered a threat in large parts of the world.

The World Health Organization (WHO) divides genital mutilation into four categories. The first involves removing the whole or parts of the clitoral nub, or *glans*. The clitoral hood is often also removed. One explanation that has often been given is the perception that the clitoris can grow into a kind of penis if it is not removed, but there's no getting away from the fact that by removing or damaging the clitoris, you're removing the principal source of women's sexual pleasure and it is an attempt to control women's sexuality. Even so, some women may retain part of their sensation and capacity to have orgasms, because the clitoral complex mainly lies beneath the surface of the skin.˙ Other women find that the scar tissue produced in the clitoris creates constant pain.

The second form of genital mutilation involves cutting away the inner labia, often combined with various forms of damage to the clitoris. The

---

*   In the book *Bonk – the curious coupling of science and sex*, Mary Roach talks about the meetings between the researcher Marie Bonaparte and Egyptian women who had suffered genital mutilation but still masturbated by stimulating the scarred clitoris.

inner labia grow when we reach puberty, in tandem with the sexual awakening of our teenage years. Perhaps people saw a connection between growth in the genitals and interest in sex. By removing the labia, they maintain the illusion of childish innocence.

The third form of female genital mutilation is the one that often gets most attention, because it's the most aggressive alteration of the genitals. In this case, the outer labia are sewn together so all that's left is a small hole above the entrance to the vagina. Most often the inner labia and the clitoris are cut away at the same time. Both urine and menstrual blood seep out of this artificial opening. One Norwegian Somali woman we met told us what a shock it was to pee in a public toilet in Norway for the first time – the Norwegian women peed like elephants! She was used to spending up to 20 minutes emptying her bladder, so sparse was her urine flow. The same problem can arise during menstruation, when the blood can accumulate in the vagina. That makes it a hot-bed of bacteria, exposing women to genital and urinary-tract infections.

The constructed hole is often too small for sexual intercourse, and therefore serves as a kind of guarantee that the woman hasn't had vaginal intercourse before she gets married. Of course, problems arise when she's due to have sex for the first time and risks having to be opened up with scissors or a knife, or being split open with the man's penis. Some women have a big enough hole to have penetrative sex, but must be opened further before they can give birth. The scar tissue around the vagina is unable to expand enough to let a baby through. If they are not opened, they risk suffering uncontrolled tears, creating the potential for heavy bleeding and damage to the rectum.

The last form of genital mutilation is a miscellaneous group that includes all the damage to the genitals that is not included in the other three groups. This can, for example, include sticking hot needles into the clitoris – a kind of ritual killing of the woman's sexuality.

All forms of genital mutilation can cause long-term problems of the genitals. In addition, the procedure itself is linked to a major risk of infections and bleeding, not to mention psychological trauma. There are good reasons why genital mutilation is strictly forbidden in large parts of the world. All forms of female genital mutilation that can lead to long-term damage of the genitals are punishable, even if the girl or woman wants it herself. Neither is it permissible to take a child overseas to have it done elsewhere.

However, there is no prohibition on being genitally mutilated. If you have previously been mutilated and have problems, you can get help. At the hospital, the doctors can carry out reconstructive surgery to try and normalise the function of your genitals. They can't give you back the genitals you were born with, but they can minimise your daily problems.

DESIGNER GENITALS – WHY WE PUT OUR VULVAS UNDER THE KNIFE

There's nothing new about women (and men) choosing to alter their appearance through surgery. Breast enhancements, nose jobs, liposuction, facelifts – some people go a long way to fulfil their aesthetic ideals. However, altering your vulva through intimate surgery is a relatively new trend.

The term intimate surgery covers all forms of surgical alteration of the external sex organs. This may involve injecting fat, smoothing out and removing fat, reducing and expanding. A lot is possible, but the most common form is labioplasty. This is plastic surgery on the labia and it's the inner labia in particular that are subjected to surgery, to make them shorter.

We view the growing trend of intimate surgery as problematic. And no, we're not writing this section because we like looking down on women who make their own choices, or because we think that women don't have the right to decide for themselves what to do with their bodies. Of course, you should decide for yourself – this is about something else. We're writing this section because we're afraid a group of young women are opting for intimate surgery on the basis of a misunderstanding. In our experience, women with normal, healthy genitals are choosing intimate surgery because they think there's something wrong with them. This misunderstanding must be corrected and to do that we need to go back to anatomy.

We make a distinction between medical and aesthetic reasons for choosing labioplasty. There's a difference between wanting to have a nose job because you have difficulty breathing through your nose and because you don't like the way it looks. In the same way, there's a difference between trimming your labia because you're struggling with pain or difficulty having intercourse, and because you don't think your genitals look nice. The length of your inner labia is only a medical issue if they cause you problems. This doesn't necessarily mean that there's anything wrong with wanting to have surgery for aesthetic reasons, but if you are going to choose to take this step it's important that the choice you make is based on knowledge, not misunderstandings.

Many women think their inner labia should always be hidden, entirely packed away inside the outer labia, but it's normal for the inner labia of adult women to protrude a long way beyond their outer labia. In fact, there's no single way women are supposed to look down there. What we do have in common are the various parts that combine to form our vulva: the inner and outer labia, the clitoris, the urinary opening and the vaginal opening. But these parts look different from one woman to the next – there is an unbelievable number of variants. Even so, the belief that the inner labia should be short and hidden is surprisingly strong among many women. In an Australian study that interviewed women between 18 and 28, all the women picked out an image of the hairless vulva with concealed inner labia when they were asked what society's 'ideal vulva' was.[108]

Where does precisely this idea come from, since there are so many wonderful, varied genitals? As with other forms of body-image pressure, we might consider the ideals of popular culture, porn culture and so on. At any rate, they may be part of the problem. What is particularly problematic when it comes to aesthetic ideals about the vulva is that it's difficult to confirm whether these are rooted in reality or whether they are unrealistic and overly homogeneous. Once a person has established a belief that normal genitals can only have short labia, this belief will be stronger than the idea that all normal bellies are flat. After all, we see bellies all over the place, every day; we know that they come in all shapes and sizes so it's easy to knock down that idea. However, we don't often have the chance to look between a woman's legs, especially now that young women and girls opt to keep their bathing costumes and knickers on in communal showers because they're afraid of being seen naked. Being naked is no longer natural. Being naked is all too often about sex, and many women connect displaying their bodies with shame.

We believe the misunderstanding surrounding the inner labia arises in part because of a critical gap in the school curriculum when it comes to pubertal development. Like the rest of the body, the female genitals change a great deal in puberty, but we cannot personally remember having been told at any time precisely what happens to the genitals in puberty. At school, we heard about how the penis grows, we heard about how the breasts grow and we heard about the different parts of the body that gradually become covered in hair. We learnt an awful lot, but we didn't learn what happens to the inner labia when we pass from childhood to adulthood.

The fact is that all girl children have genitals whose outer labia cover the inner labia. In other words, we all become familiar with and accustomed to genitals that are formed in this way while we are children. But in puberty the inner labia begin to grow. For many women, they will become so long that they protrude a good way below the outer labia, and they are often uneven in terms of thickness, folded and crinkled.

If your outer labia have always covered your inner labia, it can come as a shock if this suddenly changes, especially if nobody's warned you that it's going to happen and told you that it's normal. The feeling that something is wrong is reinforced if the friends you confide in happen not to have visible inner labia. After all, both types are quite normal.

In other words, some women believe the only normal or 'correct' genitals are the ones shaped like those we all have as children. If young girls and women had learnt as early as infant school that their genitals would change, and if they'd got to know more about what they might look like between the legs once they were adults, perhaps we might not have seen the increase in intimate surgery that we're seeing today. If we'd known that the genitals could take on an incredible number of forms, the vast majority of which are normal and healthy, fewer women would have gone under the knife as a result of a misunderstanding at any rate.

It's important to remember what the inner labia do and what it can mean to trim them. Because the inner labia have a sexual function. They're full of nerve endings and it feels good to touch them. When you cut your labia, you're removing an important and sensitive part of your genitals, and all surgery involves risk. In the worst case, it's possible there will be scar tissue that may be unsightly and cause permanent pain. That's why you should always think carefully before opting for an operation. Is the problem so great that the procedure is worth the risk?

AFTERWORD

What a journey! We hope you've learnt a lot and had a few surprises, as we most certainly have. Female genitals are fantastic. We really hope you're proud to have them. We also hope we've lit a spark in you, making you more aware of what lies between your legs, and that you've become curious and interested in your own genitals. As with all knowledge, there's always more to be had. What's more, medicine is a profession in a constant process of development. What we write about today may be outdated within a month. We never stop learning.

Unfortunately for many, their genitals are a source of mystery and shame. There's a whole world of genital problems and even though our sophisticated reproductive system is designed to put up with a lot, sometimes we face dilemmas and disease – although at least we don't have to worry about being kicked in the balls. Genital problems can feel especially intimate and shameful. Few people speak openly about these issues, the way they talk about throat infections or slipped discs, leaving many women to feel alone and anxious when things aren't the way they usually are. We hope this book has given you the knowledge you need to visit your doctor with your head held high and that perhaps it's given you a bit more confidence, so you'll know when you need to worry and when you can chill out.

We also hope you've abandoned some of the negative thoughts you may have had about your genitals or your sex life. We've met a lot of women who feel abnormal because they don't have orgasms solely through vaginal penetration, or because they think they have genital herpes or a vulva that looks nothing like the illustrations in an anatomy book. As you'll know after reading this book, this is all very, very common.

In our sexualised daily lives, it can sometimes be easy to forget that our bodies are about more than appearance and performance, and that a naked body isn't always about sex. It's easy to base your self-worth on what you get up to in bed and, not least, the way you look. What we perceive as our shortcomings often become all-consuming. Your sex life should be on your own terms. The important thing is to learn to enjoy yourself and your own body, just the way you are, both alone and with one partner or three. Not everybody gets to do everything, and not everybody looks the same. When it comes down to it, a body is just a body, but it's valuable because it's the only one you'll ever have.

Acknowledgements

We'd like to thank some specially selected people. Marius Johansen has done a fantastic job of quality-assuring the medical aspect of the text, as well as being a brilliant guy and a brilliant doctor. We hope this won't be our last collaboration. Other wonderful professionals have also contributed their specialist knowledge. Thank you to Kjartan Moe, Trond Diseth, Kari Ormstad, Sveinung W. Sørbye, Jorun Thørring, Anne Lise Helgesen, Anders Røyneberg, Eszter Vanki, Berit Austveg and Reidun Førde for the conversations, read-throughs and comments. We must also thank the professors at University of Oslo Medical Faculty who, without knowing it, have given us the answers we were wondering about during lectures or in patient conversations between classes. We must stress that any mistakes in this book are our responsibility entirely.

We would also like to thank our former and current colleagues at Medisinernes Seksualopplysning Oslo, Stiftelsen SUSS-telefon, Sex og samfunn and Olafiaklinikken for creating good, stimulating learning environments. We are also unbelievably grateful to our dear friends and colleagues who have read and discussed this with us throughout the writing process – and called us out when we've got tangled up in incomprehensible explanations.

Thanks to all of you who read our blog and those of you who've offered suggestions for topics, asked sensible questions and cheered us on. We wrote this book for you.

An especially big thank you to our editor Nazneen Khan-Østrem at Aschehoug. It makes us so happy to discuss everything from periods to punk rock with you. And it's given us such a sense of security knowing that you were watching our backs. Thank you to TegneHanne, Hanne Sigbjørnsen, who has drawn the best illustrations we could imagine. It's been a gift having such a funny nurse on our team.

And now, at last, there's no getting away from our families.

From Nina: this book was conceived at around the same time that Mads came into the world. It wouldn't have been possible without the most patient and considerate boyfriend I could wish for, Fredrik. You're a whole lot of man per square metre. Mads, you're my little ray of sunshine and I'm sure you'll be horribly embarrassed when you read Mummy's book someday. I'll try not to talk too much about lady parts at the dinner table. Mum, Dad and Helch – you are the best family a person could wish for.

From Ellen: thanks to Mum, Dad and Helge, the world's best family, who have patiently listened to long and pretty intense monológues about hymens, vulval pains, herpes and other such dross – sometimes in public and inappropriate places. Thanks also to Grandfather, who compared us to Karl Evang, women's sexual health pioneer in Norway. I love you all beyond measure. Most of all I want to thank Henning, for more reasons than I feel inclined to write down.

NOTES

PREFACE
1. Vigsnæs, M.K., Spets, K. and Quist, C. 2016 [updated 15 September 2016]. 'Politiet slår alarm: Grenseløs sexkultur blant barn og unge', *VG+* < http://pluss.vg.no/2016/0 8/20/2508/2508_23770417>

2. Bergo, I.G. and Quist, C. 2016. 'Kunnskapsministeren om sexkulturen blant unge: – Skolen må ta mer ansvar', *VG+* <http://www.vg.no/nyheter/innenriks/kunnskapsministeren-om-sexkulturen-blant-unge-skolen-maa-ta-mer-ansvar/a/23770735>

THE GENITALS
1. Boston University School of Medicine. 2002. 'Female Genital Anatomy', *Sexual Medicine* <http://www.bumc.bu.edu/sexualmedicine/physicianinformation/female-genital-anatomy>

2. Kilchevsky, A., Vardi, Y., Lowenstein, L. and Gruenwald, I. 2012. 'Is the Female G-Spot Truly a Distinct Anatomic Entity?' *The Journal of Sexual Medicine*, 9(3): 719–726.

3. Buisson, O., Foldes, P., Jannini, E. and Mimoun, S. 2010. 'Coitus as Revealed by Ultrasound in One Volunteer Couple', *The Journal of Sexual Medicine*, 7(8): 2750–2754.

4. Darling, C.A., Davidson, J.K. Sr and Conway-Welch, C. 1990. 'Female ejaculation: perceived origins, the Grafenberg spot/area, and sexual responsiveness', *Archives of Sexual Behavior*, 19(1): 29–47.

5. O'Connell, H.E. and DeLancey, J.O. 2005. 'Clitoral anatomy in nulliparous, healthy, premenopausal volunteers using unenhanced magnetic resonance imaging', *The Journal of Urology*, 173(6): 2060–2063; O'Connell, H.E., Sanjeevan, K.V. and Hutson, J.M. 2005. 'Anatomy of the clitoris', *The Journal of Urology*, 174(4), pt 1: 1189–1195; Pauls, R.N. 2015, 'Anatomy of the clitoris and the female sexual response', *Clinical Anatomy*, 28(3): 376–384.

6. Lloyd, J., Crouch, N.S., Minto, C.L., Liao, L.M. and Creighton, S.M. 2005. 'Female genital appearance: "normality" unfolds', *BJOG*, 112(5): 643–646.

7. Di Marino, V. and Lepidi, H. 2014. *Anatomic Study of the Clitoris and the Bulbo-Clitoral Organ* (Springer International Publishing): 91.

8. Maravilla, K.A., Heiman, J.R., Garland, P.A., Cao, Y., Carter, B.T., Peterson, W.O., et al. 2003. 'Dynamic MR Imaging of the Sexual Arousal Response in Women', *Journal of Sex & Marital Therapy*, 29: 71–6.

9. Karacan, I., Rosenbloom, A. and Williams, R. 1970. 'The clitoral erection cycle during sleep', *Journal of Sleep Research*.

10. Fisher, C., Cohen, H.D., Schiavi, R.C., Davis, D., Furman, B., Ward, K., et al. 1983. 'Patterns of female sexual arousal during sleep and waking: Vaginal thermo-conductance studies', *Archives of Sexual Behavior*, 12(2): 97–122.

11. Nesheim, B.-I. 2009. 'Deflorasjon', *Store Medisinske Leksikon* <https://sml.snl.no/deflorasjon>

12. Smith, A. 2011. 'The prepubertal hymen', *Australian Family Physician*, 40(11): 873.

13. Berenson, A., Heger, A. and Andrews, S. 1991. 'Appearance of the Hymen in Newborns', *Pediatrics*, 87(4): 458–465.

14. Whitley, N. 1978. 'The first coital experience of one hundred women', *Journal of Obstetric, Gynecologic, and Neonatal Nursing*, 7(4): 41–45; Hägstad, A.J. 1990. 'Mödomen – mest myt!' *Läkartidningen*, 87(37): 2857–2858.

15. Zariat, I. 2016 [updated 28 August 2016]. 'Rystende jomfrusjekk', *Ytring* (NRK) <https://www.nrk.no/ytring/rystende -jomfrusjekk-1.13106033>

16. Independent Forensic Expert Group. 2015. 'Statement on virginity testing', *Journal of Forensic and Legal Medicine*, 33: 121–124.

17. Adams, J.A., Botash, A.S. and Kellogg, N. 2004. 'Differences in hymenal morphology between adolescent girls with and without a history of consensual sexual intercourse', *Archives of Pediatrics & Adolescent Medicine*, 158(3): 280–285; Kellogg, N.D., Menard, S.W. and Santos, A. 2004. 'Genital anatomy in pregnant adolescents: "normal" does not mean "nothing happened"', *Pediatrics*, 113: 67–69.

18. McCann, J., Miyamoto, S., Boyle, C. and Rogers, K. 2007. 'Healing of hymenal injuries in prepubertal and adolescent girls: a descriptive study', *Pediatrics*, 119(5): 1094–1106.

19. Berenson, A.B., Chacko, M.R., Wiemann, C.M., Mishaw, C.O., Friedrich, W.N. and Grady, J.J. 2002. 'Use of Hymenal Measurements in the Diagnosis of Previous Penetration', *Pediatrics*, 109(2): 228–235.

20. Myhre, A.K., Borgen, G. and Ormstad, K. 2006. 'Seksuelle overgrep mot prepubertale barn', *Tidsskrift for Den norske legeforening*, 126(19): 2511.

21. Hasselknippe, O. and Stokke, O. 2006 [updated 19 October 2011]. 'Volvat slutter å selge jomfruhinner', *Aftenposten* <http://www.aftenposten.no/norge/Volvat-slutter-a-selge-jomfruhinner-423873b.html>

22. Førde, R. 2002. 'Operativ rekonstruksjon av jomfruhinne', *Tidsskrift for Den norske legeforening*.

23. The Artificial Hymen Kit. 2016. *The Hymen Shop* <http://www.hymenshop.com>

24. Telegraph. 2009. 'Egyptians want to ban fake virginity kit', *Telegraph* <http://www.telegraph.co.uk/news/worldnews/africaandindianocean/egypt/6264741/Egyptians-want-to-ban-fake-virginity-kit.html>

25. Paus, R. and Cotsarelis, G. 1999. 'The biology of hair follicles', *The New England Journal of Medicine*, 341(7): 491–7.

26. Olsen, E.A. 1999. 'Methods of hair removal', *Journal of the American Academy of Dermatology*, 40: 143–55; 56–57.

27. Paus and Cotsarelis: 491–7.
28. Shenenberger, D.W. 2016. 'Removal of unwanted hair,' *UpToDate* <https://uptodate. com/contents/removal-of-unwanted-hair>
29. Goldstein, B.G. and Goldstein, A.O. 2016. 'Pseudofolliculitis barbae,' *UpToDate* <https://www.uptodate.com/contents/pseudofolliculitis-barbae>
30. Murakami, H. 2005. *Kafka on the Shore* (London: Vintage)
31. Wallace, W.H.B and Kelsey, T.W. 2010. 'Human Ovarian Reserve from Conception to the Menopause,' *PLOS ONE*, 5(1): e8722.
32. Ibid.
33. Tanbo, T.G. 2016. E-mail from M.D. Tom Gunnar Tanbo, former consultant at the Section for Reproductive Medicine, Gynaecology department, OUS, Oslo University Hospital.

DISCHARGE, PERIODS AND OTHER GORE

1. Sobel, J.D. 2016. 'Patient education: Vaginal discharge in adult women (Beyond the Basics),' *UpToDate* <https://www.uptodate.com/contents/vaginal-discharge-in-adult-women-beyond-the-basics>
2. Dyall-Smith, D. 2016. 'Trimethylaminuria,' *DermNet New Zealand* <http://www. dermnetnz.org/topics/trimethylaminuria>
3. Emera, D., Romero, R. and Wagner, G. 2012. 'The evolution of menstruation: A new model for genetic assimilation,' *BioEssays*, 34(1): 26–35.
4. Frank, L. 10 June 2016. 'Blodig Uenighet,' *Morgenbladet*.
5. McClintock, M.K. 1971. 'Menstrual synchrony and suppression,' *Nature*; vol. 229(5282): 244.
6. Turke, P.W. 1984. 'Effects of ovulatory concealment and synchrony on protohominid mating systems and parental roles,' *Ethology and Sociobiology*, 5(1): 33–34.
7. Arden, M., Dye, L. and Walker, A. 1999. 'Menstrual synchrony: awareness and subjective experiences,' *Journal of Reproductive and Infant Psychology*, 17(3): 255–265.
8. Trevathan, W.R., Burleson, M.H., Gregory, W.L. 1993. 'No evidence for menstrual synchrony in lesbian couples,' *Psychoneuroendocrinology*, 18(5): 425–35.
9. Yang, Z. and Schank, J.C. 2006. 'Women do not synchronize their menstrual cycles,' *Human Nature*, 17(4): 433–447.
10. Dillner, L. 2016 [updated 15 September 2016]. 'Do women's periods really synchronise when they live together?' *Guardian* <https://www.theguardian.com/lifeandstyle/2016/aug/15/periods-housemates-menstruation-synchronise>
11. Wikipedia. 2016 [updated 21 September 2016]. 'Sanitary napkin,' *Wikipedia* <https://en.wikipedia.org/wiki/Sanitary_napkin>
12. NEL – Norsk elektronisk legehåndbok. 2014 [updated 22 January 2014]. 'Toksisk sjokksyndrom (TSS),' *NEL – Norsk elektronisk legehåndbok.* <https://legehandboka. no/handboken/kliniske-kapitler/infeksjoner/tilstander-og-sykdommer/bakteriesykdommer/toksisk-sjokk-syndrome>
13. Mitchell, M.A., Bisch, S., Arntfield, S. and Hosseini-Moghaddam, S.M. 2015. 'A

confirmed case of toxic shock syndrome associated with the use of a menstrual cup,'
The Canadian Journal of Infectious Diseases & Medical Microbiology, 26(4): 218–220.

14. NEL – Norsk elektronisk legehåndbok. 2015 [updated 6 September 2015].
'Premenstruelt syndrom,' *NEL – Norsk elektronisk legehåndbok* <https://
legehandboka.no/handboken/kliniske-kapitler/gynekologi/tilstander-og-sykdommer/
menstruasjonsproblemer/premenstruelt-syndrome>

15. NEL – Norsk elektronisk legehåndbook, 'Premenstruelt syndrom.'

16. Yonkers, K.A., O'Brien, P.M.S. and Eriksson, E. 2008. 'Premenstrual syndrome,' *The
Lancet*, 371(9619): 1200–1210.

17. Grady-Weliky, T.A. 2003. 'Premenstrual Dysphoric Disorder,' *New England Journal of
Medicine*, 348(5): 433–438.

18. NEL – Norsk elektronisk legehåndbook, 'Premenstruelt syndrom.'

19. Wilcox, A.J., Weinberg, C.R., Baird, D.D. 1995. 'Timing of sexual intercourse in
relation to ovulation – effects on the probability of conception, survival of the
pregnancy and sex of the baby,' *New England Journal of Medicine*, 333(23): 1517–1521.

SEX

1. Træen, B., Stigum, H., Magnus, P. 2003. 'Rapport fra seksualvaneundersøkelsene i
1987, 1992, 1997 og 2002,' *Folkehelseinstituttet* (Statens institutt for folkehelse).

2. Træen, B., Spitznogle, K. and Beverfjord, A. 2004. 'Attitudes and use of pornography
in the Norwegian population 2002,' *Journal of Sex Research*, 41(2): 193–200.

3. The Lancet, 'Table 3: Sexual partners, practices, behaviours, and attitudes reported
by women in Natsal-3, by age group,' *The Lancet* <http://www.thelancet.com/action/
showFullTableImage?tableId=tbl3&pii=S0140673613620358>

4. Mercer, C.H., Tanton, C., Prah, P., Erens, B., Sonnenberg, P., Clifton, S., et al. 2013.
'Changes in sexual attitudes and lifestyles in Britain through the life course and over
time: findings from the National Surveys of Sexual Attitudes and Lifestyles (Natsal),'
The Lancet, 382(9907): 1781–1794.

5. Marston, C. and Lewis, R. 2014. 'Anal heterosex among young people and implications
for health promotion: a qualitative study in the UK,' *BMJ Open*, 4(8): e004996.

6. Christopher, F.S. and Sprecher, S. 2000. 'Sexuality in Marriage, Dating, and Other
Relationships: A Decade Review,' *Journal of Marriage and Family*, 62(4): 999–1017.

7. Bernard, M.L.R. 2015 [updated 30 March 2015]. 'How Often Do Queer Women Have
Sex?' *Autostraddle* <http://autostraddle.com/how-often-do-lesbians-have-sex-283731>

8. Stabell, K., Mortensen, B. and Træen, B. 2008. 'Samleiefrekvens: Prevalens og
prediktorer i et tilfeldig utvalg norske gifte og samboende heteroseksuelle par,'
Journal of the Norwegian Psychological Association, 45: 683–694.

9. Klussman, D. 2002. 'Sexual motivation and the duration of partnership,' *Archives of
Sexual Behavior*, 31(3): 275–287.

10. Murray, S.H. and Milhausen, R.R. 2012. 'Sexual desire and relationship duration in

young men and women,' *Journal of Sex & Marital Therapy*, 38(1): 28–40; Rao, K.V. and Demaris, A. 1995. 'Coital frequency among married and cohabiting couples in the United States,' *Journal of Biosocial Science*, 27(2): 135–150.

11. Bernard.

12. Stabell, Mortensen and Træen, 2008: 683–694.

13. Muise, A., Schimmack, U. and Impett, E.A. 2016. 'Sexual frequency predicts greater well-being, but more is not always better,' *Social Psychological and Personality science*, 7(4): 295–302.

14. Christopher and Sprecher; Sprecher, S. 2002. 'Sexual satisfaction in premarital relationships: associations with satisfaction, love, commitment, and stability,' *Journal of Sex Research*, 39(3): 190–196; Haavio-Mannila, E. and Kontula, O. 1997. 'Correlates of increased sexual satisfaction,' *Archives of Sexual Behavior*, 26(4): 399–419.

15. Frederick, A., Lever, J., Gillespie, B.J. and Garcia, J.R. 2016. 'What Keeps Passion Alive? Sexual Satisfaction Is Associated With Sexual Communication, Mood Setting, Sexual Variety, Oral Sex, Orgasm and Sex Frequency in a National U.S. Study,' *Journal of Sex Research*: 1–16; MacNeil, S. and Byers, E.S. 2005. 'Dyadic assessment of sexual self-disclosure and sexual satisfaction in heterosexual dating couples,' *Journal of Social and Personal Relationships*, 22(2): 169–181; Montesi, J.L., Fauber, R.L., Gordon, E.A. and Heimberg, R.G. 2011. 'The specific importance of communicating about sex to couples' sexual and overall relationship satisfaction,' *Journal of Social and Personal Relationships*, 28(5): 591–609.

16. Stabell, Mortensen and Træen.

17. Richters, J., Visser, R., Rissel, C. and Smith, A. 2006. 'Sexual practices at last heterosexual encounter and occurrence of orgasm in a national survey,' *Journal of Sex Research*, 43(3): 217–226.

18. Mitchell, K.R., Mercer, C.H., Ploubidis, G.B., Jones, K.G., Datta, J., Field, N., et al. 2013. 'Sexual function in Britain: findings from the third National Survey of Sexual Attitudes and Lifestyles (Natsal-3),' *The Lancet*, 382(9907): 1817–1829.

19. Basson, R. 2006. 'Sexual Desire and Arousal Disorders in Women,' *New England Journal of Medicine*, 354(14): 1497–1506; Shifren, J.L. 2016 [updated 4 April 2016]. 'Sexual dysfunction in women: Epidemiology, risk factors, and evaluation,' *UpToDate* <https://uptodate.com/contents/sexual-dysfunction-in-women-epidemiology-risk-factors-and-evaluation>

20. Basson, R., Leiblum, S., Brotto, L., Derogatis, L., Fourcroy, J., Fugl-Meyer, K., et al. 2003. 'Definitions of women's sexual dysfunction reconsidered: advocating expansion and revision,' *Journal of Psychosomatic Obstetrics and Gynaecology*, 24(4): 221–229; Brotto, L.A., Petkau, A.J., Labrie, F. and Basson, R. 2011. 'Predictors of sexual desire disorders in women,' *Journal of Sexual Medicine*, 8(3): 742–753.

21. Nagoski, E. 2015. *Come as you are – the surprising new science that will transform your sex life* (New York: Simon and Schuster Paperbacks).

22. Ibid.

23. Ibid.

24. Ibid.; Roach, M. 2008. *BONK – the Curious Coupling of Science and Sex* (New York: W. W. Norton and Company).

25. Chivers, M.L., Seto, M.C., Lalumiere, M.L., Laan, E. and Grimbos, T. 2010. 'Agreement of self-reported and genital measures of sexual arousal in men and women: a meta-analysis,' *Archives of Sexual Behavior*, 39(1): 5–56.

26. Ibid.

27. Ibid.

28. Roach.

29. Basson, R., McInnes, R., Smith, M.D., Hodgson, G. and Koppiker, N. 2002. 'Efficacy and safety of sildenafil citrate in women with sexual dysfunction associated with female sexual arousal disorder,' *Journal of Women's Health & Gender-based Medicine*, 11(4): 367–377.

30. Shifren, J.L. 2016 [updated 19 May 2016]. 'Sexual dysfunction in women: Management,' *UpToDate* <https://www.uptodate.com/content/sexual-dysfunction-in-women-management>

31. Davis S., Papalia M-A., Norman R.J., O'Neill S., Redelman M., Williamson M., et al. 2008. 'Safety and efficacy of a testosterone metered-dose transdermal spray for treating decreased sexual satisfaction in premenopausal women: a randomized trial,' *Annals of Internal Medicine*, 148(8): 569–577.

32. Ibid.

33. Brotto, Petkau, Labrie and Basson.

34. Clayton, A.H., Althof, S.E., Kingsberg, S., DeRogatis, L.R., Kroll, R., Goldstein, I., et al. 2016. 'Bremelanotide for female sexual dysfunctions in premenopausal women: a randomized placebo-controlled dose-finding trial,' *Women's Health*, 12(3): 325–337.

35. Shifren.

36. Bradford, A. and Meston, C. 2007. 'Correlates of placebo response in the treatment of sexual dysfunction in women: a preliminary report,' *The Journal of Sexual Medicine*, 4(5): 1345–1351.

37. Nagoski.

38. Meston C.M., Levin R.J., Sipski M.L., Hull E.M., and Heiman J.R. 2004. 'Women's orgasm,' *Annual Review of Sex Research*, 15: 173–257.

39. Mah K. and Binik Y.M. 2001. 'The nature of human orgasm: a critical review of major trends,' *Clinical Psychology Review*, 21(6): 823–856.

40. Nagoski.

41. Mah and Binik.

42. Wikipedia. 2016 [updated 8 September 2016]. 'Masturbate-a-thon,' *Wikipedia* <https://en.wikipedia.org/wiki/Masturbate-a-thon>

43. Puppo V. 2011. 'Embryology and anatomy of the vulva: The female orgasm and women's sexual health.' *European Journal of Obstetrics and Gynecology and Reproductive Biology*, 154(1): 3–8.

44. Wallen K. and Lloyd E.A. 2011. 'Female sexual arousal: Genital anatomy and orgasm in intercourse,' *Hormones and Behavior*, 59(5): 780–792.

45. Korda J.B., Goldstein S.W. and Sommer F. 2010. 'Sexual Medicine History: The History of Female Ejaculation,' *The Journal of Sexual Medicine*, 7(5): 1965–1975.

46. Rosen R. 2014 [updated 4 December 2014]. 'No female ejaculation, please, we're British: a history of porn and censorship,' *Independent* <http://www.independent.co.uk/life-style/health-and-families/features/no-female-ejaculation-please-we-re-british-a-history-of-porn-and-censorship-9903054.html>

47. Pollen J.J. and Dreilinger A. 1984. 'Immunohistochemical identification of prostatic acid phosphatase and prostate specific antigen in female periurethral glands,' *Urology*, 23(3): 303–304; Wimpissinger F., Stifter K., Grin W. and Stackl W. 2007. 'The female prostate revisited: perineal ultrasound and biochemical studies of female ejaculate,' *Journal of Sexual Medicine*, 4(5): 1388–1393.

48. Wimpissinger, Stifter, Grin and Stackl.

49. Salama S., Boitrelle F., Gauquelin A., Malagrida L., Thiounn N. and Desvaux P. 2015. 'Nature and Origin of 'Squirting' in Female Sexuality,' *The Journal of Sexual Medicine*, 12(3): 661–666.

50. Pastor Z. 2013. 'Female ejaculation orgasm vs. coital incontinence: a systematic review,' *Journal of Sexual Medicine*, 10(7): 1682–1691.

51. Laqueur T. 1992. *Making Sex: Body and Gender from the Greeks to Freud* (Boston: Harvard University Press).

52. Ibid.

53. Freud, S. 1905. *Three essays on the theory of sexuality*.

54. Levin R.J. 2015. 'Recreation and procreation: A critical view of sex in the human female,' *Clinical Anatomy*, 28(3): 339–354.

55. Angel K. 2010. 'The history of "female sexual dysfunction" as a mental disorder in the 20th century,' *Current Opinion in Psychiatry*, 23(6): 536.

56. Roach.

57. Wallen and Lloyd; Oakley S.H., Vaccaro C.M., Crisp C.C., Estanol M., Fellner A.N., Kleeman S.D., et al. 2014. 'Clitoral size and location in relation to sexual function using pelvic MRI,' *The Journal of Sexual Medicine*, 11(4): 1013–1022.

58. Strömquist L. 2014. 'Kunskapens frukt,' *Galago* <http://galago.se/bocker/kunskapens-frukt>

59. Garcia J.R., Lloyd E.A., Wallen K. and Fisher H.E. 2014. 'Variation in orgasm occurrence by sexual orientation in a sample of U.S. singles,' *Journal of Sexual Medicine*, 11(11): 2645–2652.

60. Nagoski.

61. Mitchell, Mercer, Ploubidis, Jones, Datta, Field, et al.

62. Dunn K.M., Cherkas L.F. and Spector T.D. 2005. 'Genetic influences on variation in female orgasmic function: a twin study,' *Biology Letters*, 1(3): 260–263; Dawood K., Kirk K.M., Bailey J.M., Andrews P.W. and Martin N.G. 2005. 'Genetic and environmental influences on the frequency of orgasm in women,' *Twin Research and Human Genetics*, 8(1): 27–33.

63. Armstrong E.A., England P. and Fogarty A.C. 2012. 'Accounting for women's orgasm and sexual enjoyment in college hookups and relationships,' *American Sociological Review*, 77(3): 435–462.

64. Kohlenberg R.J. 1974. 'Directed masturbation and the treatment of primary orgasmic dysfunction.' *Archives of Sexual Behavior*, 3(4): 349–356.

65. Bradford A. 2016. 'Treatment of female orgasmic disorder,' *UpToDate* <https://uptodate.com/contents/treatment-of-female-orgasmic-disorder>

66. Eichel E.W., Eichel J.D. and Kule S. 1988. 'The technique of coital alignment and its relation to female orgasmic response and simultaneous orgasm,' *Journal of Sex & Marital Therapy*, 14(2): 129–141; Pierce A.P. 2000. 'The coital alignment technique (CAT): an overview of studies,' *Journal of Sex and Marital Therapy*, 26(3): 257–268.

67. Rosenbaum T.Y. 2007. 'Reviews: Pelvic Floor Involvement in Male and Female Sexual Dysfunction and the Role of Pelvic Floor Rehabilitation in Treatment: A Literature Review,' *The Journal of Sexual Medicine*, 4(1): 4–13.

68. Lorenz T.A. and Meston C.M. 2014. 'Exercise improves sexual function in women taking antidepressants: results from a randomized crossover trial,' *Depression and Anxiety*, 31(3): 188–195.

69. Roach.

CONTRACEPTION

1. Johansen, M. 2016. 'P-piller,' *Emetodebok for seksuell helse* (Oslo: Sex og samfunn).
2. Johansen, M. 2016. 'P-ring,' *Emetodebok for seksuell helse* (Oslo: Sex og samfunn).
3. Johansen, M. 2016. 'P-plaster,' *Emetodebok for seksuell helse* (Oslo: Sex og samfunn).
4. Johansen, M. 2016. 'P-stav,' *Emetodebok for seksuell helse* (Oslo: Sex og samfunn).
5. Johansen, M. 2016. 'Hormonspiral,' *Emetodebok for seksuell helse* (Oslo: Sex og samfunn).
6. Johansen, M. 2016. 'Gestagen p-piller,' *Emetodebok for seksuell helse* (Oslo: Sex og samfunn).
7. Johansen, M. 2016. 'Minipiller,' *Emetodebok for seksuell helse* (Oslo: Sex og samfunn).
8. Johansen, M. 2016. 'P-sprøyte,' *Emetodebok for seksuell helse* (Oslo: Sex og samfunn).
9. Jennings, V. 2016. 'Fertility awareness-based methods of pregnancy prevention,' *UpToDate* <https://www.uptodate.com/contents/fertility-awareness-based-methods-of-pregnancy-prevention>
10. Johansen, M. 2016. 'Kobberspiral,' *Emetodebok for seksuell helse* (Oslo: Sex og samfunn).
11. Dean, G. and Goldberg, A.B. 2016 [updated 15 September 2016]. 'Intrauterine contraception: Devices, candidates, and selection,' *UpToDate* <https://www.uptodate.com/contents/intrauterine-contraception-devices-candidates-and-selection>

12. Maltau, J.M., Molne, K. and Nesheim, B.-I. 2015. *Obstetrikk og gynekologi*, 3rd edition (Oslo: Gyldendal Akademisk): 313–314.

13. Ibid.

14. Johansen, M. 2016. 'Nødprevensjon: Levonorgestrel,' *Emetodebok for seksuell helse* (Oslo: Sex og samfunn).

15. Bordvik, M. 2016 [updated 7 June 2016]. 'P-pille-bruk kan ødelegge effekten av angrepille,' *Dagens Medisin* <http://www.dagensmedisin.no/artikler/2016/07/06/angrepille-kan-odelegge-p-pille-effekt>

16. Johansen, M. 'Nødprevensjon'.

17. Ibid.

18. WHO. 2015. Family planning/Contraception. *WHO* <http://www.who.int/mediacentre/factsheets/fs351/en>; Johansen M. 2016. 'Prevensjonsmidler,' *Emetodebok for seksuell helse* (Oslo: Sex og samfunn).

19. Karlsen, S.G., Jonassen, T.H. and Suvatne, S.S. 2015 [updated 26 June 2015]. 'Anbefaler naturalig prevensjon og påstår at den er 99.9% sikker,' *Dagbladet* <http://www.dagbladet.no/2015/06/29/kjendis/blogg/prevensjon/caroline_berg_eriksen/lege/39902645>

20. Maltau, Molne and Nesheim.

21. Juvkam, K.H. and Gudim, H.B. 2013. 'Medikamentell forskyvning av menstruasjon,' *Tidsskrift for Den norske legeforening*, 133: 166–168.

22. Legemiddehåndboken. 2016 [updated 13 September 2016]. 'Perorale gestagener,' *Norsk Legemiddelhåndbok* <http://legemiddelhandboka.no/legemidler/?frid=lk-03-endokr-7205>

23. Rosenberg, M.J. and Waugh, M.S. 1998. 'Oral contraceptive discontinuation: a prospective evaluation of frequency and reasons,' *American Journal of Obstetrics and Gynecology*, 179(3): 577–582.

24. Ibid.

25. Barsky, A.J., Saintfort, R., Rogers, M.P. and Borus, J.F. 2002. 'Non-specific medication side-effects and the nocebo phenomenon,' *JAMA*, 287(5): 622–627.

26. Peipert, J.F. and Gutmann, J. 1993. 'Oral contraceptive risk assessment: a survey of 247 educated women,' *Obstetrics & Gynecology*, 82(1): 112–117.

27. Grimes, D.A. and Schulz, K.F. 2011. 'Nonspecific side-effects of oral contraceptives: nocebo or noise?' *Contraception*, 83(1): 5–9.

28. Johansen, 'Prevensjonsmidler;' Martin, K.A. and Douglas, P.S. 2016 [updated 22 August 2016]. 'Risk and side-effects associated with estrogen-progestin contraceptives,' *UpToDate* <https//www.uptodate.com/contents/risks-and-side-effects-associated-with-estrogen-progestin-contraceptives>

29. NEL – Norsk elektronisk legehåndbok. 2015 [updated 28 December 2015]. 'Melasma'. *NEL – Norsk elektronisk legehåndbok* <https://legehandboka.no/handboken/kliniske-kapitler/hud/tilstander-og-sykdommer/pitmenterte-lesjoner/melasma-kloasma>

30. Gallo, M.F., Grimes, D.A., Schulz, K.F. and Helmerhorst, F.M. 2004. 'Combination estrogen-progestin contraceptives and body weight: systematic review of randomized controlled trials,' *Obstetrics & Gynecology*, 103(2): 359–373.

31. Moen, M.H. 2013. 'Selvvalgt menstruasjon,' *Tidsskrift for Den norsk legeforening*, 133: 131.

32. Johansen, M. 2016. 'Hormonspiral,' *Emetodebok for seksuell helse* (Oslo: Sex og samfunn).

33. Charlton, B.M., Rich-Edwards, J.W., Colditz, G.A., Missmer, S.A., Rosner, B.A., Hankinson, S.E., et al. 2014. 'Oral contraceptive use and mortality after 36 years of follow-up in the Nurses' Health Study: prospective cohort study,' *BMJ*, 349: g6356.

34. Kaunitz, A.M. 2016. 'Patient education: hormonal methods of birth control (Beyond the Basics),' *UpToDate* <https://www.uptodate.com/contents/hormonal-methods-of-birth-control-beyond-the-basics?source=see_link>

35. Heit, J.A., Kobbervig, C.E., James, A.H., Petterson, T.M., Bailey, K.R. and Melton, L.J. 2005. 'Trends in the incidence of venous thromboembolism during pregnancy or postpartum: a 30-year population-based study,' *Annals of Internal Medicine*, 143(10): 697–706.

36. Lidegaard, O., Lokkegaard, E., Jensen, A., Skovlund, C.W. and Keiding, N. 2012. 'Thrombotic stroke and myocardial infarction with hormonal contraception,' *The New England Journal of Medicine*, 366(24): 2257–2266.

37. Martin and Douglas.

38. Hannaford, P.C., Selvaraj, S., Elliott, A.M., Angus, V., Iversen, L. and Lee, A.J. 2007. 'Cancer risk among users of oral contraceptives: cohort data from the Royal College of General Practitioners' oral contraception study,' *BMJ*, 335(7621): 651.

39. Martin and Douglas.

40. Beral, V., Doll, R., Hermon, C., Peto, R. and Reeves, G. 2008. 'Ovarian cancer and oral contraceptives: collaborative reanalysis of data from 45 epidemiological studies including 23,257 women with ovarian cancer 87,303 controls,' *The Lancet*, 371(9609): 303–314.

41. Vessey, M. and Painter, R. 2006. 'Oral contraceptive use and cancer. Findings in a large cohort study, 1968–2004,' *British Journal of Cancer*, 95(3): 385–389.

42. Appleby, P., Beral, V., Berrington de Gonzalez, A., Colin, D., Franceschi, S., Goodhill, A., et al. 2007. 'Cervical cancer and hormonal contraceptives: collaborative reanalysis of individual data for 16,573 women with cervical cancer and 35,509 women without cervical cancer from 24 epidemiological studies,' *The Lancet*, 370(9599): 1609–1621.

43. Martin and Douglas.

44. Stanislaw, H. and Rice, F.J. 1988. 'Correlation between sexual desire and menstrual cycle characteristics,' *Archives of sexual behavior*, 17(6): 499–508; Caruso, S., Agnello, C., Malandrino, C., Lo Presti, L., Cicero, C. and Cianci, S. 2014. 'Do hormones influence women's sex? Sexual activity over the menstrual cycle,' *Journal of Sexual Medicine*, 11(1): 211–221.

45. Bellis, M.A. and Baker, R.R. 1990. 'Do females promote sperm competition? Data for humans', *Animal Behaviour*, 40(5): 997–999.

46. Grimes and Schulz; Lindh, I., Blohm, F., Andersson-Ellstrom, A. and Milsom, I. 2009. 'Contraceptive use and pregnancy outcome in three generations of Swedish female teenagers from the same urban population', *Contraception*, 80(2): 163–169; Brunner Huber, L.R., Hogue, C.J., Stein, A.D., Drews, C., Zieman, M., King, J., et al. 2006. 'Contraceptive use and discontinuation: findings from the contraceptive history, initiation, and choice study', *American Journal of Obstetrics and* Gynecology, 194(5): 1290–1295.

47. Grimes and Schulz.

48. O'Connell, K., Davis, A.R. and Kerns, J. 2007. 'Oral contraceptives: Side-effects and depression in adolescent girls', *Contraception*, 75(4): 299–304; Redmond, G., Godwin, A.J., Olson, W. and Lippman, J.S. 1999. 'Use of placebo controls in an oral contraceptive trial: methodological issues and adverse event incidence', *Contraception*, 60(2): 81–85.

49. Graham C.A. and Sherwin B.B. 1993. 'The relationship between mood and sexuality in women using an oral contraceptive as a treatment for premenstrual symptoms', *Psychoneuroendocrinology*, 18(4): 273–281.

50. Graham, C.A., Ramos, R., Bancroft, J., Maglaya, C. and Farley, T.M. 1995. 'The effects of steroid contraceptives on the well-being and sexuality of women: a double-blind, placebo-controlled, two-centre study of combined and progestogen-only methods', *Contraception*, 52(6): 363–369.

51. Gingnell, M., Engman, J., Frick, A., Moby, L., Wikström, J., Fredrikson, M., et al. 2013. 'Oral contraceptive use changes in brain activity and mood in women with previous negative affect on the pill – a double-blinded, placebo-controlled randomized trial of a levonorgestrel-containing combined oral contraceptive', *Psychoneuroendocrinology*, 38(7): 1133–1144.

52. Jacobi, F., Wittchen, H.U., Holting, C., Hofler, M., Pfister, H., Muller, N., et al. 2004. 'Prevalence, co-morbidity and correlates of mental disorders in the general population: results from the German Health Interview and Examination Survey (GHS)', *Psychological Medicine*, 34(4): 597–611.

53. Joffe, H., Cohen, L.S. and Harlow, B.L. 2003. 'Impact of oral contraceptive pill use on premenstrual mood: predictors of improvement and deterioration', *American Journal of Obstetrics and Gynecology*, 189(6): 1523–1530.

54. Duke, J.M., Sibbritt, D.W. and Young, A.F. 2007. 'Is there an association between the use of oral contraception and depressive symptoms in young Australian women?' *Contraception*, 75(1): 27–31.

55. Keyes, K.M., Cheslack-Postava, K., Westhoff, C., Heim, C.M., Haloosim, M., Walsh, K., et al. 2013. 'Association of hormonal contraceptive use with reduced levels of depressive symptoms: National study of sexually active women in the United States', *American Journal of Epidemiology*, 178(9): 1378–1388.

56. Toffol, E., Heikinheimo, O., Koponen, P., Luoto, R. and Partonen, T. 2011. 'Hormonal contraception and mental health: results of a population-based study,' *Human Reproduction*, 26(11): 3085–3093.

57. Skovlund, C., Mørch, L., Kessing, L. and Lidegaard, Ø. 2016. 'Association of hormonal contraception with depression,' *JAMA Psychiatry*, 73(11): 1154–1162.

58. Malmborg, A., Persson, E., Brynhildsen, J. and Hammar, M. 2016. 'Hormonal contraception and sexual desire: a questionnaire-based study of young Swedish women,' *The European Journal of Contraception & Reproductive Healthcare*, 21(2): 158–167.

59. Pastor, Z., Holla, K. and Chmel, R. 2013. 'The influence of combined oral contraceptives on female sexual desire: a systematic review,' *The European Journal of Contraception & Reproductive Healthcare*, 18(1): 27–43.

60. Davis, Papalia, Norman, O'Neill, Redelman, Williamson, et al.

61. Burrows, L.J., Basha, M. and Goldstein, A.T. 2012. 'The effects of hormonal contraceptives on female sexuality: a review,' *Journal of Sexual Medicine*, 9(9): 2213–2223.

62. Cheung, E. and Free, C. 2004. 'Factors influencing young women's decision making regarding hormonal contraceptives: a qualitative study,' *Contraception*, 71(6): 426–431.

63. Lidegaard, O., Lokkegaard, E., Svendsen, A.L. and Agger, C. 2009. 'Hormonal contraception and risk of venous thromboembolism: National follow-up study,' *BMJ*, 339: b2890.

64. Johansen, M. 2016. 'Misoppfatninger om prevensjon,' *Emetodebok for seksuell helse* (Oslo: Sex og samfunn).

65. Bagwell, M.A., Thompson, S.J., Addy, C.L., Coker, A.L. and Baker, E.R. 1995. 'Primary infertility and oral contraceptive steroid use,' *Fertility and Sterility*, 63(6): 1161–1166.

66. Mansour, D., Gemzell-Danielsson, K., Inki, P. and Jensen, J.T. 2011. 'Fertility after discontinuation of contraception: a comprehensive review of the literature,' *Contraception*, 84(5): 465–477.

67. UNDP/UNFPA/WHO/World Bank Special Programme of Research, Development and Research Training in Human Reproduction (HRP). 2012. 'Unsafe abortion incidence and mortality – Global and regional levels in 2008 and trends,' *WHO*.

68. Singh, S., Maddow-Zimet, I. 2016. 'Facility-based treatment for medical complications resulting from unsafe pregnancy termination in the developing world, 2012: a review of evidence from 26 countries,' *BJOG*, 123: 1489–1498.

69. Bjørge, L., Løkeland, M. and Oppegaard, K.S. 2015. 'Provosert abort,' *Veileder i Gynekologi 2015* (Norsk gynekologisk forening).

70. Cedars, M.I. and Anaya, Y. 2016 [updated 3 June 2016]. 'Intrauterine adhesions,' *UpToDate* <https:www.uptodate.com/contents/uterine-adhesions>

TROUBLE DOWN BELOW

1. NEL – Norsk elektronisk legehåndbok. 2014 [updated 21 July 2014]. 'Sekundær amenoré,' *NEL – Norsk elektronisk legehåndbok* <https:///legehandboka.no/ handboken/kliniske-kapitler-gynekologi/symptomer-og-tegn/amenore-sekundar>

2. Ibid.
3. Dawood, M.Y. 2006. 'Primary dysmenorrhea: advances in pathogenesis and management,' *Obstetrics and Gynecology*, 108(2): 428–441.
4. Ibid.
5. Ibid.
6. Rapkin, A.J., et al. 'Pelvic Pain and Dysmenorrhea,' Berek, J.S. (ed.). 2012. *Berek and Novak's Gynecology*, 15th edition. (Philadelphia: Lippincott Williams and Wilkins): 482.
7. Johansen, M. 2016. 'Menstruasjon,' *Emetodebok for seksuell helse* (Oslo: Sex og samfunn).
8. Ibid.
9. Rapkin, A.J., et al.
10. Hornstein, M.D., Gibbons, W.E. 2016. 'Pathogenesis and treatment of infertility in women with endometriosis,' *UpToDate*, <https://www.uptodate.com/contents/treatment-of-infertility-in-women-with-endometriosis>
11. Kisic, J., Opøien, H.K., Ringen, I.M., Veddeng, A. and Langebrekke, A. 2015. 'Endometriose,' *Veileder i Gynekologi 2015* (Norsk gynekologisk forening).
12. Rapkin, A.J., et al., 2012: 485.
13. Wilson, E.E. 'Polycystic Ovarian Syndrome and Hyperandrogenism,' Hoffman, B.L., Schorge, J.O., Schaffer, J.I., Halvorsen, L.M., Bradshaw, K.D., Cunningham, F.G., (eds). 2012. *Williams Gynecology*, 2nd edition (New York: McGraw Hill Medical).
14. Goodarzi, M.O. 2016 [updated 20 June 2016]. 'Polycystic ovary syndrome. Best Practice,' *BMJ* <http://bestpractice.bmj.com/best-practice-monograph/141/follow-up/complications.html>
15. Legro, R.S., Barnhart, H.X., Schlaff, W.D., Carr, B.R., Diamond, M.P., Carson, S.A., et al. 2007. 'Clomiphene, metforin, or both for infertility in the polycystic ovary syndrome,' *New England Journal of Medicine*, 356(6): 551–566.
16. Hardiman, P., Pillay, O.S., Atiomo, W. 2003. 'Polycystic ovary syndrome and endometrial carcinoma,' *The Lancet*, 361(9371): 1810–1812.
17. Haoula, Z., Salman, M., Atiomo, W. 2012. 'Evaluating the association between endometrial cancer and polycystic ovary syndrome,' *Human Reproduction*, 27(5): 1327–1331.
18. Goodarzi, 2016.
19. Goodarzi, 2016.
20. Wilson, 2012.
21. Goodarzi, 2016.
22. Goodarzi, 2016.
23. Heinzman, A.B., Hoffman, B.L. 'Pelvic mass,' Hoffman, B.L., Schorge, J.O., Schaffer, J.L., Halvorsen, L.M., Bradshaw, K.D. and Cunningham, F.G., (eds). 2012. *Williams Gynecology*, 2nd edition (New York: McGraw Hill Medical).
24. Heinzman and Hoffman, 2012.

25. Klatsky, P.C., Tran, N.D., Caughey, A.B. and Fujimoto, V.Y. 2008. 'Fibroids and reproductive outcomes: a systematic literature review from conception to delivery,' *American Journal of Obstetrics and Gynecology*, 198(4): 357–366.

26. Tulandi, T. 2016 [updated 24 November 2015]. 'Reproductive issues in women with uterine leiomyomas (fibroids),' *UpToDate* <https://www.uptodate.com/contents/reproductive-issues-in-women-with-uterine-leiomyomas-fibroids>

27. Pritts, E.A., Parker, W.H. and Olive, D.L. 2009. 'Fibroids and infertility: an updated systematic review of the evidence,' *Fertility and sterility*, 91(4): 1215–1223.

28. Pritts, Parker and Olive, 2009.

29. Klatsky, Tran, Caughey and Fujimoto, 2008.

30. Tulandi, 2016.

31. Stewart, E.A. 2016 [updated 29 May 2015]. 'Epidemiology, clinical manifestations, diagnosis, and natural history of uterine leiomyomas (fibroids),' *UpToDate* <https://www.uptodate.com/contents/epidemiology-clinical-manifestations-diagnosis-and-natural-history-of-uterine-leiomyomas-fibroids>

32. Stewart, E.G. 2016 [updated 30 January 2015]. 'Clinical manifestations and diagnosis of generalized vulvodynia,' *UpToDate* <https://www.uptodate.com/contents/clinical-manifestations-and-diagnosis-of-generalized-vulvodynia>

33. Stewart, 2016.

34. Iglesia, C. 2016 [updated 25 May 2015]. 'Clinical manifestations and diagnosis of localized vulvar pain syndrome (formerly vulvodynia, vestibulodynia, vulvar vestibulitis, or focal vulvitis),' *UpToDate* <https://www.uptodate.com/contents/clinical-manifestations-and-diagnosis-of-localized-vulvar-pain-syndrome-formerly-vulvodynia-vestibulitis-or-focal-vulvitis>

35. Johansen, M. 2016. 'Vanlige sexologiske problemer hos kvinner,' *Emetodebok for seksuell helse* (Oslo: Sex og samfunn).

36. Farmer, M.A., Taylor, A.M., Bailey, A.L., Tuttle, A.H., MacIntyre, L.C., Milagrosa, Z.E., et al. 2011. 'Repeated Vulvovaginal Fungal Infections Cause Persistent Pain in a Mouse Model of Vulvodynia,' *Science Translational Medicine*, 3(101): 101ra91.

37. Helgesen, A.L. 2015 [updated 15 May 2015]. 'Når samleiet gjør vondt,' *Forskning.no*. <http://forskning.no/blogg/kvinnehelsebloggen/nar-samleiet-gjor-vondt>; Tympanidis, P., Casula, M., Yiangou, Y., Terenghi, G., Dowd, P. and Anand, P. 2004. 'Increased vanilloid receptor VR1 innervation in vulvodynia,' *European Journal of Pain*, 8(2): 129–133; Tympanidis, P., Terenghi, G., Dowd, P. 2003. 'Increased innervation of the vulval vestibule in patients with vulvodynia,' *British Journal of Dermatology*, 148(5): 1021–1027.

38. Khandker, M., Brady, S.S., Vitonis, A.F., Maclehose, R.F., Stewart, E.G. and Harlow, B.L. 2011. 'The influence of depression and anxiety on risk of adult onset vulvodynia,' *Journal of Women's Health*, 20(10): 1445–1451.

39. Reed, B.D., Haefner, H.K., Punch, M.R., Roth, R.S., Gorenflo, D.W. and Gillespie, B.W.

2000. 'Psychosocial and sexual functioning in women with vulvodynia and chronic pelvic pain. A comparative evaluation,' *The Journal of Reproductive Medicine*, 45(8): 624–632.

40. NEL – Norsk elektronisk legehåndbok. 2015. 'Smerte og ubehag i vulva,' *NEL – Norsk elektronisk legehåndbok* <https://legehandboka.no/handboken/kliniske-kapitler/gynekologi/symptomer-og-tegn/smerte-og-ubehag-i-vulva>

41. Stewart, E.G. 2016 [updated 18 November 2015]. 'Differential diagnosis of sexual pain in women,' *UpToDate* <https://www.uptodate.com/contents/differential-diagnosis-of-sexual-pain-in-women>

42. Bjørnstad, S. 2015 [updated 9 March 2015]. 'Jeg bruker aldri kondom, jeg ser om jenter har en kjønnssykdom,' *Side2* <http://www.side2.no/underholdning/--jeg-bruker-aldri-kondom-jeg-ser-om-jenter-har-en-kjnnssykdom/8551263.html>

43. UNAIDS. 2016. Fact Sheet 2016. *UNAIDS*.

44. Folkehelseinstituttet. 2016 [updated 15 March 2016]. 'Nedgang i hivtilfeller i Norge i 2015,' *FHI* <https://www.fhi.no/nyheter/2016/nedgang-i-hivtilfeller-i-norge-i-20>

45. Folkehelseinstituttet. 2015. 'Klamydia og lymfogranuloma venerum (LGV) i Norge 2014,' *FHI*.

46. Folkehelseinstituttet. 2015. 'Gonoré og syfilis i Norge 2014,' *FHI*.

47. Moi, H., Maltau, J.M. 2013. *Seksuelt overførbare infeksjoner og genitale hudsykdommer*, Third edition (Oslo: Gyldendal Akademisk).

48. NEL – Norsk elektronisk legehåndbok. 2016. 'Genital klamydiainfeksjon hos kvinner,' *NEL – Norsk elektronisk legehåndbok* <https://legehandboka.no/handboken/kliniske-kapitler/gynekologi/tilstander-og-sykdommer/infeksjoner/klamydiainfeksjon-hos-kvinner>

49. Jensen, J.S., Cusini, M., Gomberg, M., Moi, H. 2016. '2016 European guideline on Mycoplasma genitalium infections,' *Journal of the European Academy of Dermatology and Venereology*.

50. Ross, J. 2016: [updated 19 February 2015]. 'Pelvic inflammatory disease: pathogenesis, microbiology, and risk factors,' *UptoDate* <https://www.uptodate.com/contents/pelvic-inflammatory-disease-pathogenesis-microbiology-and-risk-factors>

51. Sweet, R.L. 2012. 'Pelvic inflammatory disease: current concepts of diagnosis and management,' *Current Infectious Disease Reports*, 14(2): 194–203.

52. Johansen, M. 2016. 'Infeksjoner,' *Emetodebok for seksuell helse* (Oslo: Sex og samfunn).

53. Moi and Maltau, 2013.

54. Ibid.

55. Ibid.

56. Ibid.

57. Ibid.

58. Ibid.

59. Sobel, J.D. 2016. 'Candida vulvovaginitis,' *UpToDate* <https://www.uptodate.com/contents/candida-vulvovaginitis>

60. NEL – Norsk elektronisk legehåndbok. 2016 [updated 2 June 2016]. 'Candida vaginitt,' *NEL – Norsk elektronisk legehåndbok* <https://legehandboka.no/handboken/kliniske-kapitler/gynekologi/tilstander-og-sykdommer/infeksjoner/candida-vaginitt>

61. Friedman, M. 2015 [updated 24 November 2015]. 'This Woman Is Making Sourdough Bread Using Yeast From Her Vagina,' *Cosmopolitan* <http://www.cosmopolitan.com/sex-love/news/a49782/zoe-stavri-sourdough-bread-vagina-yeast>

62. Sobel, 2016, 'Candida vulvovaginitis.'

63. Ferris, D.G., Nyirjesy, P., Sobel, J.D., Soper, D., Pavletic, A. and Litaker, M.S. 2002. 'Over-the-counter antifungal drug misuse associated with patient-diagnosed vulvovaginal candidiasis,' *Obstetrics & Gynecology*, 99(3): 419–425.

64. Sobel, 2016, 'Candida vulvovaginitis.'

65. Lopez, J.E.M. 2015 [updated 16 March 2015]. 'Candidiasis (vulvovaginal),' *BMJ – Clinical Evidence* <http://clinicalevidence.bmj.com/x/systematic-review/0815/overview.html>

66. Sobel, 2016, 'Candida vulvovaginitis.'

67. NEL – Norsk elektronisk legehåndbok. 2016 [updated 6 July 2016]. 'Ukomplisert cystitt hos kvinner,' *NEL – Norsk elektronisk legehåndbok* <https://legehandboka.no/handboken/kliniske-kapitler/nyrer-og-urinveier/tilstander-og-sykdommer/infeksjoner/urinveisinfeksjon-hos-kvinner-ukomplisert>

68. Jepson, R.G., Williams, G. and Craig, J.C. 2012. 'Cranberries for preventing urinary tract infections,' *The Cochrane Library*.

69. NEL – Norsk elektronisk legehåndbok, 2016, 'Ukomplisert cystitt hos kvinner.'

70. Weiss, B.D. 2005. 'Selecting medications for the treatment of urinary incontinence,' *American Family Physician*, 71(2): 315–322.

71. NEL – Norsk elektronisk legehåndbok. 2015 [updated 8 September 2015]. 'Stressinkontinens,' *NEL – Norsk elektronisk legehåndbok* <https://legehandboka.no/handboken/kliniske-kapitler/nyrer-og-urinveier/tilstander-og-sykdommer/lekkasjeproblemer/stressinkontinens>

72. Glazener, C.M., Herbison, G.P., Wilson, P.D., MacArthur, C., Lang, G.D., Gee, H., et al. 2001. 'Conservative management of persistent postnatal urinary and faecal incontinence: randomised controlled trial,' *BMJ*, 323(7313): 593.

73. NEL – Norsk elektronisk legehåndbok, 2015, 'Stressinkontinens.'

74. O'Halloran, T., Bell, R.J., Robinson, P.J. and Davis, S.R. 2012. 'Urinary incontinence in young nulligravid women: a cross-sectional analysis,' *Ann Intern Med*, 157(2): 87–93.

75. Simeonova, Z., Milsom, I., Kullendorff, A.M., Molander, U. and Bengtsson, C. 1999. 'The prevalence of urinary incontinence and its influence on the quality of life in women from an urban Swedish population,' *Acta Obstetricia et Gynecologica Scandinavica*, 78(6): 546–551.

76. NEL – Norsk elektronisk legehåndbok, 2015, 'Stressinkontinens.'

77. NEL – Norsk elektronisk legehåndbok. 2016 [updated 7 March 2016]. 'Urgeinkontinens hos kvinner,' *NEL – Norsk elektronisk legehåndbok* <https://

legehandboka.no/handboken/kliniske-kapitler/nyrer-og-urinveier/tilstander-og-sykdommer/lekkasjeproblemer/urgeinkontinens-hos-kvinner>

78. NEL – Norsk elektronisk legehåndbok, 2016, 'Urgeinkontinens hos kvinner.'

79. Riss, S., Weiser, F.A., Schwameis, K., Riss, T., Mittlbock, M., Steiner, G., et al. 2012. 'The prevalence of hemorrhoids in adults,' International Journal of Colorectal Disease, 27(2): 215–220.

80. Griffith, W.F., Werner, C.L. 'Preinvasive Lesions of the Lower Genital Tract,' Hoffman, B.L., Schorge, J.O., Schaffer, J.I., Halvorsen, L.M., Bradshaw, K.D., Cunningham, F.G., (eds). 2012. Williams Gynecology, 2nd edition (New York: McGraw Hill Medical).

81. Cancer Research UK. 'Cervical cancer incidence,' Cancer Research UK <http://www.cancerresearchuk.org/health-professional/cancer-statistics/statistics-by-cancer-type/cervical-cancer?_ga=2.67947093.574968211.1507304868-1505854318.1507304868#heading-Zero>

82. Public Health England. 2015. 'NHS cervical screening (CSP) programme,' Public Health England <https://www.gov.uk/topic/population-screening-programmes/cervical>

83. Östör, A.G. 1993. 'Natural history of cervical intraepithelial neoplasia: a critical review,' International Journal of Gynecological Pathology, 12(2): 186.

84. Folkehelseinstituttet. 23 April 2014. 'Vaksinasjonsdekning i prosent (fullvaksinerte) per 31.12.2014 16-åringer (f. 1998),' FHI.

85. Statens Serum Institut. 2016. 'Human papillomavirus-vaccine (HPV) 1, vaccinationstilslutning,' Statens Serum Institut (Danmark).

86. Statens legemiddelverk. 2016. 'Meldte mistenkte bivirkninger av HPV-vaksine (Gardasil) - oppdaterte bivirkningstall per 31. desember 2015,' Statens legemiddelverk; Feiring, B., Laake, I., Bakken, I.J., Greve-Isdahl, M., Wyller, V.B., Håberg, S.E., Magnus, P., Trogstad, L. 2017. 'HPV vaccination and risk of chronic fatigue syndrome/myalgic encephalomyelitis: A nationwide register-based study from Norway,' Vaccine, 35(33): 4203–4212. <https://doi.org/10.1016/j.vaccine.2017.06.031>

87. European Medicines Agency. 5 November 2015. 'Review concludes evidence does not support that HPV vaccines cause CRPS or POTS,' European Medicines Agency.

88. Hviid, A., Svanström H., Scheller N.M., Grönlund O., Pasternak B., Arnheim-Dahlström L. 2017. 'Human papillomavirus vaccination of adult women and risk of autoimmune and neurological diseases,' Journal of Internal Medicine <https://doi.org/10.1111/joim.12694>

89. Zuckerberg, M. 2015 [updated 31 July 2015]. 'Priscilla and I have some exciting news: we're expecting a baby girl!' Facebook <https://www.facebook.com/photo.php?fbid=10102276573729791&set=a.529237706231.2034669.4&type=1&theater>

90. Hasan, R., Baird, D.D., Herring, A.H., Olshan, A.F., Jonsson Funk, M.L. and Hartmann, K.E. 2010. 'Patterns and predictors of vaginal bleeding in the first trimester of pregnancy,' Annals of Epidemiology, 20(7): 524–531.

91. Ræder, M.B., Wollen, A.-L., Braut, R. and Glad, R. 2015. 'Spontanabort,' *Veileder i Gynekologi 2015* (Norsk gynekologisk forening).

92. Tulandi, T. and Al-Fozan H.M. 2016; [updated 7 November 2016]. 'Spontaneous abortion: Risk factors, etiology, clinical manifestations, and diagnostic evaluation,' *UpToDate* <https://www.uptodate.com/contents/spontaneous-abortion-risk-factors-etiology-clinical-manifestations-and-diagnostic-evaluation>

93. Ibid.

94. Bardos, J., Hercz, D., Friedenthal, J., Missmer, S.A. and Williams, Z. 2015. 'A national survey on public perceptions of miscarriage,' *Obstetrics and Gynecology*, 125(6): 1313–1320.

95. Nybo Andersen, A.M., Wohlfahrt, J., Christens, P., Olsen, J. and Melbye, M. 2000. 'Maternal age and fetal loss: population based register linkage study,' *BMJ*, 320(7251): 1708–1712.

96. Pineles, B.L., Park, E. and Samet J.M. 2014. 'Systematic review and meta-analysis of miscarriage and maternal exposure to tobacco smoke during pregnancy,' *American Journal of Epidemiology*, 179(7): 807–823.

97. Chatenoud, L., Parazzini, F., di Cintio, E., Zanconato, G., Benzi, G., Bortolus, R., et al. 1998. 'Paternal and maternal smoking habits before conception and during the first trimester: relation to spontaneous abortion,' *Annals of Epidemiology*, 8(8): 520–526.

98. Tulandi and Al-Fozan.

99. Oster, E. 2013. *Expecting better – why the conventional pregnancy wisdom is wrong and what you really need to know* (New York: Penguin Press).

100. Andersen, A.-M.N., Andersen, P.K., Olsen, J., Grønbæk, M. and Strandberg-Larsen, K. 2012. 'Moderate alcohol intake during pregnancy and risk of fetal death,' *International Journal of Epidemiology*, 41(2): 405–413.

101. Nisenblat, V., Norman, R.J. 2016 [updated 24 August 2016]. 'The effects of caffeine on reproductive outcomes in women,' *UpToDate* <https://www.uptodate.com/contents/the-effects-of-caffeine-on-reproductive-outcomes-in-women>

102. Rumbold, A., Middleton, P., Crowther, C.A. 2005. 'Vitamin supplementation for preventing miscarriage,' *The Cochrane Library*, 2: Cd004073.

103. Taylor, A. 2003. 'Extent of the problem,' *BMJ*, 327(7412): 434.

104. Folkehelseinstituttet. 2015 [updated 19 November 2015]. 'Fødselsstatistikk for 2014,' *FHI* <https://www.fhi.no/nyheter/2015/fodselsstatistikkfor-2014-publiser>

105. Dunson, D.B., Baird, D.D. and Colombo, B. 2004. 'Increased infertility with age in men and women,' *Obstetrics and Gynecology*, 103(1): 51–56.

106. Rothman, K.J., Wise, L.A., Sorensen, H.T., Riis, A.H., Mikkelsen, E.M. and Hatch, E.E. 2013. 'Volitional determinants and age-related decline in fecundability: a general population prospective cohort study in Denmark,' *Fertility and Sterility*. 99(7): 1958–1964.

107. Nybo Andersen, Wohlfahrt, Christens, Olsen and Melbye.

108. Roach.

109. Howarth, C., Hayes, J., Simonis, M., Temple-Smith, M. 2016. '"Everything's neatly tucked away": young women's views on desirable vulval anatomy,' *Culture, Health & Sexuality*: 1–16.

Bibliography

Adams, J.A., Botash, A.S. and Kellogg, N. 2004. 'Differences in hymenal morphology between adolescent girls with and without a history of consensual sexual intercourse,' *Archives of Pediatrics & Adolescent Medicine*, 158(3): 280–285.

Andersen, A-M.N., Andersen, P.K., Olsen, J., Grønbæk, M. and Strandberg-Larsen, K. 2012. 'Moderate alcohol intake during pregnancy and risk of fetal death,' *International Journal of Epidemiology*, 41(2): 405–413.

Angel K. 2010. 'The history of "female sexual dysfunction" as a mental disorder in the 20th century,' *Current Opinion in Psychiatry*, 23(6): 536.

Appleby, P., Beral, V., Berrington de Gonzalez, A., Colin, D., Franceschi, S., Goodhill, A., et al. 2007. 'Cervical cancer and hormonal contraceptives: collaborative reanalysis of individual data for 16,573 women with cervical cancer and 35,509 women without cervical cancer from 24 epidemiological studies,' *The Lancet*, 370(9599): 1609–1621.

Arden, M., Dye, L. and Walker, A. 1999. 'Menstrual synchrony: awareness and subjective experiences,' *Journal of Reproductive and Infant Psychology*, 17(3): 255–265.

Armstrong E.A., England P. and Fogarty A.C. 2012. 'Accounting for women's orgasm and sexual enjoyment in college hookups and relationships,' *American Sociological Review*, 77(3): 435–462.

Bagwell, M.A., Thompson, S.J., Addy, C.L., Coker, A.L. and Baker, E.R. 1995. 'Primary infertility and oral contraceptive steroid use,' *Fertility and Sterility*, 63(6): 1161–1166.

Bardos, J., Hercz, D., Friedenthal, J., Missmer, S.A. and Williams Z. 2015. 'A national survey on public perceptions of miscarriage,' *Obstetrics and Gynecology*, 125(6): 1313–1320.

Barsky, A.J., Saintfort, R., Rogers, M.P. and Borus, J.F. 2002. 'Non-specific medication side-effects and the nocebo phenomenon,' *JAMA*, 287(5): 622–627.

Basson, R. 2006. 'Sexual Desire and Arousal Disorders in Women,' *New England Journal of Medicine*, 354(14): 1497–1506.

Basson, R., Leiblum, S., Brotto, L., Derogatis, L., Fourcroy, J., Fugl-Meyer, K., et al. 2003. 'Definitions of women's sexual dysfunction reconsidered: advocating expansion and revision,' *Journal of Psychosomatic Obstetrics and Gynaecology*, 24(4): 212–219.

Basson, R., McInnes, R., Smith, M.D., Hodgson, G. and Koppiker, N. 2002. 'Efficacy and safety of sildenafil citrate in women with sexual dysfunction associated with female sexual arousal disorder,' *Journal of Women's Health & Gender-based Medicine*, 11(4): 367–377.

Bellis, M.A. and Baker, R.R. 1990. 'Do females promote sperm competition? Data for humans,' *Animal Behaviour*, 40(5): 997–999.

Beral, V., Doll, R., Hermon, C., Peto, R. and Reeves, G. 2008. 'Ovarian cancer and oral contraceptives: collaborative reanalysis of data from 45 epidemiological studies including 23,257 women with ovarian cancer 87,303 controls,' *The Lancet*, 371(9609): 303–314.

Berenson, A., Heger, A. and Andrews, S. 1991. 'Appearance of the Hymen in Newborns,' *Pediatrics*, 87(4): 458–465.

Berenson, A.B., Chacko, M.R., Wiemann, C.M., Mishaw, C.O., Friedrich, W.N. and Grady, J.J. 2002. 'Use of Hymenal Measurements in the Diagnosis of Previous Penetration,' *Pediatrics*, 109(2): 228–235.

Bergo, I.G. and Quist, C. 2016. 'Kunnskapsministeren om sexkulturen blant unge: – Skolen må ta mer ansvar,' *VG+* <http://www.vg.no/nyheter/innenriks/kunnskapsministerenom-sexkulturen-blant-unge-skolen-maa-ta-mer-ansvar/a/23770735>

Bernard, M.L.R. 2015 [updated 30 March 2015]. 'How Often Do Queer Women Have Sex?' *Autostraddle* <http://autostraddle.com/how-often-do-lesbianshave-sex-283731>

Bjørge, L., Løkeland, M. and Oppegaard, K.S. 2015. 'Provosert abort,' *Veileder i Gynekologi 2015* (Norsk gynekologisk forening).

Bjørnstad, S. 2015 [updated 9 March 2015]. 'Jeg bruker aldri kondom, jeg ser om jenter har en kjønnssykdom,' *Side2* <http://www.side2.no/underholdning/--jegbruker-aldri-kondom-jeg-ser-om-jenter-har-en-kjnnssykdom/8551263.html>

Bordvik, M. 2016 [updated 7 June 2016]. 'P-pille-bruk kan ødelegge effekten av angrepille,' *Dagens Medisin* <http://www.dagensmedisin.no/artikler/2016/07/06/angrepille-kan-odelegge-p-pille-effekt>

Boston University School of Medicine. 2002. 'Female Genital Anatomy,' *Sexual Medicine* <http://www.bumc.bu.edu/sexualmedicine/physicianinformation/female-genital-anatomy>

Bradford, A. and Meston, C. 2007. 'Correlates of placebo response in the treatment of sexual dysfunction in women: a preliminary report,' *The Journal of Sexual Medicine*, 4(5): 1345–1351.

Bradford A. 2016. 'Treatment of female orgasmic disorder,' *UpToDate* <https://uptodate.com/contents/treatment-of-female-orgasmic-disorder>

Brotto, L.A., Petkau, A.J., Labrie, F. and Basson, R. 2011. 'Predictors of sexual desiredisorders in women,' *Journal of Sexual Medicine*, 8(3): 742–753.

Brunner Huber, L.R., Hogue, C.J., Stein, A.D., Drews, C., Zieman, M.,King, J., et al. 2006. 'Contraceptive use and discontinuation: findings from thecontraceptive history, initiation, and choice study,' *American Journal of Obstetrics and Gynecology*, 194(5): 1290–1295.

Buisson, O., Foldes, P., Jannini, E. and Mimoun, S. 2010. 'Coitus as Revealed by Ultrasound in One Volunteer Couple,' *The Journal of Sexual Medicine*, 7(8): 2750–2754.

Burrows, L.J., Basha, M. and Goldstein, A.T. 2012. 'The effects of hormonal contraceptives on female sexuality: a review,' *Journal of Sexual Medicine*, 9(9): 2213–2223.

Cancer Research UK. 'Cervical cancer incidence,' *Cancer Research UK* <http://www.cancerresearchuk.org/health-professional/cancer-statistics/statistics-by-cancer-type/cervical-cancer?_ga=2.67947093.574968211.1507304868-1505854318.1507304868#heading-Zero>

Caruso, S., Agnello, C., Malandrino, C., Lo Presti, L., Cicero, C. and Cianci, S. 2014. 'Do hormones influence women's sex? Sexual activity over the menstrual cycle,' *Journal of Sexual Medicine*, 11(1): 211–221.

Cedars, M.I. and Anaya, Y. 2016 [updated 3 June 2016]. 'Intrauterine adhesions,' *UpToDate* <https:www.uptodate.com/contents/uterine-adhesions>

Charlton, B.M., Rich-Edwards, J.W., Colditz, G.A., Missmer, S.A., Rosner, B.A., Hankinson, S.E., et al. 2014. 'Oral contraceptive use and mortality after 36 years of follow-up in the Nurses' Health Study: prospective cohort study,' *BMJ*, 349: g6356.

Chatenoud, L., Parazzini, F., di Cintio, E., Zanconato, G., Benzi, G., Bortolus, R., et al. 1998. 'Paternal and maternal smoking habits before conception and during the first trimester: relation to spontaneous abortion,' *Annals of Epidemiology*, 8(8): 520–526.

Cheung, E. and Free, C. 2004. 'Factors influencing young women's decision making regarding hormonal contraceptives: a qualitative study,' *Contraception*, 71(6): 426–431.

Chivers, M.L., Seto, M.C., Lalumiere, M.L., Laan, E., Grimbos, T. 2010. 'Agreement of self-reported and genital measures of sexual arousal in men and women: a metaanalysis,' *Archives of Sexual Behavior*, 39(1): 5–56.

Christopher, F.S. and Sprecher, S. 2000. 'Sexuality in Marriage, Dating, and Other Relationships: A Decade Review,' *Journal of Marriage and Family*, 62(4): 999–1017.

Clayton, A.H., Althof, S.E., Kingsberg, S., DeRogatis, L.R., Kroll, R., Goldstein, I., et al. 2016. 'Bremelanotide for female sexual dysfunctions in premenopausal women: a randomized placebo-controlled dose-finding trial,' *Women's Health*, 12(3): 325–337.

Darling, C.A., Davidson, J.K. Sr and Conway-Welch, C. 1990. 'Female ejaculation: perceived origins, the Grafenberg spot/area, and sexual responsiveness,' *Archives of Sexual Behavior*, 19(1): 29–47.

Davis S., Papalia M-A., Norman R.J., O'Neill S., Redelman M., Williamson M., et al. 2008. 'Safety and efficacy of a testosterone metered-dose transdermal spray for treating decreased sexual satisfaction in premenopausal women: a randomized trial,' *Annals of Internal Medicine*, 148(8): 569–577.

Dawood K., Kirk K.M., Bailey J.M., Andrews P.W. and Martin N.G. 2005. 'Genetic and environmental influences on the frequency of orgasm in women,' *Twin Research and Human Genetics*, 8(1): 27–33.

Dawood, M.Y. 2006. 'Primary dysmenorrhea: advances in pathogenesis and management,' *Obstetrics and Gynecology*, 108(2): 428–441.

Dean, G. and Goldberg, A.B. 2016 [updated 15 September 2016]. 'Intrauterine contraception: Devices, candidates, and selection,' *UpToDate* <https://www.uptodate.com/contents/intrauterine-contraception-devices-candidates-and-selection>

Di Marino, V. and Lepidi, H. 2014. *Anatomic Study of the Clitoris and the BulboClitoral Organ* (Springer International Publishing).

Dillner, L. 2016 [updated 15/09/2016]. 'Do women's periods really synchronise when they live together?' *Guardian* <https://www.theguardian.com/lifeandstyle/2016/aug/15/periods-housemates-menstruation-synchronise>

Duke, J.M., Sibbritt, D.W. and Young, A.F. 2007. 'Is there an association between the use of oral contraception and depressive symptoms in young Australian women?' *Contraception*, 75(1): 27–31.

Dunn K.M., Cherkas L.F., Spector T.D. 2005. 'Genetic influences on variation in female orgasmic function: a twin study,' *Biology Letters*, 1(3): 260–263.

Dunson, D.B., Baird, D.D. and Colombo, B. 2004. 'Increased infertility with age in men and women,' *Obstetrics and Gynecology*, 103(1): 51–56.

Dyall-Smith, D. 2016. 'Trimethylaminuria,' *DermNet New Zealand* <http://www.dermnetnz.org/topics/trimethylaminuria>

Eichel E.W., Eichel J.D. and Kule S. 1988. 'The technique of coital alignment and its relation to female orgasmic response and simultaneous orgasm,' *Journal of Sex & Marital Therapy*, 14(2): 129–141.

Emera, D., Romero, R. and Wagner, G. 2012. 'The evolution of menstruation: A new model for genetic assimilation,' *BioEssays*, 34(1): 26–35.

European Medicines Agency. 5 November 2015. 'Review concludes evidence does not support that HPV vaccines cause CRPS or POTS,' *European Medicines Agency.*

Farmer, M.A., Taylor, A.M., Bailey, A.L., Tuttle, A.H., MacIntyre, L.C., Milagrosa, Z.E., et al. 2011. 'Repeated Vulvovaginal Fungal Infections Cause Persistent Pain in a Mouse Model of Vulvodynia,' *Science Translational Medicine*, 3(101).

Ferris, D.G., Nyirjesy, P., Sobel, J.D., Soper, D., Pavletic, A. and Litaker, M.S. 2002. 'Over-the-counter antifungal drug misuse associated with patient-diagnosed vulvovaginal candidiasis,' *Obstetrics & Gynecology*, 99(3): 419–425.

Fisher, C., Cohen, H.D., Schiavi, R.C., Davis, D., Furman, B., Ward, K., et al. 1983. 'Patterns of female sexual arousal during sleep and waking: Vaginal thermoconductance studies,' *Archives of Sexual Behavior*, 12(2): 97–122.

Folkehelseinstituttet. 2015 [updated 19 November 2015]. 'Fødselsstatistikk for 2014,' *FHI* <https://www.fhi.no/nyheter/2015/fodselsstatistikkfor-2014-publiser>

Folkehelseinstituttet. 2015. 'Gonoré og syfilis i Norge 2014,' *FHI.*

Folkehelseinstituttet. 2015. 'Klamydia og lymfogranuloma venerum (LGV) i Norge 2014,' *FHI.*

Folkehelseinstituttet. 2016 [updated 15 March 2016]. 'Nedgang i hivtilfeller i Norge i 2015,' *FHI* <https://www.fhi.no/nyheter/2016/nedgang-i-hivtilfeller-i-norge-i-20>

Folkehelseinstituttet. 23 April 2014. 'Vaksinasjonsdekning i prosent (fullvaksinerte) per 31.12.2014 16-åringer (f. 1998),' *FHI.*

Førde, R. 2002. 'Operativ rekonstruksjon av jomfruhinne,' *Tidsskrift for Den norske legeforening.*

Frank, L. 10 June 2016. 'Blodig Uenighet,' *Morgenbladet.*

Frederick, A., Lever, J., Gillespie, B.J. and Garcia, J.R. 2016. 'What Keeps Passion Alive? Sexual Satisfaction Is Associated With Sexual Communication, Mood Setting, Sexual Variety, Oral Sex, Orgasm and Sex Frequency in a National U.S. Study,' *Journal of Sex Research*: 1–16.

Freud, S. 1905. *Three essays on the theory of sexuality.*

Friedman, M. 2015 [updated 24 November 2015]. 'This Woman Is Making Sourdough Bread Using Yeast From Her Vagina,' *Cosmopolitan* <http://www.cosmopolitan.com/sex-love/news/a49782/zoe-stavri-sourdough-bread-vagina-yeast>

Gallo, M.F., Grimes, D.A., Schulz, K.F. and Helmerhorst, F.M. 2004. 'Combination estrogen-progestin contraceptives and body weight: systematic review of randomized controlled trials,' *Obstetrics & Gynecology*, 103(2): 359–373.

Garcia J.R., Lloyd E.A., Wallen K. and Fisher H.E. 2014. 'Variation in orgasm occurrence by sexual orientation in a sample of U.S. singles,' *Journal of Sexual Medicine*, 11(11): 2645–2652.

Gingnell, M., Engman, J., Frick, A., Moby, L., Wikstrom, J., Fredrikson, M., et al. 2013. 'Oral contraceptive use changes in brain activity and mood in women with previous negative affect on the pill – a double-blinded, placebo-controlled randomized trial of a levonorgestrel-containing combined oral contraceptive,' *Psychoneuroendocrinology*, 38(7): 1133–1144.

Glazener, C.M., Herbison, G.P., Wilson, P.D., MacArthur, C., Lang, G.D., Gee, H., et al. 2001. 'Conservative management of persistent postnatal urinary and faecal incontinence: randomised controlled trial,' *BMJ*, 323(7313): 593.

Goldstein, B.G. and Goldstein, A.O. 2016. 'Pseudofolliculitis barbae,' *UpToDate* <https://www.uptodate.com/contents/pseudofolliculitis-barbae>

Goodarzi, M.O. 2016 [updated 20 June 2016]. 'Polycystic ovary syndrome. Best Practice,' *BMJ* <http://bestpractice.bmj.com/best-practice-monograph/141/follow-up/complications.html>

Grady-Weliky, T.A. 2003. 'Premenstrual Dysphoric Disorder,' *New England Journal of Medicine*, 348(5): 433–438.

Graham, C.A., Ramos, R., Bancroft, J., Maglaya, C. and Farley, T.M. 1995. 'The effects of steroid contraceptives on the well-being and sexuality of women: a doubleblind, placebo-controlled, two-centre study of combined and progestogen-only methods,' *Contraception*, 52(6): 363–369.

Graham C.A. and Sherwin B.B. 1993. 'The relationship between mood and sexuality in women using an oral contraceptive as a treatment for premenstrual symptoms,' *Psychoneuroendocrinology*, 18(4): 273–281.

Griffith, W.F., Werner, C.L. 'Preinvasive Lesions of the Lower Genital Tract,' Hoffman, B.L., Schorge, J.O., Schaffer, J.I., Halvorsen, L.M., Bradshaw, K.D., Cunningham, F.G., (eds). 2012. *Williams Gynecology*, 2nd edition (New York: McGraw Hill Medical).

Grimes, D.A. and Schulz, K.F. 2011. 'Nonspecific side-effects of all contraceptives: nocebo or noise?' *Contraception*, 83(1): 5–9.

Haavio-Mannila, E. and Kontula, O. 1997. 'Correlates of increased sexual satisfaction,' *Archives of Sexual Behavior*, 26(4): 399–419.

Hägstad, A.J. 1990. 'Mödomen – mest myt!' *Läkartidningen*, 87(37): 2857–2858.

Hannaford, P.C., Selvaraj, S., Elliott, A.M., Angus, V., Iversen, L. and Lee, A.J. 2007. 'Cohort data from the Royal College of General Practitioners' oral contraception study,' *BMJ*, 335(7621): 651.

Hardiman, P., Pillay, O.S., Atiomo, W. 2003. 'Polycystic ovary syndrome and endometrial carcinoma,' *The Lancet*, 361(9371): 1810–1812.

Hasan, R., Baird, D.D., Herring, A.H., Olshan, A.F., Jonsson Funk, M.L. and Hartmann, K.E. 2010. 'Patterns and predictors of vaginal bleeding in the first trimester of pregnancy,' *Annals of Epidemiology*, 20(7): 524–531.

Hasselknippe, O. and Stokke, O. 2006 [updated 19/10/2011]. 'Volvat slutter å selge jomfruhinner,' *Aftenposten* <http://www.aftenposten.no/norge/Volvat-slutter-a-selgejomfruhinner-423873b.html>

Haoula, Z., Salman, M., Atiomo, W. 2012. 'Evaluating the association between endometrial cancer and polycystic ovary syndrome,' *Human Reproduction*, 27(5): 1327–1331.

Heinzman, A.B., Hoffman, B.L. 'Pelvic mass,' Hoffman, B.L., Schorge, J.O., Schaffer, J.L., Halvorsen, L.M., Bradshaw, K.D. and Cunningham, F.G., (eds). 2012. *Williams Gynecology*, 2nd edition (New York: McGraw Hill Medical).

Heit, J.A., Kobbervig, C.E., James, A.H., Petterson, T.M., Bailey, K.R. and Melton, L.J. 2005. 'Trends in the incidence of venous thromboembolism during pregnancy or postpartum: a 30-year population-based study,' *Annals of Internal Medicine*, 143(10): 697–706.

Helgesen, A.L. 2015 [updated 15 May 2015]. 'Når samleiet gjør vondt,' *Forskning.no*. <http://forskning.no/blogg/kvinnehelsebloggen/nar-samleiet-gjor-vondt>

Hornstein, M.D., Gibbons, W.E. 2016 [updated 10 October 2013]. 'Pathogenesis and treatment of infertility in women with endometriosis,' *UpToDate* <https://www.uptodate.com/contents/treatment-of-infertility-in-women-with-endometriosis>

Howarth, C., Hayes, J., Simonis, M., Temple-Smith, M. 2016. 'Everything's neatly tucked away': young women's views on desirable vulval anatomy,' *Culture, Health & Sexuality*: 1–16.

Iglesia, C. 2016 [updated 25 May 2015]. 'Clinical manifestations and diagnosis of localized vulvar pain syndrome (formerly vulvodynia, vestibulodynia, vulvar vestibulitis, or focal vulvitis),' *UpToDate* <https://www.uptodate.com/contents/clinical-manifestations-and-diagnosis-of-localized-vulvar-pain-syndrome-formerlyvulvodynia-vestibulitis-or-focal-vulvitis>

Independent Forensic Expert Group. 2015. 'Statement on virginity testing,' *Journal of Forensic and Legal Medicine*, 33: 121–124.

Jacobi, F., Wittchen, H.U., Holting, C., Hofler, M., Pfister, H., Muller, N., et al. 2004. 'Prevalence, co-morbidity and correlates of mental disorders in the general population: results from the German Health Interview and Examination Survey (GHS),' *Psychological Medicine*, 34(4): 597–611.

Jennings, V. 2016. 'Fertility awareness-based methods of pregnancy prevention,' *UpToDate* <https://www.uptodate.com/contents/fertility-awareness-based-methodsof-pregnancy-prevention>

Jensen, J.S., Cusini, M., Gomberg, M., Moi, H. 2016. '2016 European guideline on Mycoplasma genitalium infections,' *Journal of the European Academy of Dermatology and Venereology*.

Jepson, R.G., Williams, G. and Craig, J.C. 2012. 'Cranberries for preventing urinary tract infections,' *The Cochrane Library*.

Joffe, H., Cohen, L.S. and Harlow, B.L. 2003. 'Impact of oral contraceptive pill use on premenstrual mood: predictors of improvement and deterioration,' *American Journal of Obstetrics and Gynecology*, 189(6): 1523–1530.

Johansen, M. 2016. *Emetodebok for seksuell helse* (Oslo: Sex og samfunn).

Juvkam, K.H. and Gudim, H.B. 2013. 'Medikamentell forskyvning av menstruasjon,' *Tidsskrift for Den norske legeforening*, 133: 166–168.

Karacan, I., Rosenbloom, A. and Williams, R. 1970. 'The clitoral erection cycle during sleep,' *Journal of Sleep Research*.

Karlsen, S.G., Jonassen, T.H. and Suvatne, S.S. 2015 [updated 26 June 2015]. 'Anbefaler naturalig prevensjon og påstår at den er 99.9% sikker,' *Dagbladet* <http://www.dagbladet. no/ 2015/06/29/kjendis/blogg/prevensjon/caroline_berg_eriksen/lege/39902645>

Kaunitz, A.M. 2016. 'Patient education: hormonal methods of birth control (Beyond the Basics),' *UpToDate* <https://www.uptodate.com/contents/hormonal-methods-ofbirth-control-beyond-the-basics?source=see_link>

Kellogg, N.D., Menard, S.W. and Santos, A. 2004. 'Genital anatomy in pregnant adolescents: "normal" does not mean "nothing happened",' *Pediatrics*, 113: 67–69.

Keyes, K.M., Cheslack-Postava, K., Westhoff, C., Heim, C.M., Haloosim, M., Walsh, K., et al. 2013. 'Association of hormonal contraceptive use with reduced levels of depressive symptoms: National study of sexually active women in the United States,' *American Journal of Epidemiology*, 178(9): 1378–1388.

Khandker, M., Brady, S.S., Vitonis, A.F., Maclehose, R.F., Stewart, E.G. and Harlow, B.L. 2011. 'The influence of depression and anxiety on risk of adult onset vulvodynia,' *Journal of Women's Health*, 20(10): 1445–1451.

Kilchevsky, A., Vardi, Y., Lowenstein, L. and Gruenwald, I. 2012. 'Is the Female G-Spot Truly a Distinct Anatomic Entity?' *The Journal of Sexual Medicine*, 9(3): 719–726.

Kisic, J., Opøien, H.K., Ringen, I.M., Veddeng, A. and Langebrekke, A. 2015. 'Endometriose,' *Veileder i Gynekologi 2015* (Norsk gynekologisk forening).

Klatsky, P.C., Tran, N.D., Caughey, A.B. and Fujimoto, V.Y. 2008. 'Fibroids and reproductive outcomes: a systematic literature review from conception to delivery,' *American Journal of Obstetrics and Gynecology*, 198(4): 357–366.

Klussman, D. 2002. 'Sexual motivation and the duration of partnership,' *Archives of Sexual Behavior*, 31(3): 275–287.

Kohlenberg R.J. 1974. 'Directed masturbation and the treatment of primary orgasmic dysfunction.' *Archives of Sexual Behavior*, 3(4): 349–356.

Korda J.B., Goldstein S.W. and Sommer F. 2010. 'Sexual Medicine History: The History of Female Ejaculation,' *The Journal of Sexual Medicine*, 7(5): 1965–1975.

Laqueur T. 1992. *Making Sex: Body and Gender from the Greeks to Freud* (Boston: Harvard University Press).

Legemiddelhåndboken. 2016 [updated 13 September 2016]. 'Perorale gestagener,' *Norsk Legemiddelhåndbok* <http://legemiddelhandboka.no/legemidler/?frid=lk-03-endokr-7205>

Legro, R.S., Barnhart, H.X., Schlaff, W.D., Carr, B.R., Diamond, M.P., Carson, S.A., et al. 2007. 'Clomiphene, metforin, or both for infertility in the polycystic ovary syndrome,' *New England Journal of Medicine*, 356(6): 551–566.

Levin R.J. 2015. 'Recreation and procreation: A critical view of sex in the human female,' *Clinical Anatomy*, 28(3): 339–354.

Lidegaard, O., Lokkegaard, E., Jensen, A., Skovlund, C.W. and Keiding, N. 2012. 'Thrombotic stroke and myocardial infarction with hormonal contraception,' *The New England Journal of Medicine*, 366(24): 2257–2266.

Lidegaard, O., Lokkegaard, E., Svendsen, A.L. and Agger, C. 2009. 'Hormonal contraception and risk of venous thromboembolism: National follow-up study,' *BMJ*, 339: b2890.

Lindh, I., Blohm, F., Andersson-Ellstrom, A. and Milsom, I. 2009. 'Contraceptive use and pregnancy outcome in three generations of Swedish female teenagers from the same urban population,' *Contraception*, 80(2): 163–169.

Lloyd, J., Crouch, N.S., Minto, C.L., Liao, L.M. and Creighton, S.M. 2005. 'Female genital appearance: "normality" unfolds,' *BJOG*, 112(5): 643–646.

Lopez, J.E.M. 2015 [updated 16 March 2015]. 'Candidiasis (vulvovaginal),' *BMJ – Clinical Evidence* <http://clinicalevidence.bmj.com/x/systematic-review/0815/overview.html>

Lorenz T.A. and Meston C.M. 2014. 'Exercise improves sexual function in women taking antidepressants: results from a randomized crossover trial,' *Depression and Anxiety*, 31(3): 188–195.

MacNeil, S., Byers, E.S. 2005. 'Dyadic assessment of sexual self-disclosure and sexual satisfaction in heterosexual dating couples,' *Journal of Social and Personal Relationships*, 22(2): 169–181.

Mah K. and Binik Y.M. 2001. 'The nature of human orgasm: a critical review of major trends,' *Clinical Psychology Review*, 21(6): 823–856.

Malmborg, A., Persson, E., Brynhildsen, J. and Hammar, M. 2016. 'Hormonal contraception and sexual desire: a questionnaire-based study of young Swedish women,' *The European Journal of Contraception & Reproductive Healthcare*, 21(2): 158–167.

Mansour, D., Gemzell-Danielsson, K., Inki, P., Jensen, J.T. 2011. 'Fertility after discontinuation of contraception: a comprehensive review of the literature,' *Contraception*, 845(5): 465–477.

Maravilla, K.A., Heiman, J.R., Garland, P.A., Cao, Y., Carter, B.T., Peterson, W.O., et al. 2003. 'Dynamic MR Imaging of the Sexual Arousal Response in Women,' *Journal of Sex & Marital Therapy*, 29: 71–6.

Marston, C. and Lewis, R. 2014. 'Anal heterosex among young people and implications for health promotion: a qualitative study in the UK,' *BMJ Open*, 4(8): e004996.

Martin, K.A. and Douglas, P.S. 2016 [updated 22 August 2016]. 'Risk and side-effects associated with estrogen-progestin contraceptives,' *UpToDate* <https//www.uptodate.com/contents/risks-and-side-effectsassociated-with-estrogen-progestin-contraceptives>

McCann, J., Miyamoto, S., Boyle, C. and Rogers, K. 2007. 'Healing of hymenal injuries in prepubertal and adolescent girls: a descriptive study,' *Pediatrics*, 119(5): 1094–1106.

McClintock, M.K. 1971. 'Menstrual synchrony and suppression,' *Nature*, 229(5282): 244.

Mercer, C.H., Tanton, C., Prah, P., Erens, B., Sonnenberg, P., Clifton, S., et al. 2013. 'Changes in sexual attitudes and lifestyles in Britain through the life course and over time: findings from the National Surveys of Sexual Attitudes and Lifestyles (Natsal),' *The Lancet*, 382(9907): 1781–1794.

Meston C.M., Levin R.J., Sipski M.L., Hull E.M., Heiman J.R. 2004. 'Women's orgasm,' *Annual Review of Sex Research*, 15: 173–257.

Mitchell, K.R., Mercer, C.H., Ploubidis, G.B., Jones, K.G., Datta, J., Field, N., et al. 2013. 'Sexual function in Britain: findings from the third National Survey of Sexual Attitudes and Lifestyles (Natsal-3),' *The Lancet*, 382(9907): 1817–1829.

Mitchell, M.A., Bisch, S., Arntfield, S. and Hosseini-Moghaddam, S.M. 2015. 'A confirmed case of toxic shock syndrome associated with the use of a menstrual cup,' The Canadian Journal of Infectious Diseases & Medical Microbiology, 26(4): 218–220.

Moen, M.H. 2013. 'Selvvalgt menstruasjon,' *Tidsskrift for Den norsk legeforening*, 133(2): 131.

Moi, H., Maltau, J.M. 2013. *Seksuelt overførbare infeksjoner og genitale hudsykdommer*, Third edition (Oslo: Gyldendal Akademisk).

Montesi, J.L., Fauber, R.L., Gordon, E.A. and Heimberg, R.G. 2011. 'The specific importance of communicating about sex to couples' sexual and overall relationship satisfaction,' *Journal of Social and Personal Relationships*, 28(5): 591–609.

Maltau, J.M., Molne, K. and Nesheim, B-I. 2015. *Obstetrikk og gynekologi*, 3rd edition (Oslo: Gyldendal Akademisk): 313–314.

Muise, A., Schimmack, U., Impett, E.A. 2016. 'Sexual frequency predicts greater well-being, but more is not always better,' *Social Psychological and Personality Science*, 7(4): 295–302.

Murakami, H. 2005. *Kafka on the Shore* (London: Vintage).

Murray, S.H. and Milhausen, R.R. 2012. 'Sexual desire and relationship duration in young men and women,' *Journal of Sex & Marital Therapy*, 38(1): 28–40.

Myhre, A.K., Borgen, G. and Ormstad, K. 2006. 'Seksuelle overgrep mot prepubertale barn,' *Tidsskrift for Den norske legeforening*, 126(19): 2511.

Nagoski, E. 2015. *Come as you are – the surprising new science that will transform your sex life* (New York: Simon and Schuster Paperbacks).

NEL – Norsk elektronisk legehåndbok. 2014. *NEL – Norsk elektronisk legehåndbok* <https://legehandboka.no/handboken>

NEL – Norsk elektronisk legehåndbok. 2015. *NEL – Norsk elektronisk legehåndbok* <https://legehandboka.no/handboken>

NEL – Norsk elektronisk legehåndbok. 2016. *NEL – Norsk elektronisk legehåndbok* <https://legehandboka.no/handboken>

Nesheim, B-I. 2009. 'Deflorasjon,' *Store Medisinske Leksikon* <https://sml.snl.no/deflorasjon>

Nisenblat, V., Norman, R.J. 2016 [updated 24 August 2016]. 'The effects of caffeine on reproductive outcomes in women', *UpToDate* <https://www.uptodate.com/contents/the-effects-of-caffeine-on-reproductive-outcomes-in-women>

Nybo Andersen, A.M., Wohlfahrt, J., Christens, P., Olsen, J. and Melbye, M. 2000. 'Maternal age and fetal loss: population based register linkage study', *BMJ*, 320(7251): 1708–1712.

Oakley, S.H., Vaccaro, C.M., Crisp, C.C., Estanol, M., Fellner, A.N., Kleeman, S.D., et al. 2014. 'Clitoral size and location in relation to sexual function using pelvic MRI', *The Journal of Sexual Medicine*, 11(4): 1013–1022.

O'Connell, H.E. and DeLancey, J.O. 2005. 'Clitoral anatomy in nulliparous, healthy, premenopausal volunteers using unenhanced magnetic resonance imaging', *The Journal of Urology*, 173(6): 2060–2063.

O'Connell, H.E., Sanjeevan, K.V. and Hutson, J.M. 2005. 'Anatomy of the clitoris', *The Journal of Urology*, 174(4), pt 1: 1189–1195.

O'Connell, K., Davis, A.R. and Kerns, J. 2007. 'Oral contraceptives: Side-effects and depression in adolescent girls', *Contraception*, 75(4): 299–304.

O'Halloran, T., Bell, R.J., Robinson, P.J. and Davis, S.R. 2012. 'Urinary incontinence in young nulligravid women: a cross-sectional analysis', *Ann Intern Med*, 157(2): 87–93.

Olsen, E.A. 1999. 'Methods of hair removal', *Journal of the American Academy of Dermatology*, 40: 143–55.

Oster, E. 2013. *Expecting better – why the conventional pregnancy wisdom is wrong and what you really need to know* (New York: Penguin Press).

Östör, A.G. 1993. 'Natural history of cervical intraepithelial neoplasia: a critical review', *International Journal of Gynecological Pathology*, 12(2): 186.

Pastor Z. 2013. 'Female ejaculation orgasm vs. coital incontinence: a systematic review', *Journal of Sexual Medicine*, 10(7): 1682–1691.

Pastor, Z., Holla, K. and Chmel, R. 2013. 'The influence of combined oral contraceptives on female sexual desire: a systematic review', *The European Journal of Contraception & Reproductive Healthcare*, 18(1): 27–43.

Paul, R. and Cotsarelis, G. 1999. 'The biology of hair follicles', *The New England Journal of Medicine*, 341(7): 491–7.

Pauls, R.N. 2015, 'Anatomy of the clitoris and the female sexual response', *Clinical Anatomy*, 28(3): 376–384.

Peipert, J.F. and Gutmann, J. 1993. 'Oral contraceptive risk assessment: a survey of 247 educated women', *Obstetrics & Gynecology*, 82(1): 112–117.

Pierce A.P. 2000. 'The coital alignment technique (CAT): an overview of studies', *Journal of Sex and Marital Therapy*, 26(3): 257–268.

Pineles, B.L., Park, E. and Samet J.M. 2014. 'Systematic review and meta-analysis of miscarriage and maternal exposure to tobacco smoke during pregnancy', *American Journal of Epidemiology*, 179(7): 807–823.

Pollen J.J. and Dreilinger A. 1984. 'Immunohistochemical identification of prostatic acid phosphatase and prostate specific antigen in female periurethral glands,' *Urology*, 23(3): 303–304.

Pritts, E.A., Parker, W.H. and Olive, D.L. 2009. 'Fibroids and infertility: an updated systematic review of the evidence,' *Fertility and Sterility*, 91(4): 1215–1223.

Public Health England. 2015. 'NHS cervical screening (CSP) programme,' *Public Health England* <https://www.gov.uk/topic/population-screening-programmes/cervical>

Puppo V. 2011. 'Embryology and anatomy of the vulva: The female orgasm and women's sexual health.' *European Journal of Obstetrics and Gynecology and Reproductive Biology*, 154(1): 3–8.

Ræder, M.B., Wollen, A-L., Braut, R. and Glad, R. 2015. 'Spontanabort,' *Veileder i Gynekologi 2015* (Norsk gynekologisk forening).

Rao, K.V. and Demaris, A. 1995. 'Coital frequency among married and cohabiting couples in the United States,' *Journal of Biosocial Science*, 27(2): 135–150.

Rapkin, A.J., et al. 'Pelvic Pain and Dysmenorrhea,' Berek, J.S. (ed.). 2012. *Berek and Novak's Gynecology*, 15th edition. (Philadelphia: Lippincott Williams and Wilkins): 482.

Redmond, G., Godwin, A.J., Olson, W. and Lippman, J.S. 1999. 'Use of placebo controls in an oral contraceptive trial: methodological issues and adverse event incidence,' *Contraception*, 60(2): 81–85.

Reed, B.D., Haefner, H.K., Punch, M.R., Roth, R.S., Gorenflo, D.W. and Gillespie, B.W. 2000. 'Psychosocial and sexual functioning in women with vulvodynia and chronic pelvic pain. A comparative evaluation,' *The Journal of Reproductive Medicine*, 45(8): 624–632.

Richters, J.; Visser, R., Rissel, C. and Smith, A. 2006. 'Sexual practices at last heterosexual encounter and occurrence of orgasm in a national survey,' *Journal of Sex Research*, 43(3): 217–226.

Riss, S., Weiser, F.A., Schwameis, K., Riss, T., Mittlbock, M., Steiner, G., et al. 2012. 'The prevalence of hemorrhoids in adults,' *International Journal of Colorectal Disease*, 27(2): 215–220.

Roach, M. 2008. *BONK – the Curious Coupling of Science and Sex* (New York: W. W. Norton and Company).

Rosen R. 2014 [updated 4 December 2014]. 'No female ejaculation, please, we're British: a history of porn and censorship,' *Independent* <http://www.independent. co.uk/life-style/health-and-families/features/no-female-ejaculation-please-we-rebritish-a-history-of-porn-and-censorship-9903054.html>

Rosenbaum T.Y. 2007. 'Reviews: Pelvic Floor Involvement in Male and Female Sexual Dysfunction and the Role of Pelvic Floor Rehabilitation in Treatment: A Literature Review,' *The Journal of Sexual Medicine*, 4(1): 4–13.

Rosenberg, M.J. and Waugh, M.S. 1998. 'Oral contraceptive discontinuation: a prospective evaluation of frequency and reasons,' *American Journal of Obstetrics and Gynecology*, 179(3): 577–582.

Ross, J. 2016: [updated 19 February 2015]. 'Pelvic inflammatory disease: pathogenesis, microbiology, and risk factors,' *UptoDate* <https://www.uptodate.com/contents/pelvic-inflammatory-disease-pathogenesis-microbiology-and-risk-factors>

Rothman, K.J., Wise, L.A., Sorensen, H.T., Riis, A.H., Mikkelsen, E.M., Hatch, E.E. 2013. 'Volitional determinants and age-related decline in fecundability: a general population prospective cohort study in Denmark,' *Fertility and Sterility*, 99(7): 1958–1964.

Rumbold, A., Middleton, P., Crowther, C.A. 2005. 'Vitamin supplementation for preventing miscarriage,' *The Cochrane Library*, 2: Cd004073.

Salama S., Boitrelle F., Gauquelin A., Malagrida L., Thiounn N. and Desvaux P. 2015. 'Nature and Origin of "Squirting" in Female Sexuality,' *The Journal of Sexual Medicine*, 12(3): 661–666.

Shenenberger, D.W. 2016. 'Removal of unwanted hair,' *UpToDate* <https://uptodate.com/contents/removal-of-unwanted-hair>

Shifren, J.L. 2016 [updated 4 April 2016]. 'Sexual dysfunction in women: Epidemiology, risk factors, and evaluation,' *UpToDate* <https://uptodate.com/contents/sexual-dysfunction-in-women-epidemiology-riskfactors-and-evaluation>

Singh, S., Maddow-Zimet, I. 2016. 'Facility-based treatment for medical complications resulting from unsafe pregnancy termination in the developing world, 2012: a review of evidence from 26 countries,' *BJOG*, 123: 1489–1498.

Skovlund, C., Mørch, L., Kessing, L., Lidegaard, Ø. 2016. 'Association of hormonal contraception with depression,' *JAMA Psychiatry*, 73(11): 1154–1162.

Simeonova, Z., Milsom, I., Kullendorff, A.M., Molander, U. and Bengtsson, C. 1999. 'The prevalence of urinary incontinence and its influence on the quality of life in women from an urban Swedish population,' *Acta Obstetricia et Gynecologica Scandinavica*, 78(6): 546–551.

Sobel, J.D. 2016. 'Candida vulvovaginitis,' *UpToDate* <https://www.uptodate.com/contents/candida-vulvovaginitis>

Sobel, J.D. 2016. 'Patient education: Vaginal discharge in adult women (Beyond the Basics),' *UpToDate* <https://www.uptodate.com/contents/vaginal-discharge-in-adultwomen-beyond-the-basics>

Smith, A. 2011. 'The prepubertal hymen,' *Australian Family Physician*, 40(11): 873.

Sprecher, S. 2002. 'Sexual satisfaction in premarital relationships: associations with satisfaction, love, commitment, and stability,' *Journal of Sex Research*, 39(3): 190–196.

Stabell, K., Mortensen, B. and Træen, B. 2008. 'Samleiefrekvens: Prevalens og prediktorer i et tilfeldig utvalg norske gifte og samboende heteroseksuelle par,' *Journal of the Norwegian Psychological Association*, 45: 683–694.

Stanislaw, H and Rice, F.J. 1988. 'Correlation between sexual desire and menstrual cycle characteristics,' *Archives of sexual behavior*, 17(6): 499–508.

Statens legemiddelverk. 2016. 'Meldte mistenkte bivirkninger av HPV-vaksine (Gardasil) - oppdaterte bivirkningstall per 31. desember 2015,' *Statens legemiddelverk*.

Statens Serum Institut. 2016. 'Human papillomavirus-vaccine (HPV) 1, vaccinationstilslutning,' *Statens Serum Institut* (Danmark).

Stewart, E.G. 2016 [updated 30 January 2015]. 'Clinical manifestations and diagnosis of generalized vulvodynia,' *UpToDate* <https://www.uptodate.com/contents/clinicalmanifestations-and-diagnosis-of-generalized-vulvodynia>

Stewart, E.G. 2016 [updated 18 November 2015]. 'Differential diagnosis of sexual pain in women,' *UpToDate* <https://www.uptodate.com/contents/differentialdiagnosis-of-sexual-pain-in-women>

Strömquist L. 2014. 'Kunskapens frukt,' *Galago* <http://galago.se/bocker/kunskapens-frukt>

Sweet, R.L. 2012. 'Pelvic inflammatory disease: current concepts of diagnosis and management,' *Current Infectious Disease Reports*, 14(2): 194–203.

Tanbo, T.G. 2016. E-mail from M.D. Tom Gunnar Tanbo, former consultant at the Section for Reproductive Medicine, Gynaecology department, OUS, Oslo University Hospital.

Taylor, A. 2003. 'Extent of the problem,' *BMJ*, 327(7412): 434.

The Artificial Hymen Kit. 2016. *The Hymen Shop* <http://www.hymenshop.com>

The Lancet, 'Table 3: Sexual partners, practices, behaviours, and attitudes reported by women in Natsal-3, by age group,' *The Lancet* <http://www.thelancet.com/action/showFullTableImage?tableId=tbl3&pii=S0140673613620358>

Telegraph. 2009. 'Egyptians want to ban fake virginity kit,' *Telegraph* <http://www.telegraph.co.uk/news/worldnews/africaandindianocean/egypt/6264741/Egyptians-want-to-ban-fake-virginity-kit.html>

Toffol, E., Heikinheimo, O., Koponen, P., Luoto, R. and Partonen, T. 2011. 'Hormonal contraception and mental health: results of a population-based study,' *Human Reproduction*, 26(11): 3085–3093.

Træen, B., Spitznogle, K. and Beverfjord, A. 2004. 'Attitudes and use of pornography in the Norwegian population 2002,' *Journal of Sex Research*, 41(2): 193–200.

Træen, B., Stigum, H., Magnus: 2003. 'Rapport fra seksualvaneundersøkelsene i 1987, 1992, 1997 og 2002,' *Folkehelseinstituttet* (Statens institutt for folkehelse).

Trevathan, W.R., Burleson, M.H., Gregory, W.L. 1993. 'No evidence for menstrual synchrony in lesbian couples,' *Psychoneuroendocrinology*, 18(5): 425–35.

Tulandi, T. 2016 [updated 24 November 2015]. 'Reproductive issues in women with uterine leiomyomas (fibroids),' *UpToDate* <https://www.uptodate.com/contents/reproductive-issues-in-women-with-uterine-leiomyomas-fibroids>

Tulandi, T. and Al-Fozan H.M. 2016 [updated 7 November 2016]. 'Spontaneous abortion: Risk factors, etiology, clinical manifestations, and diagnostic evaluation,' *UpToDate* <https://www.uptodate.com/contents/spontaneous-abortion-risk-factorsetiology-clinical-manifestations-anddiagnostic-evaluation>

Turke, P.W. 1984. 'Effects of ovulatory concealment and synchrony on protohominid mating systems and parental roles,' *Ethology and Sociobiology*, 5(1): 33–34.

Tympanidis, P., Casula, M., Yiangou, Y., Terenghi, G., Dowd, P. and Anand, P. 2004. 'Increased vanilloid receptor VRI innervation in vulvodynia,' *European Journal of Pain*, 8(2): 129–133.

Tympanidis, P., Terenghi, G., Dowd, P. 2003. 'Increased innervation of the vulval vestibule in patients with vulvodynia,' *British Journal of Dermatology*, 148(5): 1021–1027.

UNAIDS. 2016. Fact Sheet 2016. *UNAIDS*.

UNDP/UNFPA/WHO/World Bank Special Programme of Research, Development and Research Training in Human Reproduction (HRP). 2012. 'Unsafe abortion incidence and mortality – Global and regional levels in 2008 and trends,' WHO.

Vessey, M. and Painter, R. 2006. 'Oral contraceptive use and cancer. Findings in a large cohort study, 1968–2004,' British Journal of Cancer, 95: 385–389.

Vigsnæs, M.K., Spets, K. and Quist, C. 2016 [updated 15 September 2016]. 'Politiet slår alarm: Grenseløs sexkultur blant barn og unge,' VG+ < http://pluss.vg.no/2016/08/20/2 508/2508_23770417>

Wallace, W.H.B and Kelsey, T.W. 2010. 'Human Ovarian Reserve from Conception to the Menopause,' PLOS ONE, 5(1): e8722.

Wallen K. and Lloyd E.A. 2011. 'Female sexual arousal: Genital anatomy and orgasm in intercourse,' Hormones and Behavior, 59(5): 780–792.

Weiss, B.D. 2005. 'Selecting medications for the treatment of urinary incontinence,' American Family Physician, 71(2): 315–322.

Whitley, N. 1978. 'The first coital experience of one hundred women,' Journal of Obstetric, Gynecologic, and Neonatal Nursing, 7(4): 41–45.

WHO. 2015. Family planning/Contraception. WHO <http://www.who.int/mediacentre/factsheets/fs351/en>

Wikipedia. 2016 [updated 8 September 2016]. 'Masturbate-a-thon,' Wikipedia <https://en.wikipedia.org/wiki/Masturbate-a-thon>

Wikipedia. 2016 [updated 21 September 2016]. 'Sanitary napkin,' Wikipedia <https://en.wikipedia.org/wiki/Sanitary_napkin>

Wilcox, A.J., Weinberg, C.R., Baird, D.D. 1995. 'Timing of sexual intercourse in relation to ovulation–effects on the probability of conception, survival of the pregnancy and sex of the baby,' New England Journal of Medicine, 333(23): 1517–1521.

Wilson, E.E. 'Polycystic Ovarian Syndrome and Hyperandrogenism,' Hoffman, B.L., Schorge, J.O., Schaffer, J.I., Halvorsen, L.M., Bradshaw, K.D., Cunningham, F.G., (eds). 2012. Williams Gynecology, 2nd edition (New York: McGraw Hill Medical).

Wimpissinger F., Stifter K., Grin W. and Stackl W. 2007. 'The female prostate revisited: perineal ultrasound and biochemical studies of female ejaculate,' Journal of Sexual Medicine, 4(5): 1388–1393.

Yang, Z. and Schank, J.C. 2006. 'Women do not synchronize their menstrual cycles,' Human Nature, 17(4): 433–447.

Yonkers K.A., O'Brien P.M.S. and Eriksson E. 2008. 'Premenstrual syndrome,' The Lancet, 371(9619): 1200–1210.

Zariat, I. 2016 [updated 28/08/2016]. 'Rystende jomfrusjekk,' Ytring (NRK) <https://www.nrk.no/ytring/rystende -jomfrusjekk-1.13106033>

Zuckerberg, M. 2015 [updated 31 July 20150. 'Priscilla and I have some exciting news: we're expecting a baby girl!' Facebook <https://www.facebook.com/photo.php?fbid=10102276573729791&set=a.529237706231.2034669.4&type=1&theater>

INDEX

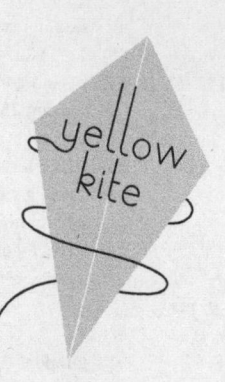

books to help you live a good life

Join the conversation and tell
us how you live a #goodlife

@yellowkitebooks
YellowKiteBooks
Yellow Kite Books
YellowKiteBooks